Geriatric Nutrition

GERIATRIC NUTRITION

Annette B. Natow, Ph.D., R.D.

Associate Professor, School of Nursing, Adelphi University
NRH Nutrition Consultants, Valley Stream, N.Y.

Jo-Ann Heslin, M.A., R.D.

Adjunct Assistant Professor, School of Nursing, Adelphi University
NRH Nutrition Consultants, Valley Stream, N.Y.

with Allen Natow

CBI

CBI Publishing Company, Inc.
51 Sleeper Street
Boston, Massachusetts 02210

Production Editor: Becky Handler
Text Designer: Becky Handler
Cover Designer: Betsy Franklin
Compositor: TKM Productions
Printer: Fairfield Graphics

Library of Congress Cataloging in Publication Data

Natow, Annette B
   Geriatric nutrition.

   Bibliography: p.
   Includes index.
   1. Aged—Nutrition.   2. Aging.   3. Geriatrics.
I. Heslin, Jo-Ann, joint author.   II. Title. [DNLM:
1. Nutrition—In old age.   QU145 N2795g]
TX361.A3N37   613.2   80-12282
ISBN 0-8436-2184-2

Printed in the United States of America

Printing (*last digit*): 9 8 7 6 5 4 3 2 1

To my mother who made all things possible.

A. B. N.

To my parents who believe good food ensures a good life.

J. H.

Contents

Foreword

The importance of maintaining good health and maximizing the health potential of the individual by promoting proper nutrition is receiving increasing emphasis as part of the comprehensive care delivered by health care professionals. The maintenance of good health and the prevention and treatment of certain diseases by diet therapy is particularly pertinent for the older adult. The elderly are often at high risk for developing a nutritional deficiency or are already suffering from a chronic illness. A significant body of knowledge is available that describes the role of certain dietary nutrients in either causing, exacerbating, or preventing certain chronic diseases. For these disorders, diet therapy is a central part of the treatment. For the older adult who may be suffering from multiple diseases, either asymptomatic or previously diagnosed, nutritional consultation and diet therapy take on major importance in the daily medical management of that individual.

Both health care professionals and the general public are increasingly aware of the role of nutrition in the pathophysiology of many diseases. Maintaining good health and maximizing the health potential of all individuals are the goals of preventive medicine. Proper eating habits and food selection, reduction of health-related risk factors, and appropriate exercise are becoming major aspects of medical care in our country. This concern has led to a focus on clinical and nutritional research of common diseases that afflict the elderly at a much higher rate than any other age group. Examples of some of these diseases under investigation are cancer, hypertension, morbid obesity, arteriosclerotic coronary artery and vessel disease, diabetes mellitus, chronic lung disease, and arthritis. The result of this research will hopefully be the reduction of the incidence of these disorders.

When evaluating the older individual for nutritional deficiencies, the clinician must be aware that eating habits and nutritional status are often a reflection of factors other than solely the physiologic condition of that individual or nutrient content in that person's diet. Some of these factors may be the ethnic and religious background of the person or couple, housing situation, or mental status of the client. For the older individual living alone, food and eating may take on significant social value in terms of maintaining relationships with family, friends, and neighbors. Improper nutrition may result from insufficient knowledge of appropriate food selection and preparation. Economic issues can also affect the nutritional status of the client in the following ways: types of food purchased, affording dentures for proper mastication, transportation for marketing, and obtaining necessary homemaking assistance.

A current trend in medical care is to approach each client in a humanistic and holistic manner. It is necessary to understand the environment and psychosocial factors affecting that person. As a result of this approach, therapeutic effectiveness is enhanced when the clinician recognizes these issues in formulating nutritional plans for the older adult. To accomplish this, a complete investigation must be made of the living situation and dietary habits of the client. Without serious consideration of these factors, unrealistic nutritional consultation may be given to the person. As a result, the client may not follow the dietary instructions, and the therapist may experience frustration without understanding the reason for this lack of cooperation.

The intent of this book is to provide a source of nutrition information for health professionals who deal with older adults. The authors discuss the important factors in the daily nutritional management of the elderly. The roles of major nutrients and trace elements are described, and the most current 1980 RDA figures have been included. The authors also cover other essential aspects of diet therapy, such as the clinical correlation between the pathophysiology of diseases and the role of nutrition, the psychosocial aspects of eating, and patient education suggestions. Because of the scope of information included in this text, this book is a valuable desk reference for the physician, nurse, nutritionist, public health worker, and other health care professionals who care for the older adult.

James D. Lomax, M.D.
Downstate Medical Center
New York, N.Y.

Acknowledgments

We would like to express our appreciation to the following individuals who helped us in our work on this book:

Dr. Ira Diamond, M.D., P.C.
   Brooklyn, New York

His experience in geriatric medicine has served as a valuable resource. We are especially grateful for his contribution of time and expertise. Also:

James D. Lomax, M.D., D.A.B.F.P.
   Assistant Professor Family Practice
   Downstate Medical Center
   State University of New York
   Brooklyn, New York

E. Neige Todhunter, Ph.D.
   Department of Biochemistry
   Vanderbilt University School of Medicine
   Nashville, Tennessee

Nicholas J. Johnnides, D.M.D.
   formerly General Practice at Peninsula Hospital Center
   Queens, New York

We are grateful for the cooperation of our colleagues in the School of Nursing, Adelphi University, and for those who shared resources with us:

Jacqueline L. Fraser, M.S., R.N.
Director, Gerontological Grant
Adelphi University
Garden City, New York

Elaine B. Jacks, M.S., R.N.
Director of Adelphi University Multidisciplinary Center on Aging (AUMCOA)
Adelphi University
Hempstead, New York

We would like to thank our families for their help, patience, and encouragement.

Laura for typing the manuscript;

Steven for proofreading;

Kristen and Karen for playing quietly while mother worked;

Harry and Joseph for their unfailing support;

and of course—Allen.

Introduction

"By increasing our knowledge and understanding of what it is like to be old, we increase our understanding of what it is to be a whole human being."

Robert Kastenbaum
Geriatric Focus, 1970

Mr. Kastenbaum's statement might well be expanded to say also that by increasing our understanding of the final stage in the life cycle, we help to ensure that this final stage will be as challenging, productive, and enjoyable as any other. This book is intended to increase the reader's understanding of the elderly from the standpoint of nutrition—that single most important environmental determinant of health. It is hoped that the reader will be able to integrate an understanding of geriatric nutrition into the mode of care of elderly persons so that life will remain a positive experience for this age group.

Aging is a continuous process, with few clear-cut divisions. As a matter of convenience only, "the elderly" in this book refers to those people over sixty years of age. Much of this book, however, may also be applicable to those over fifty years of age—those entering the second half of life. You should be aware of the biological changes experienced by the elderly so that these changes can be anticipated, and lifestyle (especially eating habits) modified accordingly.

A tremendous amount of attention is currently being focused on the elderly in the form of research, graduate-level education, and government programs. The elderly today enjoy the benefits of many more federally and locally supported projects, based on recently developed concepts and employing better-trained social workers and health professionals, than were available less than a generation ago. Still, the life of the elderly person is far from problem-free, and health problems are of major concern to many elderly persons. The 1971 White House Conference on Aging estimated that one-third to one-half of the health problems of the elderly may be related to nutrition. Nutritional care *must* be the responsibility of all those concerned with the health and well-being of the elderly.

Nutritional care encompasses nutrition education. Nutrition education programs specifically designed for the elderly are new in concept. The educator dealing with the elderly needs to use ingenuity to effectively convey information. The elderly are not too old to learn new ideas, but teaching them requires an approach distinct from that used for teaching any other age group (see Chapter 11).

In all interactions with the elderly, it is important to keep in mind that they do not constitute a homogeneous group. Individual needs should be considered, beyond the fact that the individual is a member of some arbitrarily defined group. We use this idea in our approach to nutritional intervention: treat the person, not the disease, and treat the person with moderation when possible.

Most of the information in this book is moderate rather than aggressive. A moderate approach to dietary manipulation frequently meets with success and effects change. On the other hand, severely restricted diets are difficult or impossible to successfully impose on people of any age.

There is a lack of complete information as well as disagreement on many of the topics addressed in this book. We have simply attempted to bring together many currents of thought regarding the nutriture of the elderly and to provide a balanced view of the information presently available. Geriatrics as a field is rapidly coming of age. We hope this book will serve as an introductory guide to the nutritional needs of the elderly, so that those who work with them will be more fully aware of and understanding of their needs. Toward this end, we have provided you with a wide range of theoretical and practical information as well as extensive resources. This material will help you deal more effectively with the elderly and aid you in evaluating new information as it becomes available.

Working towards the improvement of care for the aged is in a sense self-serving, since "age is a great universalizing force, something we all have in common." (Maggie Kuhn, National Convenor, Grey Panthers)

ABN
JH
AJN

Diversity of age! Diversity of need! Diversity of taste!

Moderation and simplicity are the passwords to health.

Mary Swartz Rose,
Feeding the Family (1919)

‖‖‖‖‖‖‖‖‖‖‖‖‖‖‖‖‖‖‖‖‖‖‖‖‖‖‖‖‖‖‖‖‖‖‖‖‖‖ 1

Nature of the Aging Process

In many traditional cultures, age is admired and the elderly are honored and respected for their wisdom and achievements. However, in the United States, and in other highly industrialized countries, the elderly usually retire and leave the mainstream of activity; they are generally not considered important enough to be wooed by manufacturers, merchants, or politicians. They are expected to take a back seat, now that they have made their contributions, and let the younger generation take over. Undoubtedly this will not remain true for very long, because "senior citizens"—persons aged sixty-two or over—are becoming an important political and economic force as their numbers increase.

The United States has a population with one out of every nine Americans aged sixty-five or older. Between 1900 and 1970, the total population of this country nearly tripled; the over-sixty-five population increased nearly sevenfold, and the over-sixty-five population continues to grow more rapidly than the under-sixty-five population. Also of significance is the fact that senior citizens as a group are a rapidly changing population. Each day approximately 5,000 Americans reach sixty-five, while 3,600 Americans die[1]. So, in addition to the annual increase of a half million senior citizens, there is an even more dramatic influx of senior citizens who are only recently retired, have more education, and are more at home with activism; hence they are less likely to remain silent about the inequities in how they are treated.

Projected estimates show that the fraction of elderly people in our country will be increasing through the year 2030, when the post-war baby boom infants will have joined the ranks. At that time, 18.3 percent of this nation's population will be aged sixty-five or over (see Table 1-1). This estimate, however, is based on a continued fertility rate that is somewhat higher than has been shown to be the case recently. If a lower fertility rate remains the rule in the future, then the total population of the United States will be smaller than projected and hence the proportion of elderly people will be even larger.

			(numbers in thousands)			
Year	All Ages	Number	Percent-age of All Ages	Number of Males	Number of Females	Number of Females per 100 men
1977	216,745	23,431	10.8	9,545	13,885	145
1980	222,159	24,927	11.2	10,108	14,819	147
1985	232,880	27,305	11.7	11,012	16,293	148
1990	243,513	29,824	12.3	11,999	17,824	149
1995	252,750	31,401	12.4	12,602	18,799	149
2000	260,378	31,822	12.2	12,717	19,105	150
2005	267,603	32,436	12.1	12,924	19,512	151
2010	275,333	34,837	12.7	13,978	20,858	149
2015	283,164	39,519	14.0	16,063	23,456	146
2020	290,115	45,102	15.6	18,468	26,634	144
2025	295,742	50,920	17.2	20,861	30,059	144
2030	300,349	55,024	18.3	22,399	32,624	146
2035	304,486	55,805	18.3	22,434	33,371	149
2040	308,400	54,925	17.8	21,816	33,108	152
2045	312,054	54,009	17.3	21,335	32,674	153
2050	315,622	55,494	17.6	22,055	33,439	152

TABLE 1-1   Population projections (Series 11), total and 65-plus by sex, 1977–2050.

Source: Part I Developments in Aging: 1977. A report of the Special Committee on Aging United States Senate, pursuant to S. Res. 78, Feb. 11, 77. and S. Res. 147, June 14, 77. Resolution Authorizing A Study of the Problems of the Aged and Aging Together with Additional and Supplemental Views. April 27, 1978 United States Government Printing office, Washington, D.C. 1978.

THEORIES OF AGING

The average individual's lifespan has increased over the years because of improvements in medical care and social environment. However, the maximum lifespan one can attain has increased only slightly. It is believed that man has a genetically determined potential lifespan. If reductions in all the killer diseases of later life were to occur, it is estimated that probably no more than ten years would be added to an individual's average life expectancy. This means that a greater percentage of the population would come closer to living out their maximum genetically determined lifespan. A lifespan of approximately 115 years is believed to be a fixed upper limit for humans and little is known about how to alter this genetic potential. However, research has shown that severe underfeedings of rats can extend their lifespan from a normal maximum of three years to as long as five years[2]. Thus, even the genetic determinants of lifespan may not necessarily fix the maximum length of one's life.

Researchers have long been interested in understanding the aging process. To unravel the mechanism of aging, studies have been carried out at the cellular level as well as the societal level. While the aging process is still quite poorly understood, certain currents of thought have emerged to explain many of the scientific observations that continue to be noted. Clearly, any explanation of the aging process will ultimately have to account for all these observations, and no such explanation is at hand. What follows here is a discussion of several of the more popular theories of aging (largely resulting from research at the cellular level), and also a discussion of factors that influence an individual's longevity (largely arising from population studies).

Cellular Theories

Aging has been defined as the sum total of the changes that occur in an individual, with the passage of time, from birth to death. *Senescence* more specifically refers to the degenerative changes that occur in the body after maturity has been reached and that ultimately result in death.

The changes that occur in the body after maturity are many and varied. Some are obvious to even the casual observer, such as the loss of acuity of sense perception. Other changes that occur at the tissue and cellular levels may not be as readily apparent.

It is not entirely clear what causes the age-related changes in metabolism that result in degeneration or loss of function of various parts of the body. Although it is certain that the complex process of aging cannot be explained by one simple mechanism, there are several theories that attempt to do just this. These theories focus either on derangements that occur during the formation of cellular proteins or on changes that occur in cellular proteins after they are formed. Theories include focusing on an accumulation of somatic mutations, the deterioration of collagen and elastin, the action of free radicals in the cell, dysfunction of the immune system, a decline in hormone production, an accumulation of toxins due to metabolic errors, and environmental factors, most notably nutrition.

The error theory of aging postulates that by the time a cell has multiplied a number of times, its DNA (deoxyribonucleic acid) has accumulated a number of errors and there is a gradual disruption of its ability to accurately transmit and express genetic information. The aged and error-ridden DNA directs the synthesis of defective RNA (ribonucleic acid), which in turn codes for faulty proteins. Thus the cell grows unable to function properly, as its protein content, which includes necessary enzymes, becomes increasingly abnormal. The cell may continue to survive if it can obtain the metabolites it lacks from neighboring cells or from its own faulty metabolism, but eventually cell death occurs. Recently it has been reported that there are differences in the RNA that is isolated from old and young tissues. This evidence tends to support the error theory of aging[2].

It is theorized that exposure to radiation accelerates aging by causing mutations in cells. Most of these mutations are harmful, and may occur not only after exposure to radiation but in aging nonradiated animals as well. At the present time, the somatic mutation theory is not considered to be a useful explanation of aging for various reasons, including the fact that most cells are able to repair somatic mutation damage.

Collagen, which comprises about 25 to 30 percent of the body's protein, is a major constituent of connective tissue. As the molecular composition of collagen remains static for extended periods of time, over the years there is an increased number of cross-linkages between molecules which makes the collagen increasingly rigid. This increased rigidity results in a loss of elasticity in skin and blood vessels, a loss of flexibility of muscles, and inhibition of the oxygenation of body tissues. It is further theorized that cross-linkages occur in intracellular protein, including enzymes and proteins bound to DNA in the course of aging[2]. It has been found that certain chemicals, such as nitriles and penicillamine, can slow the rate of cross-linkage. However, it is unclear whether these chemicals increase longevity.

The free radical theory relates aging to the formation of highly reactive cellular components which damage cells. These are formed from components of the cell when it is exposed to ionizing radiation. These free radicals react with unsaturated fatty acids in the cell to form highly reactive intermediates that in turn can damage cell membranes, including the membranes surrounding lysosomes which normally keep the lysosomal enzymes from attacking the rest of the cell. Free radicals also can disrupt enzyme activity and lead to the formation of lipofuscin, or aging pigment, in cells. Lipofuscin in a region of the cell tends to make that region nonfunctional. It has been proposed that antioxidants such as butyl-hyroxytoluene (BHT), vitamin E, and selenium may inhibit the aging effect of free radicals[3].

With aging there tends to be a reduction of immune function, which normally protects the body against disease and against abnormal cells which may form in the body. The aged individual's immune system tends to be less able to distinguish normal cells from abnormal ones, so abnormal cell proliferation as well as autoimmune reactions may take place[4]. Cancer and autoimmune diseases are found more frequently as one ages and are often associated with immune system dysfunction. It is not unreasonable to believe that at least part of the cell loss associated with aging is by way of autoimmune mechanisms.

Other theories of aging point to a decline in endocrine functions (elaborated in Chapter 2), an accumulation of toxins because of metabolic error, reduced effectiveness of the nervous system, and the effect of environmental factors such as stress and nutrition. The role of nutrition in aging, the most important and most easily controlled environmental factor, has been extensively studied in animals and humans.

Animal Studies

Classic studies on animals and fish fed calorie-restricted diets were carried out by Clive M. McCay beginning in the late 1920s[5,6,7]. He found that brook trout fed low-protein diets consisting of skim milk and cereal grains were retarded in their growth and outlived those trout that grew at normal rates on normal diets.

White rats have been studied to investigate the effects of calorie-restricted diets that were adequate in all nutrients. On these diets, any resultant retardation of growth could be attributed to the deficiency of calories. (See Chapters 4 and 5 for a discussion of calories and nutrients.) In one study, the underfed rats were found to be more subject to disease and convulsions than were the control rats who received normal diets, yet the rats that survived these conditions outlived the normally fed rats. An interesting finding was that in the animals with retarded growth, chronic diseases progressed more slowly and tumors developed less frequently than in rats with normal growth. Manipulation of the protein content of diets was attempted in another study by other researchers who found that they could increase a rat's life by 28 percent by feeding a high protein diet in the first four months of life and a low protein diet after that time[8].

Morris H. Ross of the Institute for Cancer Research in Philadelphia has manipulated diets so as to double the life expectancy of rats and also delay the onset of degenerative diseases. From his work, Dr. Ross developed some conclusions about the relationships between diet and length of life: that higher intakes of food, whatever the composition, resulted in shorter lifespan, with the heaviest survivors having the shortest lives; and that diets high in protein early in life and low in protein later in life increased lifespan[9]. Perhaps we have been mistaken in considering adequate that diet which allows for maximum growth and optimum health.

Animals raised on a diet which restricted tryptophan, an essential amino acid, have extended life and fertility beyond that found in controls[10]. Different forms of underfeeding have been shown to increase longevity in many animal species. Underfeeding also results in reduced incidence, and delay in onset, of certain types of disease. Nutritional manipulations have been shown to yield beneficial results when initiated in adulthood as well as during an animal's growth period. Studying various dietary manipulations on primates may provide further insight as the studies described above were performed on small laboratory animals.

Dietary manipulations of the aforementioned type cannot normally be performed on humans. Therefore, naturally occurring "experimental situations" are carefully studied when they may offer insight into how humans might tolerate similar conditions. In 1948, the National Research Council studied the island populations of Newfoundland following a four–year period of blockade and food restriction during World War II[11]. It was found that the adults were small and lean and the children showed an impaired growth rate. The young and middle-aged adults appeared older than their chronological ages. They had premature grey hair, loss of teeth, gaunt faces and wrinkled skin. It appeared that underfeeding and malnutrition had resulted in premature aging. It was unclear whether these changes were due to a simple caloric deficit, malnutrition due to a deficiency of specific nutrients, or to additional contributing factors such as long exposure to cold climates and inbreeding of the population over several centuries. While findings are not in conflict with the animal studies previously noted, any comprehensive explanation of the relationship between nutrition and aging needs to reconcile both sets of data.

The foregoing has presented some common theories of aging. Each theory, though not providing nearly a complete story, does provide some clues to the mechanism of this complex process. Manipulation of the aging process through the diet is a simple form of intervention and should be explored more fully. While we are certain that nutrition plays an important role in human growth and development, its possible preventive and therapeutic role in aging has not been fully elucidated.

FACTORS INFLUENCING LONGEVITY

While our present understanding of aging offers little more than a hint at the extreme complexity of this process, we have some understanding of those factors which are important determinants of lifespan. However, we know rather little about how these factors influence specific processes important in aging. The length of one's lifespan is determined by an interplay of genetic and environmental factors. Attributes as seemingly disparate as the presence or absence of specific disease states, one's dietary habits, personality type, intelligence, and sex have all been correlated with particular lifespans.

It is now generally accepted that man has a finite maximum lifespan. This idea is supported by numerous studies that have shown that cells replicate themselves a prescribed (probably genetically determined) number of times. This is in contrast to previously accepted work by Carrel which supported the idea that chick embryo cell explants could be kept alive indefinitely[12]. Cells taken from older animals undergo fewer cell divisions than do cells taken from younger animals. Growth potentials are significantly reduced as the age of the donor increases. Research is currently being performed to show why this happens and to learn if anything can be done to extend the number of times cells may replicate themselves. It is important to keep in mind that work done on cells outside the animal body may provide insight into some processes of aging but cannot duplicate all the factors at play on cells within the animal body.

Inheritance of specific disease states may reduce one's lifespan. For example, cells taken from diabetic donors have a reduced ability to survive and grow in culture. This would be expected as most juvenile diabetics have a reduced lifespan. Other familial diseases such as hypercholesterolemia affect longevity as well.

Though often arising from different disorders, brain impairment, called "organic brain syndrome," and incontinence have both been associated with a shortened life. Early onset of these conditions are more predictive of shortened lifespan than later onset[13].

A sedentary lifestyle places a person at increased risk of early death, while regular exercise may have a protective effect. It may also be useful to regulate one's body weight. Being overweight by 20 percent or more increases the risk of sudden death. Also, overweight individuals tend to be more prone to diabetes, gallstones, and hypertension than those of more normal weight.

Moderate use of alcohol, one or two ounces a day, may be associated with prolonged life, as recent studies show. However, excessive drinking leads to inadequate nutritional intake, liver damage, violence, or even suicide (see Chapter 8).

High intelligence is associated with longer lifespan. Among college graduates, honor students have a higher life expectancy than other graduates. Also, people listed in *Who's Who* have a lower mortality rate than others in the population. These findings may be explained by the fact that higher socioeconomic status correlates with longevity.

Studies of personality type show that those people more affected by time pressures are more vulnerable to myocardial infarction and are more likely to have serious disease. However, this applies only to persons in Western cultures. In contrast, studies performed on Druze tribesmen—Arabic-speaking people living in Israel—show that those with accommodating personalities could also develop alcoholism, have poorer health and short lives. Thus, in different cultures, or perhaps in people of different races, similar styles of behavior result in different health consequences.

Women generally live longer than men. This may be a purely biological phenomenon resulting from the "protective" effect of female hormones (or lack of male hormones) or may be of psychosocial origin. Women may be more concerned with weight control and may smoke fewer cigarettes. Certainly more research needs to be carried out before these issues are to be adequately addressed. Perhaps the new roles women are assuming will affect their lifespan in the future. It will be some time before we can conclude what effect on longevity, if any, has resulted from recent changes in women's roles in society.

Man has always quested in search of eternal youth or very long life. We often read about populations such as the Hunzas in northern Pakistan or the Georgians in the Russian Caucasus who have a high proportion of centenarians. When they and other long-lived groups are studied there appear to be few commonalities in their diets. Some eat much meat and dairy products, use tobacco, and drink alcohol. One factor all these groups do seem to have in common is a high degree of physical activity. All these groups, however, have in common a scarcity of written birth records; some of these people may not be as old as they claim[14]. The *Guinness Book of World Records* notes that the number of centenarians claimed in the Caucasus has declined rapidly, from 8,000 in 1950 to 4,500 in 1970[15]. Similar information was reported by Alexander Leaf who had overestimated the age and number of centenarians based on exaggerated claims of age among residents of Vilcabamba, Ecuador[16]. His conclusion, based on careful examination, was that individual longevity in that remote area was similar to that found throughout the rest of the world.

Thus, the idea of man's lifespan having a genetically determined upper limit is widely supported. Also widely supported is the idea that a great number of genetic and environmental factors modify this common genetic endowment. Though the interplay of the various factors is very complicated and not well understood, one general trend repeatedly emerges from study of the factors influencing longevity: the single most effective predictor of one's lifespan is the lifespan of one's biological parents.

CITED REFERENCES

1. The National Council on the Aging, Inc. February 1978. *Fact book on aging.* 1828 L. Street, N.W., Washington, D.C. 20036.
2. Shock, N. W. 1977. Biological theories of aging. In *Handbook of the psychology of aging,* eds. J. E. Birren and K. W. Schaie, p. 103. New York: Van Nostrand Reinhold Co.
3. Kent, S. 1977. Do free radicals and dietary antioxidants wage intracellular war? *Geriatrics* 32:127.
4. Krehl, W. A. 1974. The influence of nutritional environment on aging. *Geriatrics* 29:65.
5. McCay, C. M.; Sperling, G.; and Barnes, L. L. 1943. Growth, aging, chronic disease and lifespan in rats. *Arch. Biochemistry* 2:469.
6. McCay, C. M.; Crowell, M. F.; and Maynard, L. A. 1935. The effect of retarded growth upon the length of lifespan and upon the ultimate body size. *J. Nutrition* 10:63.
7. McCay, C. W., et al. 1939. Retarded growth, lifespan, ultimate body size and age changes in the albino rat after feeding diets restricted in calories. *J. Nutrition* 18:1.
8. Barrows, C. H., Jr., and Roeder, L. M. 1977. Nutrition. In *Handbook of the biology of aging,* eds. C. E. Finch and L. Hayflick. New York: Van Nostrand Reinhold Co.
9. Ross, M. H. 1976. Nutrition and longevity in experimental animals. In *Nutrition and aging,* ed. M. Winick, p. 43. New York: John Wiley and Sons.
10. Kent, S. 1976. What nutritional deprivation experiments reveal about aging. *Geriatrics* 31:141.
11. Aykroyd, W. R., et al. 1949. Medical resurvey of nutrition in Newfoundland 1948. *Canadian Medical Assoc. J.* 60(4):329.
12. Carrel, A., and Ebeling, A. H. 1923. Antagonistic growth principles of serum and their relation to old age. *J. Experimental Medicine* 38:419.
13. Eisdorfer, C. 1972. Some variables relating to longevity in

humans. *Epidemiology of aging.* U.S. Dept. Health Education and Welfare, DHEW Pub. No. (NIH) 77-711.
14. Wallace J. 1977. The biology of aging: 1976, an overview. *J. Amer. Geriatrics Soc.* 25(3):104.
15. McWinter, M. 1978. *Guinness book of world records.* New York: Bantam.
16. Leaf, A. 1973. Observations of a peripatetic gerontologist. *Nutrition Today* 8(5):4.

OTHER REFERENCES

Adams, G. 1977. *Essentials of geriatric medicine.* New York: Oxford University Press.
Brotman, H. B. 1972. The fastest growing minority: The aging. *Family Economics Review* United States Dept. of Agriculture, p. 10.
Havighurst, R. J. 1974. Understanding the elderly and the aging process. *J. Home Economics* 66:17.
Kent, S. 1976. How do we age? *Geriatrics* 31:128.
Paradise lost, a staff report. 1978. *Nutrition Today* 13(3):6.
Rosenfeld, A. 1976. *Prolongevity.* New York: Alfred A. Knopf.
Rowe, D. 1978. Aging—a jewel on the mosaic of life. *J. Amer. Dietetic Assoc.* 72:478.
Shank, R. E. 1977. Nutrition and aging. In *Epidemiology of aging,* eds. A. M. Ostfeld and D. C. Gibson. DHEW Pub. No. (NIH) 77-711, Washington D. C.
Shank, R. E. 1976. Nutritional characteristics on the elderly—An overview. In *Nutrition, longevity and aging,* ed. M. Rockstein and M. L. Sussman, p. 9. New York: Academic Press.
Strumph, N. 1978. Aging—a progressive phenomenon. *J. Gerontological Nursing* 4(2):17.
Tappel, A. L. 1967. Where old age begins. *Nutrition Today* 2(4):2.
———. 1973. Vitamin E. *Nutrition Today* 8(4):4.
Watkin, D. M. 1978. Logical basis for action in nutrition and aging. *J. Amer. Geriatrics Soc.* 26(5):193.
———. 1973. Nutrition for the aging and the aged. In *Modern nutrition in health and disease,* eds. R. S. Goodhart and M. E. Shils, p. 681. Philadelphia: Lea and Febiger.
Weg, R. B. 1978. *Nutrition and the later years.* California: The Ethel Percy Andrus Gerontology Center, University of Southern California Press.

||||||||||||||||||||||||||||||||||||||||||| 2

How Aging Affects the Body

As mentioned in the preceding chapter, aging can be defined as a change in the activity of living systems due to the passage of time. Different organs and tissues change over a period of time at varying rates, so chronological norms and physical appearances are less relevant to describing the aged than are parameters such as cell division rates or glucose rebound time. A man of forty may, for the first time in his life, need glasses to read the newspaper, while his lung function may be virtually unchanged from what it was twenty years before. On the other hand, this man's wife of forty may still have perfect vision though her lung capacity may be only 90 percent of what it was when she was twenty. Thus, not only does aging affect different organ systems in different ways but aging of specific organs also proceeds at different rates in different people.

Generally, with advancing age, there is an increased tendency of cells that normally divide to stop doing so, and there is a deterioration of specialized nondividing cells, such as nerve and muscle cells, which leads to their death. Some physiological parameters such as blood volume and red cell count are unchanged with increasing age. However, the connective tissue proteins, such as collagen, become increasingly rigid, causing blood vessels to be more resistant to flow. Therefore, blood pressure and tissue nourishment may become problems.

The organ systems of young adults are able to meet much greater demands than are ordinarily placed on them. This "reserve capacity" of most systems gradually decreases with aging. Thus, the elderly are less able than younger persons to maintain a stable body environment when subjected to stress. For example, after a load of glucose is ingested, the return of the blood sugar level to normal will take substantially longer in the elderly than it will in a twenty-year-old[1].

A gradual loss of functioning cells in most organs and tissues of the body is associated with aging, and in those cells remaining there is a gradual change of structural and functional characteristics. In aging cells, the nucleus shrinks, the Golgi bodies become fragmented, the nucleoli enlarge, and there is an increased number of intracellular vacuoles. As would be expected, the biochemistry of aged cells is different from that of younger cells. Lactate, histone, and lipofuscin levels are elevated. The activity of most enzymes gradually decreases, though the activity of some, such as monoamine oxidase, aldolase, and phosphofructokinase actually increases. Glycolytic activity increases while oxidative phosphorylation decreases, causing a decrease in adenosine triphosphate and creatine phosphate, hence a decreased basal metabolic rate in most cells, particularly those of the brain, skeletal muscle, and heart. Liver and kidney cells are not so profoundly affected.

In brief, advanced age is associated with nonuniform changes in the various body tissues. Generally, all these changes result in a loss of cells and lower energy levels of the remaining cells. This is associated with a diminished reserve capacity of most organs, slowed reaction times, and a reduced flexibility of collagen and elastin, which comprise over 40 percent of the body's protein. With this general background, we will now discuss more specifically the changes in the major organ systems that are associated with the aged.

CARDIOVASCULAR SYSTEM

After age nineteen, there is a decrease in the heart's force of contraction and stroke volume[2] amounting to about 1 percent per year. By age sixty-five, there may be a decline in cardiac output (heart rate times stroke volume) of 40 percent. The body's circulation redistributes to compensate for the decreased cardiac output so that the blood supply to the heart and brain is decreased less than is the blood supply to the kidney and liver. It should be noted that a decreased blood supply does not necessarily result in decreased function since the heart, kidney, and liver all have large functional reserves.

The functioning of the heart valves may be impaired because of fibrosis and calcification and thus become more rigid. The collagen molecules in the heart wall and peripheral vessels become increasingly cross-linked, so that all collagen tissues become increasingly rigid. Elastin tends to accumulate pigment and be degraded, also contributing to the rigidity of vessels. The rigid arteries offer increased resistance to blood flow, which contributes to the reduced amount of blood delivered to body tissues. This arterial resistance increases about 1 percent per year after maturity and results in increased blood pressure and possibly in enlargement of the heart as well.

Systolic blood pressure generally increases from age twenty to age seventy or eighty, though there is not uniform agreement on this point. Diastolic pressure increases gradually over the same time period, though again a variety of different time courses have been reported. Normal blood pressure at age twenty-five is about 120/75 while levels of approximately 160/90 are expected after age sixty-five. Those with blood pressure levels over these figures at these ages are considered to be hypertensive. However, it is difficult to define hypertension in old age. Its diagnosis should really be based on adverse effects to the eye, kidney, heart, and brain and not simply on elevated blood pressure measurements.

Reduced cardiac output limits one's capacity for physical work. More specifically, it hinders the body's ability to adjust to physical stress. Exercise of a given intensity and duration raises the heart rate and blood pressure more in old age than in youth.

RESPIRATORY SYSTEM

Aging processes in the lungs and chest bring about changes in lung volume. There is a decrease in the vital capacity, the maximal volume of air expired from full inspiration (an index of pulmonary function). This maximal breathing capacity is reduced by 40 percent between the ages of twenty and eighty. The lungs' residual volume and physiological dead space increase with age, meaning that the turnover of air in the lungs is less rapid in the elderly. These changes are due mainly to a loss in elastic recoil because of the reduced flexibility of the collagen and elastin in lung tissue. Structural changes in the lungs and vascular wall lead to decreased diffusing capacity of the respiratory membrane and to less efficient oxygen absorption.

The decreased pliability of the lungs and reduced efficiency of blood oxygenation tend to make hypoxia a significant problem for the elderly. The reduced turnover of air in the lungs, along with a decreased capacity for coughing and deep breathing, results in an increased susceptibility of elderly people to pneumonia and other respiratory illnesses. The reduced lung capacity and low efficiency of blood oxygenation along with the effect of stooped posture and weakened respiratory muscles lead to more rapid fatigue in the elderly.

RENAL SYSTEM

Renal efficiency is impaired in the elderly. The blood flow to the kidneys is reduced by an average of 55 percent between the ages of thirty-five and eighty. Some cells in the tubules and glomeruli are impaired or lost. In aged rats, a decline in the number of nephrons has been observed[3].

The aforementioned changes act to reduce the kidneys' filtration rate by one-half. Also, the capacity to secrete para-aminohippuric acid, a test of renal function, decreases, as does the capacity to reabsorb glucose and fluid. The ability to form concentrated urine may be reduced. This means that fluid intake must be carefully considered. Dehydration can result in confusion, and both dehydration and fluid retention can cause electrolyte imbalance.

Decreased renal function permits medications to remain present and active in the body of the elderly for longer periods, increasing the possibility of drug toxicity. Additionally, reduced renal function may lead to elevated blood pressure.

NEUROMUSCULAR SYSTEM

Motor function declines with age, as does physical strength. For instance, a decrease in handgrip strength is detectable as early as age thirty. The size of an elderly person's muscles is reduced and there may be degenerative changes in the joints, leading to weakness and joint stiffness. The elderly person has a reduced capacity for muscular work and requires a longer time to warm up to full working capacity. By age seventy-five the overall excitability of muscles decreases and the speed of nerve conduction is reduced by 10 percent.

NERVOUS SYSTEM

With age, there is a general slowing of responses to environmental stimuli. There is a loss of neurons with age, but the significance of this loss is unclear since there is uneven loss of neurons throughout the nervous system, with some portions of the brain exhibiting no loss at all.

The functioning of sense organs becomes impaired, affecting taste, pain, touch, heat, cold, and point-position perceptions. The numbers of olfactory receptors markedly decline, resulting in a reduced sensitivity to odors. The elderly are found to require a threshold concentration at least eleven times as great as that of young persons to perceive a wide variety of odors. There is loss of visual and auditory acuity as well.

With advanced age, a high level of intellectual activity is possible because of the functioning of adaptive mechanisms that compensate for deficiencies in the nervous system. It is generally believed that there is a decline in the functioning of the central nervous system with age. However, in many cases such a decline is due to diseases, such as Parkinson's, which are prevalent in the elderly. In healthy individuals there may simply be a slowing of function, but no actual loss. It is observed that the loss of brain cells with age is most pronounced in those with diabetes, hypertension, and alcoholism. As mentioned above, in healthy persons there is no cell loss associated with aging in many parts of the brain.

The decreased conduction velocity of neurons associated with old age results in slowed voluntary movements, slowed reflex and reaction time, and increased time necessary for decision making. Also, high blood pressure, a common problem in the elderly, is associated with a decline in memory and intellectual function. However, the reduced blood flow to the brain characteristic of advanced age does not tend to have any adverse effects if the individual is in good health. Thus, in the absence of pathological conditions, longterm memory, reasoning ability, and learning ability are not affected by old age.

ENDOCRINE SYSTEM

With aging, the amount of connective tissue in the endocrine glands increases and tends to replace secretory cells. Thus, generally, blood levels of all hormones decrease. Blood concentrations of testosterone in men and of estrogen in women decrease with old age. Blood levels of triiodothyronine are decreased also, and the functional activity of the thyroid gland diminishes. However, body tissues adapt to the lower levels of thyroid hormone and the body's normal level of hormonal regulation is preserved. Parathyroid hormone also shows a fall in blood concentration with a concomitant increase in tissue sensitivity.

Decreased glucose tolerance is apparent in the aged, as the elderly pancreas is less able to secrete insulin in response to glucose challenges. Yet, the elderly often have higher blood levels of insulin as well as a higher tissue sensitivity to insulin compared to younger adults. It has been theorized that the elderly may have increased amounts of insulin antagonists in the blood, and thus a lower *effective* blood insulin level. Indeed, the incidence of diabetes in the aged population may be overestimated because of a failure to appreciate the natural age-related changes in glucose tolerance.

It has been hypothesized that the majority of age-related endocrine changes can be due to the changing levels of specific plasma proteins involved in the transport of many hormones, so the activity of many hormones is lessened since fewer hormone molecules are reaching target tissues. As the hormone is not being transported away from the site of secretion, high local concentrations suppress further secretions.

GASTROINTESTINAL SYSTEM

Not all studies on taste and smell sensitivity in the elderly are in agreement. Different methods have produced different results[4]. Sex differences, diseases, and the effect of smoking further complicate attempts at generalization. The reduced taste and smell perception that are reported to occur with advanced age may affect the appetite and desire for food. The loss of taste buds is believed to begin at middle age and primarily affects those buds that detect sweet or salty taste. The taste buds that detect bitter or sour remain. This may explain why some elderly complain that all foods taste bitter or sour. Dentures that cover the palate further reduce taste sensation. Deficiencies of niacin, vitamin A, and zinc may cause decreased taste acuity. Deficiencies of copper and nickel are also related to changes in one's ability to taste. Disease states such as cancer and treatment such as radiotherapy, major surgery and drug therapy also alter taste acuity (see Chapter 7). A recent study showed that improved oral hygiene in the elderly improved taste perception, particularly for sweet and salty tastes[5].

One's diet is greatly affected by the loss of teeth and by ill-fitting dentures. Fifty percent of all Americans have lost all their teeth by age sixty-five[6]. A study of 100 seventy-year-olds showed that twenty-eight men and thirty-eight women had lost all their teeth, and, of these, eighty percent either did not replace them or replaced them with ill-fitting dentures[7]. Even well-fitting dentures present problems of adaptation, and dentures that fit well at one time may become loose due to atrophy of the gingiva. We have all seen people who have few or no teeth at all "gum" foods and appear to handle even hard foods, such as nuts, by mashing them with their gums. Despite these few, the loss of teeth leads to impaired chewing ability, often limits the choice of foods, and even may affect the desire to eat. Misplaced dentures—many are placed on meal trays and inadvertently discarded with meal leavings—are not always easily replaced.

With aging, there is a diminution in the secretory activity of the various sections of the gastrointestinal tract. Decreased salivary secretion may interfere with eating by causing difficulty in swallowing, which may already be impaired by slowed reflex muscular activity. Salivary secretion is reduced by the intake of tranquilizers and other drugs. (See Chapter 8, for a discussion of this problem.)

With aging, the parietal cells of the stomach lose their ability to secrete hydrochloric acid. The incidence of achlorhydria (the absence of hydrochloric acid in the stomach) increases after the age of sixty. Hydrochloric acid has several functions: it creates the proper acidity for protein digestion, it converts the inactive form of the gastric protease pepsinogen to pepsin, it increases the solubility of iron and calcium, and it acts as a bactericidal agent. The reduction of hydrochloric acid in the stomach thus may interfere with protein digestion and mineral absorption as well as contribute to proliferation of bacteria that can cause digestive upsets. The incidence of pernicious anemia is associated with reduced hydrochloric acid secretion but the reason for this association has not been clarified.

In the elderly, there is also a reduced secretion of mucus and of digestive enzymes which affect the digestion and absorption of foods. Salivary amylase, pancreatic amylase, and lipase, as well as trypsin and pepsin secretion, are all decreased. For some enzymes, the reduction begins in one's teens. The decreased production of lactase with age is very prevalent in certain groups of people. The problem of lactose intolerance as it affects one's nutritional status will be discussed elsewhere (see Chapter 4).

Generally, despite all of the above, there does *not* seem to be a marked decrease in the ability of the aged to digest most foods. However, there is some evidence that protein digestion is less efficient in the aged.

Loss of muscle tone in the stomach results in reduced gastric motility which in turn causes delayed emptying of the stomach. Along with reduced gastric motility is a reduction of hunger contractions. Indeed, there is a reduction in the motility of the entire gastrointestinal tract as well as a reduced blood supply to it and a lessened response to neural control.

Aging affects the integrity of the gastrointestinal tract. Medications such as steroids, aspirin, and reserpine, passing through a weakly motile tract, may predispose the elderly to ulcer formation. The prevalence of intestinal diverticulae also is age–related and may result in bouts of diverticulitis.

The type and numbers of intestinal microflora change with age, and more putrefactive and fever-producing bacteria are found in the intestine of the elderly than in younger people. This may cause flatulence and a greater susceptibility to food–borne illness.

D–xylose, a carbohydrate, is used to study the intestinal absorption of food. No change in the absorption of xylose is found until after age eighty[2]. However, there have been reports of impaired absorption of thiamine, folic acid, and fats in the aged. Poor absorption of fat is often linked to malabsorption of calcium because unabsorbed fat may form insoluble complexes with the calcium present in the gastrointestinal tract.

The loss of muscle tone and resultant reduction in peristalsis may contribute to constipation. (This problem will be explained more fully in Chapter 7.) A study focusing on digestive disorders in older people found the most frequent complaint to be constipation in each of two age groups: the middle-aged (45–64) and those over sixty-five[8]. However, the prevalence of the complaint was three times as great in those aged sixty-five and over than in the middle-aged group. Hence, the common use of laxatives among the elderly.

BODY COMPOSITION

All of the changes at the cellular, tissue, and organ levels described above are accompanied by changes in body composition (see Figure 2–1)[9]. During the adult years there is a progressive decrease in one's lean body mass and an increase in body fat. Studies have shown an average lean body mass of 59 kg (kilograms) at age twenty-five which decreases to 47 kg by age sixty-five to seventy. During this same time, the average amount of body fat increases from 14 to 26 kg. In other words, the proportion of body weight which is fat is 20 percent in a twenty-five-year-old and 36 percent in a sixty-five-year-old (women of age twenty-five years average 33 percent body fat and those of sixty-five average 49 percent). This indicates a decrease of 12 kg lean body mass and an increase in body fat of 12 kg. This increased amount of fat is probably not due to an increased rate of fat deposition but rather to a reduced capacity of the body to mobilize fat. Triglyceride lipases are activated by hormones. This activation has been shown to be less effective in the fat tissue of aged animals than in young animals. The biochemical basis of this is unknown.

    With age there is a decrease in the amount of body water along with a reduced oxygen consumption. The reduction in lean body mass and body water, when considered along with the aforemen-

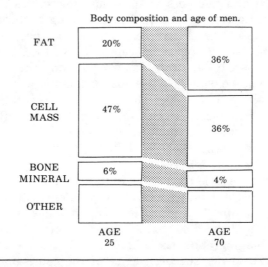

Body composition and age of men.

FAT — 20% — 36%

CELL MASS — 47% — 36%

BONE MINERAL — 6% — 4%

OTHER

AGE 25 — AGE 70

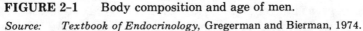

FIGURE 2–1   Body composition and age of men.

Source: *Textbook of Endocrinology,* Gregerman and Bierman, 1974.

tioned reduced basal metabolic rate of older persons, supports the idea that there are reductions in the number of cells in the bodies of aging persons.

Bone loss occurs in later life. Maximum bone density is found in women around age forty and in men around fifty. Thus, men and women begin losing bone matter after these ages. Women lose far more bone than men do—about 8 percent per decade as opposed to 3 percent per decade for men[10]. Additionally, women do not have a leveling off of this rate of bone loss as do older men. This bone loss can cause serious clinical problems in the elderly, and it does not seem to be easily corrected by nutritional means. Increasing the intake of calcium to 1.5 gm per day does not seem to entirely prevent this bone loss. (This problem will be more fully discussed in Chapter 5.) On the other hand, recent evidence suggests that getting one hour of endurance exercise four times a week is sufficient to arrest bone loss in the elderly. Such exercise may also act to lower the proportion of body fat in the elderly to that characteristic of middle-aged individuals[11].

CITED REFERENCES

1. Shock, N. W. 1970. Physiologic aspects of aging. *J. Amer. Dietetic Assoc.* 56(6):491.
2. Masoro, E. 1972. Other physiologic changes with age. In *Epidemiology of aging,* eds. A. M. Ostfeld and D. C. Gibson. DHEW Publication No. (NIH) 77–711.
3. Parsons, V. 1977. What decreasing renal function means to aging patients. *J. of Geriatrics* 32:93.
4. Engen, T. 1977. Taste and smell. In *Handbook of the psychology of aging,* eds. J. E. Birren and K. W. Schaie, p. 554. New York: Van Nostrand Reinhold Co.
5. Langdon, M. J., and Yearick, E. S. 1976. The effects of improved oral hygiene on taste perception and nutrition of the elderly. *J. of Gerontology* 31(4):413.
6. Busse, E. W. 1978. How mind, body and environment influence nutrition in the elderly. *Postgrad. Medicine* 63(3):118.
7. Masoro, E. 1976. Physiologic changes with aging. In *Nutrition and aging,* ed. M. Winick, p. 61. New York: John Wiley and Sons.
8. Shank, R. E. 1976. Nutritional characteristics of the elderly— An overview. In *Nutrition, longevity and aging,* eds. M. Rockstein and M. L. Sussman. New York: Academic Press, Inc.
9. Gregerman, R. I., and Bierman, E. L. 1974. In *Textbook of endocrinology,* ed. R. H. Williams, p. 1059. Philadelphia: W.B. Saunders Co.
10. Goldman, R., and Rockstein, M. 1975. *The physiology and pathology of human aging.* New York: Academic Press.
11. Smith, K. H.; Shephard, R. J.; and Harrison, J. E. 1977. Endurance training and body composition of the elderly. *Amer. J. Clinical Nutrition* 30:326.

OTHER REFERENCES

Adams, G. 1977. *Essentials of geriatric medicine.* Oxford: Oxford University Press.

Jones, D. A.; Dunbar, C. F.; and Jirovec, M. H. 1978. *Medical-surgical nursing. A conceptual approach.* New York: McGraw-Hill Book Company.

Mayer, J. 1974. Aging and nutrition. *J. of Geriatrics* 29:57.

Rossman, I. 1976. Human aging changes. In *Nursing and the aged,* ed. I. N. Burnside, p. 81. New York: McGraw-Hill.

Von Hahn, H. P. 1975. *Practical geriatrics.* Basel: S Harger.

|||||||||||||||||||||||||||||||||||||||||||||||| 3

Are the Aged Well Nourished?

RECOMMENDED DIETARY ALLOWANCES

Most studies that seek to determine if the elderly are well nourished use the Recommended Dietary Allowances (RDA) of the National Academy of Sciences/National Research Council as the standard of adequacy[1]. These were first published in 1943. At that time, the population was younger than at present and nutritionists were primarily concerned with the eradication of deficiency diseases. These initial recommendations set the unrealistic precedent for lumping all people over fifty-one into one group. The latest revision of the RDA, published in 1980, gives allowances for energy as calories (see Table 3–1(a)) as well as allowances for seventeen essential nutrients, as they have been established for various age and sex groups. Estimated "Safe and Adequate Daily Dietary Intakes of Additional Selected Vitamins and Minerals" are also provided for twelve nutrients (see Table 3–1(b)). For the first time, energy intakes for those over fifty are divided into two age classifications: fifty-one to seventy-five years; seventy-six plus years. This distinction is not made for the other nutrients tabulated. Table 3–1(c) shows the Recommended Dietary Allowances for adults fifty-one plus years of age.

The Food and Nutrition Board states that "The Recommended Dietary Allowances are the levels of intake of essential nutrients considered, in the judgment of the Food and Nutrition Board on the basis of available scientific knowledge, to be adequate to meet the known nutritional needs of practically all healthy persons." Thus, the recommendations for all nutrients (not including calories, which are not truly nutrients but are often considered along with them) are planned to exceed the needs of most healthy people. The recommendations are not intended to cover an individual's therapeutic needs.

Many elderly people have one or more chronic illnesses that affect their nutritional needs along with a variety of other social and psychological influences, that affect their dietary intake. Food processing, packaging, storage, and preparation have a major influence on one's choice of food. Such an influence is significant to the elderly because often their food is prepared in quantity at senior citizen centers and residences. A study done on the vitamin C content of food delivered by a "meals on wheels" program showed that destruction of vitamin C exceeded 50 percent between the time it was prepared and the time it was delivered to the recipient[2].

Mean Heights and Weights and Recommended Energy Intake

Category	Age (years)	Weight (kg)	(lb)	Height (cm)	(in)	Energy Needs (with range) (kcal)	(MJ)
Males	51–75	70	154	178	70	2400 (2000–2800)	10.1
	76 +	70	154	178	70	2050 (1650–2450)	8.6
Females	51–75	55	120	163	64	1800 (1400–2200)	7.6
	76 +	55	120	163	64	1600 (1200–2000)	6.7

TABLE 3–1(a)   The allowances for the two older age groups represent mean energy needs over these age spans, allowing for a 2% decrease in basal (resting) metabolic rate per decade and a reduction in activity of 200 kcal/day for men and women between 51 and 75 years, 500 kcal for men over 75 years and 400 kcal for women over 75. The customary range of daily energy output is shown for adults in parentheses, and is based on a variation in energy needs of ±400 kcal at any one age, emphasizing the wide range of energy intakes appropriate for any group of people.

Source: Recommended Dietary Allowances, Ninth Edition (1980, at press), reproduced with the permission of the National Academy of Sciences, Washington, D.C.

The above chart is taken from the Recommended Dietary Allowances which were at press at the time this book was ready for publication. A full discussion of the charts will be found in the ninth edition of the RDA to be published in 1980, available from the National Academy of Sciences, Washington, D.C.

Estimated Safe and Adequate Daily Dietary Intakes of Additional Selected Vitamins and Minerals[a]

	Vitamins			Trace Elements[b]						Electrolytes		
	Vitamin K (μg)	Biotin (μg)	Pantothenic Acid (mg)	Copper (mg)	Manganese (mg)	Fluoride (mg)	Chromium (mg)	Selenium (mg)	Molybdenum (mg)	Sodium (mg)	Potassium (mg)	Chloride (mg)
Age (years)												
Adults 51+	70–140	100–200	4–7	2.0–3.0	2.5–5.0	1.5–4.0	0.05–0.2	0.05–0.2	0.15–0.5	1100–3300	1875–5625	1700–5100

[a] Because there is less information on which to base allowances, these figures are not given in the main table of the RDA and are provided here in the form of ranges of recommended intakes.

[b] Since the toxic levels for many trace elements may be only several times usual intakes, the upper levels for the trace elements given in this table should not be habitually exceeded.

TABLE 3–1(b)   Daily intakes of additional vitamins and minerals.

Source: Recommended Dietary Allowances, Ninth Edition (1980, at press), reproduced with the permission of the National Academy of Sciences, Washington, D.C.

The above chart is taken from the Recommended Dietary Allowances which were at press at the time this book was ready for publication. A full discussion of the charts will be found in the ninth edition of the RDA to be published in 1980, available from the National Academy of Sciences, Washington, D.C.

Food and Nutrition Board, National Academy of Sciences-National Research Council Recommended Daily Dietary Allowances,[a] Revised 1980. Designed for the maintenance of good nutrition of practically all healthy people in the U.S.A.

	Age (years)	Weight (kg) (lbs)	Height (cm) (in)	Protein (g)	Fat-Soluble Vitamins			Water-Soluble Vitamins		
					Vitamin A (µg R.E.)[b]	Vitamin D (µg)[c]	Vitamin E (mg α T.E.)[d]	Vitamin C (mg)	Thiamin (mg)	Riboflavin (mg)
Males	51+	70 154	178 70	56	1000	5	10	60	1.2	1.4
Females	51+	55 120	163 64	44	800	5	8	60	1.0	1.2

	Water-Soluble Vitamins				Minerals					
	Niacin (mg N.E.)[e]	Vitamin B_6 (mg)	Folacin[f] (µg)	Vitamin B12 (µg)	Calcium (mg)	Phosphorus (mg)	Magnesium (mg)	Iron (mg)	Zinc (mg)	Iodine (µg)
Males	16	2.2	400	3.0	800	800	350	10	15	150
Females	13	2.0	400	3.0	800	800	300	10	15	150

[a] The allowances are intended to provide for individual variations among most normal persons as they live in the United States under usual environmental stresses. Diets should be based on a variety of common foods in order to provide other nutrients for which human requirements have been less well defined.

[b] Retinol equivalents. 1 Retinol equivalent = 1 µg retinol or 6 µg carotene. See text for calculation of vitamin A activity of diets as retinol equivalents.

[c] As cholecalciferol. 10 µg cholecalciferol = 400 I.U. vitamin D.

[d] α tocopherol equivalents. 1 mg d-α-tocopherol = 1 α T.E. See text for variation in allowances and calculation of vitamin E activity of the diet as α tocopherol equivalents.

[e] 1 NE (niacin equivalent) is equal to 1 mg of niacin or 60 mg of dietary tryptophan.

[f] The folacin allowances refer to dietary sources as determined by *Lactobacillus casei* assay after treatment with enzymes ("conjugases") to make polyglutamyl forms of the vitamin available to the test organism.

TABLE 3-1(c) Recommended daily dietary allowances.

Source: Recommended Dietary Allowances, Ninth Edition (1980, at press), reproduced with the permission of the National Academy of Sciences, Washington, D.C.

The above chart is taken from the Recommended Dietary Allowances which were at press at the time this book was ready for publication. A full discussion of the charts will be found in the ninth edition of the RDA to be published in 1980, available from the National Academy of Sciences, Washington, D.C.

Because the elderly are often not in good health and may not have access to a wide variety of food sources, the RDA may not be an appropriate benchmark of dietary adequacy for them[3]. The allowances were developed as guidelines for overall good nutrition of the population and were not intended to represent the precise nutritional needs of individuals—certainly not for elderly individuals—although they are often used for this purpose. Malnutrition does not exist in all instances when the RDAs are not met. Moreover, ingesting all the nutrients in the amounts listed in the table does not necessarily ensure optimal nutrition.

Accordingly, one must consider the intended uses of these allowances when reviewing studies which rate the nutrient intake of the elderly in comparison to the RDA or some other standard based on the RDA. Another factor that would affect findings of studies based on the RDA is that in each of the nine revisions, standards for some nutrients were changed appreciably (protein, calories, vitamin C), and thus studies based on earlier recommendations may indicate large deviations from the standard mean because of references to a standard level that is no longer considered reasonable. The 1980 revision of the RDA more precisely describes the energy needs of the elderly, taking into account the different energy needs of those fifty-one to seventy-five years and those over age seventy-six. The recommendation for the other nutrients tabulated considers all those over age fifty-one in one category.

FOOD CONSUMPTION SURVEYS

There is less information available concerning the nutrient quality of the diet eaten by the elderly than for any other age group[4]. The following is a discussion of several of the major surveys that helped assess the nutritional status of the elderly over the past twenty years.

Department of Agriculture Survey

Approximately every ten years the Consumer and Food Economics Research Division of the Agriculture Research Service of the United States Department of Agriculture conducts a household food consumption survey. The most recent one was conducted in 1977-78.

The findings from this survey are not yet available. The 1965–66 survey, based on data of a twenty-four-hour intake of 1,643 people aged sixty-five and over, showed that, as age increased, the mean intake of nutrients and calories decreased[5]. Men aged fifty-five to sixty-four had an average calorie intake of 2,465 Calories (kcal). Calorie intakes dropped to 2,051 for men aged sixty-five to seventy-four with a further reduction to 1,866 Calories for men aged seventy-five and over[10]. It is interesting to note that, though the mean amounts of all nutrients ingested declined as the subjects' age increased, the intake of only one nutrient, calcium, fell well below the RDA, and this was only in those individuals aged seventy-five and over.

For women aged fifty-five and over, thiamine intake was 87 percent, riboflavin 84 percent, and calcium 64 percent of the RDA. When the aged with low incomes were evaluated separately, it was found that those with lower incomes had less adequate diets when assessed by comparison to the RDA. It is difficult to obtain an accurate picture of how many individuals in the population have intakes of one or more nutrients that are below recommended allowances, due to the way the data of this survey are presented. Additionally, the nutrients contributed by the use of vitamin and mineral supplements were not considered as part of daily intake. As these supplements are widely used by the elderly, omitting information on the extent of their use may seriously affect the results of any survey. Additionally, as this survey did not include data from elderly persons living in institutions and rooming houses, these individuals—including many who are ill and disabled—were not included. Thus this study cannot be considered representative of all the elderly in the United States.

Ten State Nutrition Survey

The Ten State Nutrition Survey, carried out in 1968–1970 by the Center for Disease Control, focused on low income people. The populations studied were in districts with the lowest quartile of income at the time of the 1960 census. The standards for adequacy of intake of various nutrients in this survey were developed using the RDAs and data from the Food and Agriculture Organization of the World Health Organization as guides. The standards used for protein and iron are similar to the RDA but the standards for other nutrients were about 50 percent of the RDA[6].

In this survey, all individuals over sixty years were studied as one group. The sample studied included over 2,000 persons who reported food intake during a twenty-four hour period. The most prevalent nutrient deficiencies in the elderly were found to be iron in both men and women, vitamin A among Spanish-Americans of both sexes, riboflavin in black and Spanish-American people, and vitamin C, which was deficient in all males. Obesity was found more often in the women (black and white) than in the men. The percentage of obese women declined with increasing age. It was determined that the individuals surveyed aged sixty and over, as a group, consumed too little food to meet nutritional standards as determined for their age, sex and weight. The Ten State Survey reported slightly lower intakes than did the United States Department of Agriculture Food Consumption Survey.

Clinical assessments performed as part of the Ten State Survey included dental evaluations. The incidence of periodontal disease increased with age so that by age sixty-five to seventy-five over 90 percent of those surveyed had evidence of this disease. No correlations between dental disorders and plasma levels of vitamin A and serum vitamin C were found. Neither the clinical nor the biochemical evaluations suggested a high level of severe malnutrition or marked age-related nutritional deficiencies. This may lead one to doubt the validity of the RDA as a measure of nutritional adequacy of a diet.

Health and Nutrition Examination Survey

The first Health and Nutrition Examination Survey (HANES) was carried out in 1971-72[7]. Its test population was a scientifically-designed random sampling representative of the United States civilian population aged one to seventy-four years. For those over sixty, the most frequent nutritional deficits found were in dietary iron, vitamins A and C, and calcium. However, clinical signs due to deficiencies in nutrients other than iron were found only infrequently. Many poor elderly people were found to have very low caloric intakes. It was determined that 21 percent of the white population and 36 percent of the black population aged sixty and over, from the lower income groups, had daily intakes of fewer than 1,000 Calories. In spite of this, obesity was found to be associated with low income females; 25 percent or more of the lower income black and white women surveyed, aged forty-five to seventy-four, were found to be obese. A high percentage of elderly blacks had low values for hemoglobin and hematocrit, which was unrelated to iron deficiency because serum iron levels in these individuals were not low.

Other Surveys

Another survey of 680 elderly who had, or believed they had, arthritis found 65 percent overweight and 5 percent underweight[8]. (The incidence of osteoarthritis may be higher among those who are overweight than among those who are not.) The intakes of calcium and vitamin A were found to be inadequate in 57 percent and 34 percent of this population respectively. Also, 71 percent of the subjects had diets inadequate in one or more nutrients. An interesting finding of this study was that 81 percent of the subjects ate three meals daily, 17 percent ate two meals, and 3 percent ate only one meal per day.

One small survey comparing independently living elderly and nursing home residents found lower middle class elderly with a low level of education consuming slightly better diets than nursing home residents with similar backgrounds from the same geographical areas. From these studies we can see that the elderly population is likely to consume diets deficient in calories and some nutrients. However, the aforementioned studies, as well as most others done on elderly populations, have serious biases and thus cannot truly be considered to report authoritatively on all elderly people. The aged who are most likely to suffer from malnutrition are least likely to be included in these studies. Those who are bedridden or institutionalized are not included. Those who are unable to keep the records necessary for many food surveys are also not included. Even assuming a person's ability to keep records, the accuracy of listings may be suspect if there is no corroboration on the part of a third party. Many studies are based on twenty-four-hour recall (in which a person is asked to list all foods eaten in the preceding twenty-four hours), and this may be too limited a time period to accurately reflect one's eating habits and nutrient intake. Furthermore, twenty-four-hour recalls tend to underestimate the number of calories consumed[9]. In fact, studies with the elderly show that they tend to overreport small intakes and underreport large intakes. This has been referred to as "talking a good diet."

Other factors enter into assessing the adequacy of the nutrient intake of the elderly, such as the use of vitamin/mineral supplements, the question of food and drug interactions (which will be discussed in Chapter 8), and the effects of stress and illness on nutritional status (which will be discussed in Chapter 7).

Moreover, despite the frequent reporting of inadequate dietary intake of many nutrients by the elderly, there has been a relative lack of evidence demonstrating that the elderly actually suffer from nutritional deficiencies. This leads one to suspect the inappropriateness of the RDAs as standards for good nutrition in the elderly.

ASSESSMENT

A good nutritional state can be defined as a physical and mental state of health that cannot be improved by providing or withholding food. Although it is possible to draw some conclusions about an individual's nutritional state simply by observation of one's appearance, an accurate assessment of nutritional status depends on the collection and correlation of data from medical and dietary histories, anthropometric measurements, a physical examination for signs associated with nutritional deficiencies, and a biochemical assessment.

Medical and Dietary History

The nutritional state of an elderly person reflects not only his current food intake but his previous diet history as well. A nutritional assessment must include an evaluation of those factors in an individual's medical history that may affect his present nutritional state. Some of these factors are food allergies (it makes little difference if these are documented or anecdotal; in either event, food intake is affected), surgical procedures that affect one's ability to digest or to feed oneself, the existence of a disease state (such as diabetes or ulcers) which calls for a restricted diet, and physical disabilities that interfere with the obtaining, preparation, and eating of food.

Gaining information about what a person usually eats can be done in various ways. *Household food surveys* count the quantity of various foods consumed in a specified time span in a given household. This type of information is useful for determining food consumption patterns in different socio-economic groups, though it does not offer information regarding the consumption patterns of individuals.

A *diet history* of an individual elicits information about what a person eats habitually. It is qualitative rather than quantitative. A written *food record*, which is kept by an individual for a period of three days to one week, can, if it is kept accurately, give information about kinds and amounts of food eaten.

A *twenty-four-hour recall* is often employed in which a trained interviewer asks "Tell me everything that you ate in the last twenty-four hours beginning with the last food eaten." This is the most frequently used method in assessing the current nutritional intake of the elderly. It can be completed by a trained interviewer in about twenty minutes. However, estimates of food eaten may be inaccurate, foods may be forgotten, and the twenty-four-hour period used may not be representative of usual intake. As with all people, the eating habits of the elderly are often erratic, and a twenty-four-hour recall may be unreliable as an indicator of usual diet.

A skilled interviewer is the basic requirement for obtaining accurate information in a twenty-four-hour recall. The interviewer must first determine whether or not the subject is willing and able to talk about his diet. Fatigue, anxiety, and discomfort may cause the individual to be uncooperative. It is important to be sure that there is no particular problem weighing heavily on the subject's mind. For example, a person waiting for the results of a series of diagnostic tests may not be in the proper frame of mind for a diet interview.

A prepared form such as that in Figure 3-1 (the Nutritional Assessment Form, pp. 36–39) is useful in directing the flow of a dietary interview. However, the interviewer should endeavor to use a casual and conversational approach rather than adhering strictly to a predetermined design when interviewing. Especially when relaxed, the subject may offer what appears to be gratuitous, extraneous material which might include some useful clues to his nutritional intake. Thus an informal approach to the interview is best. An interviewer should avoid using questions that suggest a correct answer or which can be answered with a perfunctory "yes" or "no." It is better to say "Tell me, what was the first thing you ate this morning?" than "Do you eat cereal for breakfast?"

Nutritional Assessment Form

Name_____   Date_____

Birth date_____   Age _____

Informant_____   Telephone _____

Address_____

Race_____Ethnic Origin_____   Religion _____

Education level_____   Marital Status_____

Occupation_____   Hours of working day_____

Hours per week_____

Family Composition

Name_____   Age_____   Sex_____

_____   _____   _____

_____   _____   _____

_____   _____   _____

Housing: room_____   apartment_____   own home_____

Income: source_____

adequacy_____

Height_____   Weight _____

Has weight increased_____

Has weight decreased_____

Teeth: Good condition_____, missing____, no dentures____, dentures____

chewing ability _____good, _____fair, _____poor

Appetite: good_____ fair_____ poor_____

Indicate any problems with the following:

Sense of taste _____

Sense of smell _____

Digestion _____

Elimination _____

Vision _____

Daily Activities

Do you smoke?_____ How much?_____

Do you drink beer_____, wine_____, alcohol_____
How much?_____

(continued)

Do you take any medication?_____ What type?_____

Who prescribed?_____

Do you take vitamin/mineral supplements?_____

What type?_____

Who prescribed?_____

Do you take any food supplements such as rutin, bone meal, protein supplements?_____ What kind?_____ Why?_____

Do you exercise?_____ How often?_____

How long?_____

Do you go outdoors?_____ Daily?_____ Occasionally?_____

Hardly ever?_____

Diet Information

Have you ever been on a special diet?_____ What kind?_____

Are you on one now?_____ What kind?_____

Who prescribed the diet?_____

Do you follow the diet: all the time?_____ part of the time?_____

Hardly ever?_____

Are you allergic to any foods?_____ Which ones?_____

Who diagnosed the allergy?_____

Do you have religious prohibitions regarding foods?_____

Which foods?_____

Do you prepare all your own meals?_____

Do you do your own marketing?_____

Do you eat out?_____ Once a day?_____ Occasionally?_____

Hardly ever?_____

Where?_____

Do you eat differently on weekends?_____

How is it different?_____

How many times a day do you eat?_____

Do you eat alone?_____

Do you skip meals?_____ Which ones?_____

How often?_____

(continued)

Have you increased, decreased, or eaten about the same amount of the following foods?

Food	Increased	Decreased	Same
Margarine			
"Corn-oil"			
"Diet"			
Butter			
Milk			
Skim milk (fresh)			
or powdered			
Cooking oil			
Solid canned fat			
Bacon			
Red meat			
Fish			
Poultry			
Eggs			
Whole grain bread			
White bread			
Cooked cereal			
Dry cereal			
Coffee			
Decaffeinated coffee			
Tea			
Potatoes			
Raw vegetables			
Cooked vegetables			
Cooked fruits			
Raw fruits			
Salty snacks			
Baked goods			
Juice			
Soda			
Cocoa			

There are so many "convenience foods" on the market today, do you use them:

	Yes/frequency	No/why not? (Expensive, don't like, too large serving)
Instant milk (dried)		
TV Dinners		
Frozen main meals		
Frozen vegetables		

(continued)

	Yes/frequency	No/why not? (Expensive, don't like, too large serving)
Special reinforced milks		
Imitation sour cream		
Special margarines		
Nondairy cream		
Instant breakfasts		
Powdered orange juice		
Instant coffee		
Canned meats		
Cake-muffin mixes		
Pudding mix		
"Boxed" main meals		
Others		

FIGURE 3-1   A nutritional assessment form useful in dietary interviews.

One of the authors remembers doing a diet study with a group of elderly individuals. They were given forms in which to keep seven-day food records. On the front of the form was an example of how the records should be kept. The example listed a breakfast that would make any nutritionist's heart glow. It included orange juice, an egg, cereal, milk, and toast. Almost every participant listed exactly this breakfast on each of the seven days.

It is very important that the interviewer not ask any questions that can be construed as being unnecessary or prying. While some individuals enjoy being interviewed and will speak freely on many subjects, others naturally may feel less inclined to discuss areas that they believe to be personal. It is often possible to obtain information about sensitive subjects—such as availability of sufficient money for food—by indirect questioning about other activities.

Above all, the interviewer should allow plenty of time for the interview. It is important to give the subject time to think and respond fully to the questions. The interviewer should use terms and examples that are familiar to the subjects. If food models are available, they should be used for accurate assessment of portion size.

If the elderly individual is unable to communicate adequately, diet information may be obtained from a relative or friend. It is important to obtain information about who purchases and prepares the food because that person often controls consumption. Other information obtained should include supplemental vitamin/mineral intake, since the use of supplements often is unrelated to the amount of nutrients obtained from food. Consider also the number of meals eaten per day, food preferences and dislikes, food fads followed, food preparation facilities and knowledge, food budget, and foods consumed habitually (alcohol, candy, coffee) in addition to the usual daily diet.

Very often, the social worker, home aide, or volunteer worker who sees the elderly on a regular basis in their homes has not had the necessary training to do a complete evaluation of an individual's food intake. They can, however, identify potential nutritional problems and alert the public health nurse or nutritionist to the need for further investigation of the situation. Figure 3-2 is a checklist that would be useful for an assessment of nutritional risk in the elderly. Use of this or a similar checklist may help the home visitor identify problems that might otherwise have been overlooked[10].

Assessment of Need for Nutritional Intervention

Name _____ Referred By _____

Address _____ Telephone _____

Date of Birth _____ Male _____ Female _____

Marital Status: Single _____ Married _____ Widowed ____ Separated ____

Race: Caucasian ____ Indian ____ Black ____ Oriental ____ Spanish _____

    Other _____

Household Composition: Live Alone ____ Spouse ____ Child ____ Other ____

Local Church Affiliation _____

Local Club Affiliation _____

Have you been active in a Nutrition/Feeding Program before? _____

What kind? _____

Emergency Contact _____
                (Name)   (Address)

    (Phone)   (Relationship)

Name of local physician _____

(continued)

Do you have a refrigerator? _____ stove? _____

                kitchen? _____ kitchen privileges? _____

Estimated yearly income _____

Are you eligible for food stamps? Yes _____ No _____

Do you use food stamps? Yes _____ No _____

Are you able to grocery shop independently? Yes _____ No _____

If not, what assistance is necessary? _____

Ambulation: Full _____ Partial _____ Wheelchair _____

               Crutches _____ Cane or Walker _____ Bedfast _____

Neuromuscular problem affecting eating? Yes _____ No _____

Vision: Adequate _____ Partial _____ Blind _____

Hearing: Adequate _____ Partial _____ Hard of Hearing ____ Deaf _____

Teeth: Own in good condition _____ Dentures _____ None _____

Mental Competence: Adequate _____ Inadequate _____

Comments _____

_____

Do you take medication daily? Yes _____ No _____ What kind _____

Are you on a special diet? Yes _____ No _____

             What kind? _____

             Who prescribed it? _____

Do you usually eat alone? _____ with someone? _____

Is mealtime pleasurable? Yes _____ No _____

Recommendations: _____

FIGURE 3–2   A checklist useful for determination of nutritional risk.

Anthropometric Measurements

Height, weight, and skinfold measurements, particularly of triceps and subscapular areas, are simple procedures often utilized in nutritional assessment. Weight alone is the single most useful measurement of nutritional status. However, interpretation of weight information is not necessarily a simple matter. The standard height–weight tables used most often are those developed by the Metropolitan Life Insurance Company in 1960 (see Table 3–2). These tables give desirable weights based on the average weight for height of individuals in the population aged 25 to 29. The desirable

Weight in Pounds According to Frame (in Indoor Clothing)*

Desirable Weights for Men Aged 25 and Over

Height with Shoes 1-inch Heels		Small Frame	Medium Frame	Large Frame
Feet	Inches			
5	2	112–120	118–129	126–141
5	3	115–123	121–133	129–144
5	4	118–126	124–136	132–148
5	5	121–129	127–139	135–152
5	6	124–133	130–143	138–156
5	7	128–137	134–147	142–161
5	8	132–141	138–152	147–166
5	9	136–145	142–156	151–170
5	10	140–150	146–160	155–174
5	11	144–154	150–165	159–179
6	0	148–158	154–170	164–184
6	1	152–162	158–175	168–189
6	2	156–167	162–180	173–194
6	3	160–171	167–185	178–199
6	4	164–175	172–190	182–204

*For nude weight, deduct 5 to 7 lbs. (male).

TABLE 3–2(a)   Standard height/weight tables for men.

Source: Prepared by Metropolitan Life Insurance Company. Derived primarily from data of the Build and Blood Pressure Study, 1959, Society of Actuaries. Courtesy of Metropolitan Life Insurance Company.

weights are given for three different body frames: small, medium, and large. There is some problem defining frame size, as the method for determining it is not explained on the table, though the age of the population from which the chart is drawn should present no problem. In fact, a reliable estimate of a person's weight at age twenty-five is probably the best guide to evaluate his weight at any subsequent time. Weight gain after age twenty-five generally results from an increase in body fat. The only exception to this would be for the person who becomes physically active after this age and would thus have an increased weight from enlarged muscle mass. One complication in weight data interpretation is the possibility of fluid retention, which can result from prolonged undernutri-

Weight in Pounds According to Frame (in Indoor Clothing)*

Desirable Weights for Women Aged 25 and Over

Height with Shoes 2-inch Heels		Small Frame	Medium Frame	Large Frame
Feet	Inches			
4	10	92– 98	96–107	104–119
4	11	94–101	98–110	106–122
5	0	96–104	101–113	109–125
5	1	99–107	104–116	112–128
5	2	102–110	107–119	115–131
5	3	105–113	110–122	118–134
5	4	108–116	113–126	121–138
5	5	111–119	116–130	125–142
5	6	114–123	120–135	129–146
5	7	118–127	124–139	133–150
5	8	122–131	128–143	137–154
5	9	126–135	132–147	141–158
5	10	130–140	136–151	145–163
5	11	134–144	140–155	149–168
6	0	138–148	144–159	153–173

*For nude weight, deduct 2 to 4 lbs. (female).

TABLE 3–2(b)   Standard height/weight tables for women.

Source: Prepared by Metropolitan Life Insurance Company. Derived primarily from data of the Build and Blood Pressure Study, 1959, Society of Actuaries. Courtesy of Metropolitan Life Insurance Company.

tion and medical problems. Even if the aged individual does not appear edematous, retained fluid can add enough weight to cover up the effect of tissue wasting so that neither weight nor appearance indicates that the person is undernourished. (For a further discussion of malnutrition, see Chapter 7.) Height–weight measurements also may be misleading in an older person with osteoporotic changes which affect height or in a person who has had a loss of body parts due to trauma or surgery.

If weight is to be measured repeatedly as part of an ongoing assessment, weights should be obtained on the same scale and during the same time of the day, when the subject is wearing the same amount of clothing. Arm circumference measurement, taken on the nondominant side if possible, is a good indication of muscle mass. This measurement is made at the mid-point of the upper arm[11].

Measurement of skinfold thickness by calipers may provide more information about body fat than weight and height alone because one-half of all fat in the body is found directly under the skin. The triceps measurement is often used because of accessibility. However, the subscapular skinfold is less subject to error; it does not have to be done at a precise spot because the fat layer in that area is uniform.

Although the use of skinfold measurements has been criticized because of difficulty in replicating results, if done properly, skinfold measurements provide data which correlate well with other procedures for determining body fatness. The standards most often used for skinfold measurements are those by Seltzer and Mayer[12]. These measurements have not been standardized for people above age fifty. In the Ten State Nutrition Survey discussed above, the criterion for obesity was set at a triceps skinfold of more than 25.1 mm for women and 18.6 mm for men.

With any of the aforementioned methods of measurement, it is important to utilize standard procedure and equipment for accuracy.

Physical Signs of Nutrient Deficiency

The physical signs of nutrient deficiency are not early signs that a particular nutrient is lacking. Rather, they develop after a period of inadequate intake, during which time tissue stores are depleted and then normal metabolism is disturbed. Additionally, physical signs of deficiency are nonspecific; they may be caused by a deficiency of several nutrients or by a variety of other factors, such as exposure or lack of cleanliness. For example, mottled tooth enamel (or fluorosis) is a result of an excessively high intake of the mineral fluorine, though one might guess that this arose from poor hygiene.

Table 3-3 gives those physical signs most often associated with malnutrition[13]. It should be noted that, especially in the aged, other environmental factors can be responsible for what may appear to be a sign of nutrient deficiency. Inflamed, reddened gums, which may be due to a lack of ascorbic acid, also occur in cases of periodontal diseases. Cracks in the corners of the mouth may not necessarily be due to a B vitamin deficiency, but may be caused by ill-fitting dentures or a herpes infection.

An interesting observation has been that the elderly do not

often manifest the clinical signs of vitamin deficiency that might be expected considering their nutrient intakes. Dr. Adrian Ostfeld notes that many elderly who consume severely restricted diets such as milk and soda crackers three times a day nonetheless had no lesions of malnutrition and appeared as vigorous and healthy as those who consumed a more adequate diet[14]. No explanation was offered for this occurrence, though this may serve as further testimony of the inappropriateness of RDA values for assessing the nutrition of the elderly, as mentioned previously.

Biochemical Assessment

The laboratory assessment of blood and urine samples allows measurement of levels of nutrients, or metabolites of nutrients, circulating or excreted. Urine is routinely tested for pH, protein, glucose, and acetone, and may be tested for creatinine, thiamine, riboflavin, and n-methylnicotinamide. Blood may be tested for hemoglobin, hematocrit, total protein, serum albumin, cholesterol and triglycerides, glucose, sodium, potassium, chloride, uric acid, calcium, phosphorus, total iron, alkaline phosphatase, and less often for levels of carotene and vitamins A and C.

There is no single test to measure nutritional status, but measures such as hemoglobin, plasma ascorbate, or serum protein levels are considered important in the assessment of nutritional state[15]. However, there is not general agreement on the appropriate standards to be used, particularly for the elderly. Some researchers feel tissue saturation is optimum. Others will accept lower levels as adequate. For example, it has been postulated that hemoglobin levels presently accepted as normal may not be appropriate for black people who may "normally" have lower levels of circulating hemoglobin. Hemoglobin levels at or below the lower end of normal range are considered a natural concomitant of aging. These low values should not simply be accepted as the result of aging alone, unless all possible nutritional and other etiologies have been ruled out.

Biochemical assessment of elderly individuals may also uncover elevated levels of some nutrients. Increased levels of certain nutrients, principally of vitamins A and D, indicated by increased blood levels (in the case of vitamin A) and elevated blood calcium levels (in the case of vitamin D) may indicate toxic results of excessive intake. Elevation of serum lipid levels and its dietary treatment will be considered in Chapter 7.

Physical Signs of Malnutrition

Body Area	Normal Appearance	Signs Associated with Malnutrition
Hair	Shiny; firm; not easily plucked	Lack of natural shine; hair dull and dry; thin and sparse; hair fine, silky and straight, color changes (flag sign); can be easily plucked
Face	Skin color uniform; smooth, pink, healthy appearance; not swollen	Skin color loss (depigmentation); skin dark over cheeks and under eyes (malar and supra-orbital pigmentation); lumpiness or flakiness of skin of nose and mouth; swollen face; enlarged parotid glands; scaling of skin around nostrils (nasolabial seborrhea)
Eyes	Bright, clear, shiny; no sores at corners of eyelids; membranes a healthy pink and are moist. No prominent blood vessels or mound of tissue or sclera	Eye membranes are pale (pale conjunctivae); redness of membranes (conjunctival injection); Bitot's spots; redness and fissuring of eyelid corners (angular palpebritis); dryness of eye membranes (conjunctival xerosis); cornea has dull appearance (corneal xerosis); cornea is soft (keratomalacia); scar on cornea; ring of fine blood vessels around corner (circumcorneal injection)
Lips	Smooth, not chapped or swollen	Redness and swelling of mouth or lips (cheilosis); especially at corners of mouth (angular fissures and scars)
Tongue	Deep red in appearance; not swollen or smooth	Swelling; scarlet and raw tongue; magenta (purplish color) of tongue; smooth tongue; swollen sores; hyperemic and hypertrophic papillae; and atrophic papillae
Teeth	No cavities; no pain; bright	May be missing or erupting abnormally; gray or black spots (fluorosis); cavities (caries)
Gums	Healthy; red; do not bleed; not swollen	"Spongy" and bleed easily; recession of gums
Glands	Face not swollen	Thyroid enlargement (front of neck); parotid enlargement (cheeks become swollen)

46

Skin	No signs of rashes, swellings, dark or light spots	Dryness of skin (xerosis); sandpaper feel of skin (follicular hyperkeratosis); flakiness of skin; skin swollen and dark; red swollen pigmentation of exposed areas (pellagrous dermatosis); excessive lightness or darkness of skin (dyspigmentation); black and blue marks due to skin bleeding (petechiae); lack of fat under skin
Nails	Firm, pink	Nails are spoon-shape (koilonychia); brittle, ridged nails
Muscular and skeletal systems	Good muscle tone; some fat under skin; can walk or run without pain	Muscles have "wasted" appearance; baby's skull bones are thin and soft (craniotabes); round swelling of front and side of head (frontal and parietal bossing); swelling of ends of bones (epiphyseal enlargement); small bumps on both sides of chest wall (on ribs)—beading of ribs; baby's soft spot on head does not harden at proper time (persistently open anterior fontanelle); knock-knees or bow-legs; bleeding into muscle (musculoskeletal hemorrhages); person cannot get up or walk properly
Internal Systems: Cardiovascular	Normal heart rate and rhythm; no murmurs or abnormal rhythms; normal blood pressure for age	Rapid heart rate (above 100 tachycardia); enlarged heart; abnormal rhythm; elevated blood pressure
Gastrointestinal	No palpable organs or masses (in children, however, liver edge may be palpable)	Liver enlargement; enlargement of spleen (usually indicates other associated diseases)
Nervous	Psychological stability; normal reflexes	Mental irritability and confusion; burning and tingling of hands and feet (paresthesia); loss of position and vibratory sense; weakness and tenderness of muscles (may result in inability to walk); decrease and loss of ankle and knee reflexes

TABLE 3–3   Physical signs indicative or suggestive of malnutrition, as compared to normal appearance.

Source: Nutritional Assessment in Health Programs Part I—Methodology, Clinical Assessment of Nutrition Status, *Am. Journal of Public Health,* 63:18, Nov. 1973.

CITED REFERENCES

1. Food and Nutrition Board. 1974. *Recommended dietary allowances.* 8th ed. National Research Council, National Academy of Sciences, Washington, D.C.
2. Michelsen, O. 1976. The possible role of vitamins in the aging process. In *Nutrition, longevity and aging,* eds. M. Rockstein and M. L. Sussman, p. 123. New York: Academic Press, Inc.
3. Harper, A. E. 1978. Recommended dietary allowances for the elderly. *Geriatrics* 33:73.
4. O'Hanlon, C., and Kohrs, M. B. 1978. Dietary studies of older Americans. *Amer. J. Clinical Nutrition* 31:1257.
5. Household Food Consumption Survey, 1965–66. November 11, 1972. *Food and nutrient intake of individuals in the United States—Spring 1965.* Washington, D.C.: U.S. Department of Agriculture, Agriculture Research Service Report.
6. Dept. of Health, Education and Welfare, Health Service and Mental Health Administration, Center for Disease Control. *Ten states nutrition survey, 1968–1970.* 1972. DHEW Pub. No. (HSM) 72-8130-34. Atlanta.
7. *Anthropometric and clinical findings, preliminary findings of the first Health and Nutrition Examination Survey (HANES), U.S. 1971–1972.* 1975. DHEW Publication No. (HRA) 75-1229. U.S. Government Printing Office, Washington, D.C.
8. Tempelton, C. L. 1978. Nutrition counseling needs in a geriatric population. *Geriatrics* 33:59.
9. The validity of twenty four hour dietary recalls. 1976. *Nutrition Reviews* 34(10):310.
10. Metress, J., and Kart, C. 1978. A system for observing the potential nutritional risks of elderly people living at home. *J. Geriatric Psychiatry* 11(1):67.
11. Caly, J. C. 1977. Assessing adult's nutrition. *Amer. J. Nursing* 77(10):1605.

12. Seltzer, C. C., and Mayer, J. A. 1965. A simple criterion of obesity. *J. Postgrad. Medicine* 38:A101.
13. Nutrition assessment of the elderly. 1973. *Amer. J. Public Health Supplement* 63:68.
14. Ostfeld, A. M. Nutrition and aging-discussants perspective. In *Epidemiology of aging,* eds. A. M. Ostfeld and D. C. Gibson, p. 215. DHEW Pub. No. (NIH) 77-711.
15. Sandstead, H. H., and Pearson, W. N. 1973. Clinical evaluation of nutrition status. In *Modern nutrition in health and disease,* eds. R. S. Goodhart and M. E. Shils, p. 562. Philadelphia: Lea and Febiger.

OTHER REFERENCES

Allard, J.; Carden, P. T.; and Murray, E. January 5, 1978. Malnutrition and neglect. *Nursing Mirror,* p. 18.
Brewster, L., and Jacobson, M. F. 1978. *The changing American diet.* Washington, D.C.: Center for Science in the Public Interest.
Brown, P., et al. 1977. Dietary status of elderly people. *J. Amer. Dietetic Assoc.* 71:41.
Butterworth, C. E., and Blackburn, G. L. 1975. Hospital malnutrition. *Nutrition Today* 10(2):8.
Fisher, S.; Handricks, D. G.; and Mahoney, A. W. 1978. Nutritional assessment of senior rural Utahans by biochemical and physical measurement. *Amer. J. Clinical Nutrition* 31:667.
Luke, B. 1976. Good geriatrics, nutrition is a lifelong nursing matter. *R.N.* 39(7):24.
Madden, J. P.; Goodman, S. J., and Guthrie, H. A. 1976. Validity of the 24-hour recall. *J. Amer. Dietetic Assoc.* 68:143.
Nutritional assessment in health programs, part I—Methodology clinical assessment of nutritional status. 1973. *Amer. J. Public Health Supplement* 63:18.
Stiedemann, M.; Jansen, C.; and Harrill, I. 1978. Nutritional status of elderly men and women. *J. Amer. Dietetic Assoc.* 73:132.
Wellman, N. S. 1978. The evaluation of nutritional status. In *Nutrition and clinical care,* eds. R. J. Howard and N. H. Herbold. New York: McGraw-Hill Book Co.
Yearick, E. S. 1978. Nutritional status of the elderly, anthropometric and clinical findings. *J. Gerontology* 33(5):657.

IIIIIIIIIIIIIIIIIIIIIIIIIIIIIIIIIIIIIIIIIII 4

Energy Nutrients

More than forty different nutrients are needed to maintain life, growth, health, and vigor. These nutrients include protein, fat, carbohydrate, vitamins, and minerals. Fiber and water, which are non-nutritive substances, are also necessary as part of an optimal diet. All individuals, whatever their age, need the same nutrients. However, the amount of each nutrient that one needs depends on sex, body size, activity, condition of health, and age. While the needs for optimal nutrition in the healthy aged individual differ little from those of younger persons, it is necessary to remember that the aged constitute a much less homogeneous group than do younger persons. Each person differs from others as a result of genetic endowments coupled with the stresses of life to which he has been subjected. Each one also has specific personal attitudes toward food, and varying physical and mental conditions. For these reasons, it is wrong to generalize about what constitutes the optimum diet. Even moreso than with younger persons, dietary needs of the elderly must be individualized.

The following three chapters discuss the importance of the various nutrients, fiber, and water, including guidelines for the choosing of appropriate amounts of each in the diet. This chapter discusses energy and those nutrients that the body is able to use for energy.

ENERGY

Proper body function relies on the production of energy from the body's fuel supply—food. This energy is commonly measured as calories or kilocalories (abbreviated as C or kcal; 1 kcal = 1,000 calories), which is the amount of heat needed to raise the temperature of 1 kilogram (kg) of water 1 °C. Recently, the standard international unit kilojoule has come into use as a unit of energy. One kilocalorie is equal to 4.184 kilojoules. Kilojoules are commonly referred to as *Joules* and kilocalories are more commonly called *Calories.*

The fuel factor (average number of Calories for each gram) of each of the three energy yielding nutrients—carbohydrate, protein, and fat—is:

carbohydrate—4 Calories (or 17 Joules) per gram

protein—4 Calories (or 17 Joules) per gram

fat—9 Calories (or 37.6 Joules) per gram

These factors represent a simplification in that various carbohydrates differ slightly in the number of Calories per gram that they hold, although the average figure for ingested carbohydrates as a group is four. The same is also true of various proteins and fats, and the values listed for these are averages also. It is apparent that fat is the most concentrated source of calories in the diet.

There is no general agreement as to the ideal caloric intake for the aged individual, although it is usually recommended that an aged person's caloric level be reduced from that recommended for young adults. The National Research Council in the Recommended Dietary Allowance (see Chapter 3, Table 3-1) recommends that the energy allowance for those over fifty-one be reduced. This takes into account a 2 percent decrease in basal (resting) metabolic rate per decade, and a reduction in activity of 200 kilocalories for men and women between fifty-one and seventy-five years. For those over seventy-five, a reduction of 500 kilocalories for men and 400 kilocalories for women is recommended. The customary range of daily energy output is also given and is based on a variation in energy needs of plus or minus 400 kilocalories at any one age. This emphasizes the wide range of energy intakes appropriate for any group of people. The recommended energy intake for males is: fifty-one to seventy-five years, 2400 kilocalories; seventy-six and over, 2050 kilocalories. The recommended energy intake for females is: fifty-one to seventy-five years, 1800 kilocalories; seventy-six and over, 1600 kilocalories.

The Joint Food and Agriculture Organization, World Health Organization (FAO/WHO) Committee on Energy and Protein Requirements recommends a reduction in daily caloric intake of 5 percent for each decade between the ages of forty and fifty-nine, and a 10 percent reduction from sixty to sixty-nine years with another 10 percent reduction for those aged seventy and over.

With a reduced caloric intake, calories must be chosen carefully so that all necessary nutrients are included despite the reduction. A general recommendation is to eliminate, or severely reduce, consumption of fats and sweets. The 250 Calories obtained from a doughnut must be an occasional luxury for most of the aged because their reduced caloric intake demands that more nutritious foods be selected that provide the needed protein, vitamins, and minerals along with calories.

Eliminating most sweets and fats benefits the elderly in other ways. An impaired glucose tolerance with delayed insulin response is frequently found in the elderly, especially in older women. In addition a high fat intake may cause indigestion and may contribute to degenerative changes.

It is well to remember that 1 gm of alcohol yields about seven Calories and the consumption of alcoholic beverages may contribute appreciably to caloric intake and may displace other needed foods[1]. This problem will be covered more fully in Chapter 8.

Elderly people subsisting on insufficient calories often show fatigue, lassitude, and lack of interest in their surroundings. It is also believed that an insufficient caloric intake may contribute to premature aging. One study of the relation of calorie intake to health of 100 women aged forty to seventy years showed that those whose health was rated as "good" consumed 1,650 to 1,825 Calories a day while those whose health was rated as "poor" consumed 1,125 to 1,425 Calories a day[2]. When one's daily caloric intake is low there is an increased likelihood of other nutrient deficiencies. It is difficult to distinguish cause from effect. Perhaps a lowered caloric intake results in poor health. On the other hand, an individual in poor health is likely to consume less food. Both of these factors probably are at work.

Since one's level of activity may change from day to day, there is no exact number of calories that an individual needs to consume daily. In practice, one's intake must be adjusted to prevent one from becoming either over- or underweight. Special care must be taken to ensure that a diet low in calories includes foods that supply all essential nutrients.

PROTEIN

The very name protein (derived from the Greek word meaning "of first importance") gives an indication of the value placed on this nutrient. In fact, more than 15 percent of the average human body by weight is protein. Protein is a constituent of every cell and substance in the body except urine and bile.

There is a wide variety of proteins in the body with a wide range of specialized functions and characteristics. The body utilizes protein for growth, maintenance and repair of tissues, as well as for energy.

Protein, as found in food and in the body, is made up of combinations of twenty or more different amino acids. The type and amount of the amino acids as well as their physical arrangement determine the characteristics of the protein. In digestion, food proteins are split into their constituent amino acids by specialized enzymes which themselves are proteins. The body then uses these amino acids to build protein substances that it needs. These proteins might be structural proteins such as collagen, which makes up connective tissue, blood proteins such as albumin, muscle protein, enzymes, antibodies, hormones or nucleoproteins such as deoxyribonuclease.

Of the twenty or so amino acids used by the body, there are nine that the body cannot make in amounts sufficient to independently maintain an adequate supply. Thus these nine amino acids, termed the essential amino acids, must be obtained in food. All of these amino acids must be present at the same time in adequate amounts in order for the body to synthesize the proteins it needs. Foods containing all the essential amino acids in optimum concentrations are said to contain "complete" proteins or proteins of "high biological value." Examples of these are eggs, milk, meat, and soybeans. Mixtures of two or more foods may greatly increase their protein values as the amino acids in short supply in one of these foods may be supplemented by the amino acids in another food, such as in a mixture of rice and beans, or in a cereal served with a small amount of milk.

The other amino acids needed by the body are termed nonessential. This does not mean that they are less important to the body but rather that, given an adequate source of nitrogen, carbon, hydrogen, and oxygen, they can be readily produced in the body. The term nonessential refers to the fact that they are nonessential in the diet, though all twenty amino acids are needed by the body in its protein.

Nitrogen balance studies are used to ascertain minimum protein requirements and also to determine if an individual is gaining or losing tissue protein under various conditions of health and dietary intake. The dietary intake of protein, usually calculated from amounts listed on nutritive value food charts, is measured against the nitrogen lost in urine and feces and through the skin. When the amount of nitrogen taken in as food equals the amount of nitrogen lost through these three routes, the individual is said to be in nitrogen balance. A positive nitrogen balance means that the body is retaining more nitrogen than it is losing, as is the case during growth periods, pregnancy, and recovery from a stressful period. A negative nitrogen balance, which indicates that the body is losing more nitrogen than it retains, may occur during injury, surgery, fever, infection, or emotional stress, or during a period of inadequate protein intake[2]. From this information alone one can see the protein needs of a healthy aged individual may differ dramatically from one who is ill.

Most of the studies performed to determine the protein needs of the elderly used healthy persons as subjects. It was found that their requirements were similar to those of younger adults. These studies are not in agreement with some showing the aged to have an increased need for protein to maintain nitrogen balance and other studies showing the aged to need less protein[3]. There is, apparently, a great variation in the amount of protein needed for equilibrium among aged individuals.

The daily protein intake recommended by the National Research Council is 0.8 gm of protein per kilogram of body weight throughout adult life, which is believed to cover the needs of almost all healthy individuals. If one's intake consists primarily of protein of high biological value, the allowance is 0.6 gm/kg of body weight[4].

The FAO/WHO daily allowances are 0.57 gm/kg of body weight for adult males and 0.52 gm/kg of body weight for adult females[5]. These intakes have been found to maintain nitrogen equilibrium in most healthy elderly people during short-term studies.

As the above-mentioned recommendations are based on healthy aged, it is possible that various illnesses frequently found in the elderly may decrease one's protein absorption or increase one's protein loss. In light of the fact that old age is rarely found without concomitant disease, some recommend an intake of 1 gm/kg protein for all elderly.

All of these recommendations assume that the non-protein nutrients in one's diet are providing sufficient calories to meet energy needs. If this is not the case, more protein would be needed to maintain optimum nutrition. Many studies have shown that older people consuming fewer than 1,400 Calories a day usually have diets inadequate in calcium, iron, and vitamins. Even though sufficient protein may be provided in the 1,400 Calorie intake, since too few calories for energy are present, much of the ingested protein may be used for energy rather than to make structural and enzymatic proteins. The result is a negative nitrogen balance.

Relevant to the diet concerns of the elderly is the observation that, as the caloric content of the diet is decreased, it is advisable that an increased proportion of ingested calories be from protein. This is to say that despite a reduction of total caloric intake, protein intake must remain adequate (i.e., must undergo little or no change). Since the protein intake of a middle-aged adult should approximate 12 percent of total daily caloric intake, by using the aforementioned caloric intakes recommended for the elderly of various ages, one may arrive at similar figures relevant to the elderly (12–14 percent).

High protein intakes may be contraindicated under certain conditions. Decreased functioning or disorders of liver or kidney may necessitate a reduction in the amount of protein allowed in the diet. High dietary protein interferes with calcium absorption and may result in a negative calcium balance. This may predispose an individual to osteoporosis. A diet low in protein usually means that it is deficient in iron, riboflavin, niacin, and thiamine, since these nutrients tend to occur together in high protein foods. For further discussion of these nutrients, see Chapter 5.

Several factors cause the elderly to consume less protein than younger adults. These include the fact that often (except for dry skim milk) protein foods are more expensive than other foods. Meat may be hard to chew and swallow. Also, the preparation of many protein foods requires equipment and physical energy which may be in short supply. Additionally, many elderly reject milk from their diets although it is reasonable in cost and requires no preparation. This may be because of the discomfort associated with milk drinking due to lactose intolerance, but is more likely to be due to long standing habit.

A sufficient but not excessive amount of protein, enough to maintain nitrogen balance, must be included in the diet of elderly individuals. For ways to do this, see Appropriate Food Selection, Chapter 12.

LIPID

Lipid is a term that refers to a class of compounds including fat, fatty acids, and cholesterol. In the average American diet, lipid (commonly, though incorrectly, known as fat) contributes about 42 percent of the calories eaten daily. There are large amounts of lipid in many such foods as meats, whole milk, eggs, cheese, and nuts, as well as, more obviously, in oils, butter, and margarine. The lipid in these latter foods is referred to as visible lipid while lipid not readily apparent, such as that in milk, is termed invisible lipid. The invisible lipids contribute more than one-half of the total lipid in the average diet.

There is lipid in all animal and vegetable foods. The total amount of lipid in the Western diet has increased since early in this century. Lately, Americans have been increasing their consumption of vegetable fats, such as cooking oils and margarine, and at the same time they have been eating less animal fat, such as that from eggs, butter, and milk[4].

Fat and Fatty Acids

"Fat" is the chemical name for a type of molecule comprised of fatty acids bonded to a glycerol molecule. Fatty acids are organic acids of a variety of types. Fatty acids vary in the number of carbon atoms that they contain. Some have as few as two to four and are called short chain fatty acids; those with six to ten carbon atoms are referred to as the medium chain fatty acids, while long chain fatty acids have twelve to twenty-four carbon atoms. These carbon atom chains can be completely filled with hydrogen atoms, in which case the fatty acid is termed "saturated." Alternatively, the carbon chain may have some atoms that are not holding the maximum amount of hydrogen possible; these are termed "unsaturated." The degree of unsaturation of a fatty acid is further distinguished as either monounsaturated or polyunsaturated, referring to whether one or several carbon atoms are capable of holding more hydrogen.

Dietary fats contain mixtures of fatty acids—saturated, mono-unsaturated, and polyunsaturated. Fats from vegetable sources such as vegetable oils tend to be higher in polyunsaturated fatty acids than are the fats from animal sources. However, coconut oil, a vegetable fat, contains a high percentage of saturated fatty acids.

Cholesterol

Cholesterol is an alcohol found in all animal tissues. There is some evidence that elevated levels of cholesterol in the blood contribute to the development of atherosclerosis and are associated with an increased prevalence of cardiovascular disease. However, there is no proof of a causal relationship between cholesterol levels in the blood and cardiovascular disease. There is only a statistical correlation between the two. There is also a correlation between dietary satu-rated fat and plasma cholesterol levels. Polyunsaturated fats in the diet have been correlated with a lowered serum cholesterol level in the body while dietary saturated fats have been correlated with ele-vated serum cholesterol levels (monounsaturated fats appear to have no effect on serum cholesterol levels). Many factors enter into the etiology of cardiovascular disease and these will be discussed in Chapter 7.

Cholesterol is obtained in the diet mainly through consump-tion of eggs, meat, organ or glandular meats, whole milk, and cheese. Cholesterol is also synthesized in the body. In fact, about three times as much cholesterol is synthesized in the body as is absorbed from food. Cholesterol is essential in the body as a struc-tural component of cell membranes and plasma lipids and as a metabolic precursor of bile acids needed for digestion. Cholesterol is also a precursor of several steroid hormones and of vitamin D, which is formed in the body from 7-dehydrocholesterol.

The level of serum cholesterol generally increases with age. This increase tends to occur earlier in life in men than in women. However, women in their fifties and sixties tend to have higher serum cholesterol levels than their male counterparts[6].

Essential Fatty Acids

Linoleic acid, a polyunsaturated fatty acid, is an essential fatty acid for humans. (Arachidonic acid is sometimes classified as an essential fatty acid, but it can be made in the body from linoleic acid.) Linoleic acid is a precursor of other important molecules and must be obtained in the diet because it cannot be synthesized in the body. Essential fatty acid deficiency—which is evidenced by scaly skin, poor wound healing, and a reduced number of platelets in the blood—is rare. This deficiency has been reported in individuals who have been maintained for several weeks on fat-free total parenteral feedings (nourishments given by entry routes into the body other than the mouth).

The National Research Council recommends that 1–2 percent of one's total caloric intake be from essential fatty acids. Good food sources include the various vegetable oils such as corn, peanut, cottonseed, soybean, and safflower.

Lipids and Diet

In addition to providing essential fatty acids, fats yield a concentrated source of energy, more than double that from an equal weight of carbohydrates or protein. This is valuable for people whose energy requirements are high due to large amounts of physical activity or body stress. (For most people, who need to limit caloric intake, reducing the amount of fat eaten is desirable.) Fats are also important in the diet because they carry the fat-soluble vitamins, A, D, E, and K, from the gastrointestinal tract into the blood stream. These vitamins will be described more fully in Chapter 5.

Fat deposits, as adipose tissue, thermally insulate the body and also cushion organs. Lipids and their derivatives are found in many structural elements of the cell and in many necessary body compounds such as some hormones.

Fats give flavor to foods either when occurring naturally in a food such as meat or when added during preparation or serving of a food. Because fat remains longer in the stomach than other foods, a meal or snack that contains some fat will tend to delay the return of hunger, thus satisfying the individual longer than other types of food.

There are indications that Americans consume too much fat. Fat intake has been identified as a risk factor associated with coronary heart disease, and diets high in fat and animal protein have been identified as risk factors in the development of certain types of cancer. The incidence of obesity is also correlated with the consumption of concentrated sources of calories from foods high in fat and sugar.

The American Heart Association recommends that lipid should contribute no more than 35 percent of the calories in the diet. This would necessitate an approximate reduction of 7 percent of an average individual's intake. This suggestion is based on a realization of the need for a reduction in lipid intake, yet at the same time indicates an appreciation that most healthy Americans would not voluntarily consume a diet with a very restricted lipid content.

Nathan Pritikin, Director of the Longevity Research Institute of California, recommends a diet containing only 5-10 percent of its calories as fat and less than 100 mg of cholesterol along with other restrictions of sugar, salt, and caffeine. He believes that the present suggestions of limited restrictions are not sufficient to ensure good health. He has reported reversal of atherosclerosis in several patients maintained on his diet and exercise regimen[7]. A controlled experimental study is necessary to properly evaluate the effect of this diet modification.

The minimum amount of lipid needed by an adult is believed to be 15-25 gm a day. This would provide 135 to 225 Calories or about 10-15 percent of total energy intake. If appropriately chosen, this amount could provide all the essential fatty acids and fat-soluble vitamins needed. However, this would represent a drastic reduction in lipid intake that would not be acceptable to most individuals. A more realistic suggestion for the elderly would be to reduce lipid intake to 30-35 percent of total calories. A moderate reduction of lipid intake, down to 38-40 percent of total calories, can be achieved by cutting down on the amount of visible or separable lipid. Reducing it beyond this to 30-35 percent of total calories requires modification of food choices and methods of food preparation.

A high fat intake is undesirable for the elderly for reasons other than obesity and possible contribution to degenerative diseases. A high fat intake can cause indigestion; malabsorption may result because of a lessened efficiency of the gastrointestinal tract as well as pancreatic and liver insufficiency characteristic of old age.

CARBOHYDRATE

The third energy-yielding nutrient provides over 50 percent of the calories in the average diet in the United States, and is the primary source of energy for all people. Carbohydrate-rich foods such as crackers, breads, cereals, and sweets are low in cost when compared to most other foods. Also, they are easily stored for long periods of time without refrigeration and are easy to prepare—often ready to eat. For these reasons, the elderly may consume a great deal of carbohydrate, sometimes at the expense of protein and other nutrients. This is most likely to be so when one's primary carbohydrate source is refined sugar.

Monosaccharides   Carbohydrates refer to sugars and starches. Included in the sugar category are monosaccharides, which are single sugar units, and disaccharides, which are two sugars (two monosaccharides) complexed together. Also included are polysaccharides, which are complex carbohydrates (such as starch) made up of many units of monosaccharides.

All carbohydrates are at some time broken down to, or converted to, the monosaccharide glucose, also known as dextrose, which is the most common form of carbohydrate transported and used by the body. (The normal blood glucose level is 60 to 100 mg/100 ml; levels below 60 mg/100 ml are termed *hypoglycemia,* while levels above 100 mg/100ml indicate *hyperglycemia.*) Blood glucose levels in the elderly tend to be somewhat higher than average. This may be due largely to inefficiency of the pancreas to secrete insulin (necessary for absorption of glucose by most cells) in response to a rise in blood glucose levels. Glucose is stored as a polymer called glycogen which is easily broken back down to glucose for immediately useable energy.

Fructose, another monosaccharide, is—as its name implies—found in many fruits. It is much sweeter than glucose and is being considered as a substitute for table sugar in foods for diabetics. Fructose is absorbed from the gastrointestinal tract in an insulin-independent fashion and more slowly than glucose. Most fructose is metabolized in the liver, where insulin is needed only for the later stages of metabolism. Consequently, the ingestion of fructose by a diabetic causes only a modest rise in blood glucose level (as some fructose is converted to glucose during the absorption process). Therefore, the use of small amounts of fructose by a well-controlled diabetic does not necessitate any additional dosage of insulin. However, fructose should not be used "ad lib" by the diabetic since it is a source of both glucose and calories[8].

Other simple sugars are galactose, found primarily in milk as a constituent of lactose (see below), and mannose, found in the sap of certain trees.

Disaccharides   The most familiar disaccharide is sucrose, or table sugar, which is composed of one molecule each of glucose and fructose. Sucrose is refined from the sugar cane or sugar beet. Many fruits and vegetables contain sucrose naturally—bananas, dates, pineapples, sweet potatoes. The sugar in these foods is often termed natural, while table sugar is referred to as "unnatural." Sucrose from fruits and vegetables is chemically and nutritionally identical to refined sucrose. However, when one consumes fruits or vegetables, one is obtaining calories from the sugar as well as other needed nutrients while refined sugar provides calories alone.

The current average diet in the United States has 15–20 percent of its total calories as sucrose (a 50 percent increase over the amount used in 1910)[9]. This is over 100 lbs of sucrose used per person each year. Gelatin desserts are among those foods often served to the elderly because they are inexpensive and easily eaten. Contrary to popular belief, however, gelatin is a source of only low quality protein. It contains mainly sucrose with added artificial color and flavor. One half-cup serving of gelatin dessert provides approximately eighty calories, 95 percent of which are from the sucrose. It is interesting to note that almost one-fourth of the sugar consumed in the United States (approximately twenty-two pounds per person per year) is from soft drinks which provide only sucrose, water, artificial coloring, flavoring, and sometimes caffeine and carbon dioxide. The elderly, with lessened caloric needs, should be wary of food items such as these which displace other more nutritious sources of carbohydrate in the diet.

Other major disaccharides in the diet are maltose, formed in the breakdown of starch, and lactose, the principle sugar in milk. The presence of lactose in milk makes it an unacceptable food for some people who, because of a lack of the enzyme lactase, cannot digest lactose. Lactase is necessary to split the disaccharide lactose into its component monosaccharides prior to absorption.

In the absence of lactase, lactose passes unchanged through the digestive tract and into the large intestine where it is fermented by bacteria. The lactose and its fermentation products exert an osmotic force that draws fluid into the colon and causes diarrhea, flatulence, and cramps. There may be a loss of normally absorbable nutrients due to these gastrointestinal disturbances.

Lactose intolerance due to lactase deficiency is more common among the elderly than the young. It is estimated that this deficiency occurs in as many as 80 percent of the older individuals of many populations, especially Asians and Africans. A recent study on milk drinking habits of the elderly of various social backgrounds in Texas found that over 90 percent of blacks, Mexican-Americans, and Anglos drank milk without symptoms. Very few reported that they did not drink milk because of symptoms that might be attributed to low lactase levels[10]. This is not in agreement with other published reports on incidence of lactose intolerance. A possible explanation for this lack of agreement is that in tests for lactase activity, 50 gm of lactose dissolved in water is given to a fasting subject. A glass of milk contains only about 12 gm of lactose and milk is generally consumed along with other foods which might slow the passage of lactose through the gastrointestinal tract and thus aid in its full digestion, thereby lessening the chance of symptoms.

Some lactose intolerant individuals seem to be able to digest fermented dairy products such as yogurt and buttermilk. These products contain slightly less lactose than milk does. Small amounts of milk, up to one cup, may also be well tolerated by some individuals. There is a product available, Lact-aid, which contains an enzyme from yeast—*saccharomyces lactis* lactase—which splits the lactose in milk into its component monosaccharides, glucose and galactose. This should prove useful to those with a lactase deficiency. Soybean milk is another possibility for the lactose-intolerant individual; it contains adequate amounts of protein and many marketed brands contain no lactose.

Lactose is a basic ingredient of many varieties of tube feedings. Common side effects of these feedings include abdominal distention, cramping, and diarrhea. It has been shown that even individuals with normal lactose tolerance tests may exhibit symptoms when large amounts of lactose are fed, as may be common with some tube feedings[11]. It has been recommended that lactose be eliminated from tube feedings and there are some feedings currently available that do not contain it.

Polysaccharides   Polysaccharides include starches (which yield calories because they can be digested), as well as cellulose and other structural substances such as hemicelluloses, pectin, mucilages, gums, and lignins (which are indigestible and furnish bulk). Lignin, a woody substance, is often grouped with polysaccharides because it is found in plants bound to cellulose, though it is not truly a carbohydrate because it contains nitrogen. The indigestible carbohydrates, known as fiber, will be considered in Chapter 6.

In the United States, people are consuming fewer complex carbohydrates while the consumption of table sugar is rising, as noted above. In 1976, it was estimated that complex carbohydrates accounted for 21 percent of the calories consumed in the average diet, a substantial decrease from the 37 percent of the diet's calories from this source in 1909–1913[9].

This substitution of sugar for starch is considered to be the single greatest change in human diets over the past 150 years. This dietary change is believed to be responsible for the prevalence of dental caries and may contribute to the current incidence of diabetes and cardiovascular disease[12]. Studies show that when sucrose is substituted isocalorically for complex carbohydrates, there is an increase in the concentration of serum cholesterol and triglycerides. It is important to note here that honey, frequently extolled as a "health food," contains only minute amounts of nutrients other than carbohydrates and is essentially equivalent to table sugar in the diet. Thus it should be used no more liberally.

Persons maintained on very restricted carbohydrate intakes or carbohydrate-free diets may develop ketosis. This refers to the accumulation of ketone bodies which are formed when fatty acids are oxidized to two-carbon fragments, a point at which they may enter the pathway of normal oxidation of carbohydrates. However, in the absence of carbohydrate, complete oxidation of all the two-carbon fragments does not occur and they condense to form "ketones." These "ketones" are fairly strong acids. Some are metabolized, but the excess is excreted in urine along with the alkaline salts of sodium, calcium, and magnesium. This results in a loss of water and basic substances from the body, leading to a reduction in the pH value of the blood and a disruption of the body's acid–base balance. Ketosis is associated with symptoms which include the breakdown of body protein, increased sodium and fluid excretion, and loss of energy, and may even precipitate gout. Intakes of 50 to 100 gm of carbohydrate daily seem to prevent ketosis. Certain populations, such as Eskimos, have lived on diets practically devoid of carbohydrate and thus there is some question as to whether carbohydrate is essential in the diet. Nevertheless, carbohydrates, particularly starches, contribute to a balanced diet.

The elderly should be encouraged to consume at least 60 percent of their calories from carbohydrates, principally complex carbohydrates and not sugars. These carbohydrates should be obtained from whole grain or enriched breads and cereals, rice, potatoes, beets, peas, lentils, corn, and beans. Other vegetables, coming from the leaf, flower, or stem of a plant, contain more water and fiber and less carbohydrate than the roots, tubers, or seeds, but contribute to the carbohydrate supply as do the simple sugars and disaccharides in fruits. Canned and frozen fruits often have sugar added and these should be avoided, if possible, so that a greater portion of one's energy needs can be met by complex carbohydrate intake.

Artificial Sweeteners and Sugar Substitutes

A complete discussion of carbohydrates and nutrition requires at least brief mention of agents used to replace carbohydrates in the diet. Quite a few substances have been investigated for use as sucrose substitutes. A discussion of these follows.

Saccharin is the only artificial sweetener currently permitted in the food supply. The Food and Drug Administration is considering banning it because of reports that its ingestion causes liver tumors in rats. It is presently sold with the following warning label: "Use of this product may be hazardous to your health. This product contains saccharin, which has been determined to cause cancer in laboratory animals." The Food and Drug Administration is expected to issue a decision in 1980, on whether or not they will permit saccharin to be sold and how it will be sold.

Calcium and sodium cyclamates were banned in 1969 because they were reported to cause bladder tumors in rats. It is expected that manufacturers of these sweeteners will petition for reconsideration of their use.

Other artificial sweeteners have been studied. Aspartame is composed of two amino acids, a molecule of aspartic acid linked to one of phenylalanine[13]. It is 160 times as sweet as sugar, though its safety has been questioned and it has not yet been approved for use. Neohesperidin, derived from citrus rinds, has not shown any ill effects in animal experimentation. However, its flavor is unacceptable because it exhibits an intense sweetness which is slow in onset, followed by considerable lingering. Further investigation is needed to develop an analog of neohesperidin with the desired sweetening characteristics.

Sorbitol is an alcohol made from glucose. It is absorbed very slowly so it has little effect on blood glucose levels. For this reason it is used as a sweetener in foods manufactured for diabetics. Although not as sweet as sugar, it does provide as many calories, so it should not mistakenly be thought of as an adjunct to dieting. Large amounts of sorbitol—over two tablespoons per day—may cause osmotic diarrhea because it is absorbed so slowly from the intestine.

Mannitol is an alcohol of mannose used as a drying agent in foods. As it is poorly absorbed, mannitol supplies only one-half of the calories of an equivalent amount of glucose.

Xylitol, a sweetener found in strawberries, raspberries, and cauliflower, is also made in the body. It is approximately as sweet as fructose and is presently used as a sugar substitute in chewing gum. Test results have indicated a link between xylitol and cancer in laboratory animals. This has made future use of this sweetener questionable[14].

Fructose, sorbitol, and xylitol can all enter the cell and be metabolized to trioses in the glycolytic pathway without insulin. However, further catabolism of all three molecules requires the presence of insulin[8].

CITED REFERENCES

1. Schroeder, H. A. 1971. Nutrition. In *Cowdry's The care of the geriatric patient,* ed. F. V. Steinberg, p. 191. St. Louis: Mosby.
2. Guthrie, H. A. 1979. Introductory nutrition. 4th ed. St. Louis: Mosby.
3. Young, V. R. et al. 1976. Protein and amino acid requirements of the elderly. In *Nutrition and aging,* ed. M. Winick, p. 77. New York: J. Wiley and Sons.
4. National Research Council 1974. *Recommended dietary allowances.* 8th ed. National Research Council, National Academy of Science, Washington, D.C.
5. Joint Committee, FAO/WHO: Energy and protein requirements. 1973. WHO Tech. Rep. 522, World Health Organization, Geneva, 1973.
6. Kritchevsky, D. 1978. How aging affects cholesterol metabolism. *Postgraduate Medicine* 63(3):133.
7. Isaacs, B. November 8, 1976. Can this new diet prevent heart attacks? *New York* p. 48.
8. Brunzell, J. D. 1978. Use of fructose, xylitol, or sorbitol as a sweetener in diabetes mellitus. *Diabetes Care* 1(4):223.
9. Brewster, L., and Jacobson, M. F. 1978. *The changing American diet.* Washington, D.C.: Center for Science in the Public Interest.
10. Maris, D. C. 1978. Milk drinking by the elderly of three races. *J. Amer. Dietetic Assoc.* 72:495.
11. Walike, B. C., and Walike, J. W. 1973. Lactose content of tube feeding diets as a cause of diarrhea. *The Laryngoscope* 83(7).
12. Ahrens, R. A. 1974. Sucrose, hypertension and heart disease, an historical perspective. *Amer. J. Clinical Nutrition* 27:403.
13. Dubois, G. E.; Crosby, G. A.; and Suffron, P. 1977. Nonnutritive sweeteners: Taste-structure relationships for some new simple dehydrochalcones. *Science* 195:397.
14. McElleny, V. J. November 23, 1977. Xylitol gum cuts cavities, hurts Wrigley, *New York Times,* p. D1.

OTHER REFERENCES

Bender, A. E., and Thodana, P. V. 1970. Some metabolic effects of dietary sucrose. *Nutrition Metabolism* 12:23.

Chandler, C. A., and Marston, R. N. May–August 1976. Fat in the U.S. diet. *Nutrition Program News* U.S. Dept. of Agriculture, Washington, D.C.

Hegstead, D. M. 1976. Protein needs and possible modifications of the American diet. *J. Amer. Dietetic Assoc.* 68:317.

Mann, G. V. 1973. Relationship of age to nutrient requirements. *Amer. J. Clinical Nutrition* 26:1096.

Munro, H. N., and Young, V. R. 1978. Protein metabolism in the elderly. *Postgrad. Medicine* 63(3):143.

Selected aspects of geriatric nutrition. 1972. *Dairy Council Digest* 43(2):7.

Service, F. J. 1977. Hypoglycemia. *Contemporary Nutrition* 2(7):1.

Watkin, D. M. 1975. Nutrition for the elderly of today and tomorrow. *Nutrition News* 38(2):5.

Young, V. R. 1976. Protein metabolism and needs in elderly people. In *Nutrition, longevity and aging,* eds. M. Rockstein and M. L. Sussman, p. 67. New York: Academic Press, Inc.

|||||||||||||||||||||||||||||||||||||||||||||| 5

Vitamins and Minerals

           Vitamins and minerals include a wide variety of substances that are considered together primarily because they are all required in the diet, but only in minute amounts. Vitamins are organic (carbon-containing) compounds with a variety of biological activities. Minerals, on the other hand, are inorganic compounds of generally less chemical complexity than vitamins, though they are no less essential in the diet.

           Following is a discussion of the major vitamins and minerals important in the diet, their food sources, functions, toxicities, and signs of their deficiencies. Such information is important in assessing certain health problems and understanding which problems may be ameliorated by the addition or deletion of certain factors (vitamins, minerals, and others) in the diet. At the end of this chapter is a brief discussion of the rationale of nutrient supplementation.

VITAMINS

Vitamins are organic substances required by the body in small amounts. They must be supplied in the diet or in food supplements because they cannot be synthesized in the body in sufficient amounts to maintain health. They are not used primarily as sources of energy or as structural material, but rather perform specific functions as regulators of metabolism. Each vitamin acts as a cofactor in a wide variety of reactions involving other nutrients and vitamins. Because of these metabolic interrelationships, a deficiency of one vitamin may affect the metabolism of others.

The number of necessary substances supplied by cellular synthesis tends to vary inversely with the complexity of the organism. Man depends on the environment for some nutrients that lower forms of life (such as microorganisms) can synthesize for themselves. Vitamins are examples of substances required by higher species. They are not chemically related but are grouped together primarily by custom.

After the earliest discoveries of vitamins, only two types of accessory food factors were distinguished: fat-soluble A and water-soluble B. The discovery of vitamin C, another water-soluble substance, confused this simple division, as did the realization that fat-soluble A also contained vitamin D. Still, the distinction between fat-soluble and water-soluble vitamins remains a useful one. There are major differences between each vitamin group as well as some similarity of the properties of all vitamins in each group.

The fat-soluble vitamins A, D, E and K are found dissolved in the fats of animals and plants. They are absorbed from the gastrointestinal tract along with other fats, so anything interfering with fat absorption may produce a deficiency of fat-soluble vitamins even though they may be plentifully supplied. Fat-soluble vitamins are not easily excreted from the body, but are stored in the liver and other tissues. Because they are not readily excreted, there is the danger of excessive accumulation of fat-soluble vitamins, particularly vitamins A and D, with resultant toxic effects.

Water-soluble vitamins include the B vitamins and ascorbic acid (vitamin C). Most of these are precursors for substances involved in energy metabolism. They are not stored in the body in large quantities and are easily excreted in the urine. Because of this, toxic accumulations of water-soluble vitamins are generally not thought to be a problem. Recently, however, ingestion of large quantities of these vitamins, particularly vitamin C, has become commonplace and has been found to produce undesirable effects in the body.

FAT-SOLUBLE VITAMINS

Vitamin A

The role of vitamin A in vision is central, as its chemical name, retinol (the alcohol form of the vitamin), indicates. The vitamin exists in aldehyde (retinal) and acid (retinoic acid) forms as well as in the alcohol form. All three forms are biologically active, but some have specific functions not common to the others (i.e., the acid form is not useful in the visual cycle).

Vitamin A is necessary to regenerate the pigment rhodopsin, a complex of protein (opsin) and retinol, needed for vision in dim light. Night blindness results from a deficiency of vitamin A. A serious lack of the vitamin may lead to disintegration of the cornea of the eye and blindness, which indicates that it is also necessary for the maintenance of normal epithelial cells. Vitamin A was once called the anti-infection vitamin because when epithelial tissue in the respiratory tract is maintained intact it is a defense against infection. A hardening and drying of such cells occurs when there is a deficiency of vitamin A.

In animals, a deficiency of vitamin A leads to abnormal bone development. It has been hypothesized that there is a common metabolic factor in the effect of vitamin A on cartilage, bone, and epithelium, but this has not yet been elucidated.

The active vitamin A in the diet is derived from animal and vegetable sources. The preformed vitamin is found primarily in animal foods, although there is a small amount in spinach. Some of the yellow-colored pigments in plant foods—the carotenoids—are precursors of vitamin A; they can be converted to this vitamin in the body. Beta-carotene, most readily converted to vitamin A of all the carotenoids, and some other carotenes are therefore referred to as provitamin A. Not all yellow-colored pigments can be converted to vitamin A, however. Lycopene, found in watermelon and tomatoes, and xanthophyll in corn have no vitamin A activity.

The vitamin A requirement was formerly expressed in International Units (I.U.). One I.U. is 0.3 mcg of retinol, 0.6 mcg of beta-carotene, or 1.2 mcg of other carotenes. Equal numbers of I.U. of the various vitamin A forms are not functionally equivalent, because only about one-third of the carotenes ingested are absorbed and of this only one-half are converted to the vitamin. Thus, carotenes are utilized with only one-sixth the efficiency of vitamin A. In order to more easily express the vitamin activity of food, more recent daily allowance recommendations are expressed in retinol equivalents (R.E.). One R.E. is 1 mcg of retinol, 6 mcg of beta-cartene, or 12 mcg of other carotenes. This system takes into account both the preformed vitamin and its provitamins. The Recommended Dietary Allowance of 1,000 and 800 R.E. respectively for the male and female over fifty-one years assumes that the American diet provides one-half of total vitamin A activity as retinol and one-half as provitamin A carotenoids.

Whole milk, eggs, butter, liver, and kidney are good sources of the preformed vitamin, while provitamin A is found in yellow and green leafy vegetables—carrots, squash, peppers, collards, and spinach (the green pigment chlorophyll masks the yellow carotenes present). The more deeply colored varieties of vegetables contain more of the provitamin. Often skim milk and margarine are fortified with vitamin A as well as with vitamin D.

Well-nourished adults have been found to have large stores of retinol in their liver, enough to supply needs for this vitamin for years without any dietary intake. This may not be true of all elderly persons, who may have deficiencies because of restricted diets, or impaired ability to store vitamins, due to liver disease, or to convert provitamins to vitamin A, as may occur in diabetes mellitus. Habitual use of mineral oil may interfere with absorption of vitamin A. Laxatives, inadequate bile excretion, pancreatic insufficiency, sprue, ulcerative colitis, or antibiotic use may also hinder its absorption. Protein malnutrition results in poor absorption of vitamin A. Cholestyramine, a drug used to lower blood cholesterol levels, also interferes with the absorption of the vitamin.

It has been reported that rats given four times the minimum amount of vitamin A had their lifespan extended by 10 percent, but that intakes of eight times the minimum amount decreased their lifespan[1]. The intake of vitamin A which causes toxicity in adults has been determined to be daily intakes of approximately 600,000 International Units, although severe liver degeneration has been reported with daily doses of 100,000 units for only six weeks. Studies with rats suggest that older rats can tolerate higher chronic intoxication doses than can younger animals[2]. It has not been determined whether aged humans are as likely to suffer the effects of excessive vitamin A intake as children. Symptoms of intoxication include loss of appetite, loss of hair, blurred vision, dry, itching skin, and enlargement of the liver and spleen. The symptoms usually disappear when the excessive vitamin intake is discontinued, although there have been some reports of residual effects.

Excessive intakes of food rich in carotenes may cause yellowing of skin (though not of the sclera of the eye), especially in uncontrolled diabetics, although this discoloration has not been found to be harmful. Such excessive intakes are more likely to occur in vegetarians who eat large amounts of green and yellow vegetables and in individuals who habitually pulverize vegetables to juice. One may, for example, drink, in one glass of carrot juice, the equivalent of four or five carrots, a much greater quantity than one would be likely to consume if whole carrots were eaten instead.

Because of the potential for vitamin A toxicity, it is advisable to limit intake of the vitamin to approximately the recommended allowance and certainly no more than five times that amount unless there is a medical indication and blood values are closely monitored[2].

Vitamin D

Vitamin D functions in the metabolism of calcium and phosphorus. It is necessary for normal bone formation. The absorption of calcium and phosphorus from the intestine is promoted by the vitamin, as is the deposition of calcium in bone. Vitamin D also promotes the reabsorption of phosphate by the kidneys.

Cholecalciferol, the natural form of vitamin D (also formed in the skin by the action of ultraviolet light on the provitamin 7-dehydrocholesterol), is converted into its active form by two separate hydroxylations, one in the kidney and one in the liver. The resultant metabolite has been commonly called a hormone because it is formed in the skin, kidney, and liver, and acts on other organs—the intestine, kidney, and bones. Vitamin D has been found to improve calcium absorption and balance in postmenopausal women with small fractures.

Caused by a deficiency of vitamin D, *rickets* is a disease of children in which the bones are softened, demineralized, and deformed. Deficient adults develop a softening of bones termed *osteomalacia.*

Osteomalacia is a common disorder in elderly women. It has been believed that a deficiency of dietary vitamin D is not a usual cause of osteomalacia in people living in developed countries but rather that the deficiency occurs as a complication of intestinal malabsorption, gastric surgery, and renal disorders. Renal disease can interfere with the hydroxylation of vitamin D in the kidney, which converts the vitamin into its active form. Recently it has been hypothesized that the many cases of osteomalacia in the elderly are due to an insufficient dietary intake of vitamin D and a lack of exposure to sunlight[3].

Osteomalacia is often confused with osteoporosis. The demineralization of osteoporosis typically begins in the spine, while in osteomalacia the demineralization tends to occur in the peripheral skeleton. In osteoporosis, pain occurs in conjunction with fractures only (usually in a vertebra or femur), while in osteomalacia the pain is diffuse and continuous, resulting from strain on soft bone rather than from fractures[4].

Most foods, except for those which are fortified with vitamin D, are poor sources of the vitamin. Butter, eggs, liver, and fish are the major dietary sources in addition to fortified milk, margarine, and some cereals. Most individuals synthesize sufficient amounts of the vitamin in their skin to maintain health. It has been estimated that Caucasian skin of 20 sq cm area can synthesize about 10 mcg of vitamin D daily if there is adequate exposure to sunlight. This is an amount sufficient to prevent rickets in infants. Heavily pigmented skin, however, may screen out as much as 95 percent of the sun's ultraviolet rays, and thus may synthesize less vitamin D.

It has been reported that elderly persons who have long stays in the hospital as well as those who are housebound may have inadequate intakes of vitamin D. One dietary survey of fifty-six female patients over age sixty-five showed that none of these people had a dietary intake of as much as 100 I.U. a day, which is half of the RDA. Additionally, they received no ultraviolet light irradiation since the light of wavelengths necessary for the synthesis of vitamin D are screened out by glass windowpanes[3]. As low levels of plasma 25-hydroxycholecalciferol were found in these patients after low but usually adequate supplements of vitamin D, it was suspected that factors other than a supply of the vitamin contributed to the low serum levels.

Poor absorption of the vitamin due to any interference with fat absorption can contribute to low serum levels of vitamin D and cause the development of osteomalacia in the elderly, as can an impaired ability to convert the vitamin to its active metabolite. Prolonged treatment with sedatives and anticonvulsants may accelerate metabolism of vitamin D and contribute to development of osteomalacia. (See Chapter 8 for additional information.)

It is important to ensure adequate intake of vitamin D in the elderly since the most common dietary source, fortified milk, may not be ingested regularly in sufficient amounts by elderly persons. The Recommended Dietary Allowance is 5 mcg (200 I.U.) for adults. Formerly there was no RDA for adults as it was assumed they had sufficient exposure to sunlight. This may not be the case with many adults, especially the elderly. Insufficient exposure, coupled with low dietary intake and inadequate conversion of the vitamin precursor to its active form, may require that an elderly person obtain adequate amounts of vitamin D in the diet through fortified foods or supplementation.

Vitamin D is highly toxic in small amounts. Individuals apparently vary in their need for this vitamin due to genetic factors as well as due to the calcium and phosphorus content of their diets. It has been concluded that most people can ingest up to 2,000 I.U. (50 mcg) daily without toxic effects. Doses larger than this have caused hypercalcemia in infants. Massive doses of 150,000 I.U. (3,750 mcg) to 500,000 I.U. (12,500 mcg) daily for the treatment of rheumatoid arthritis have led to toxic effects, including calcification of the kidney, heart, and other organs, hypercalcemia, loss of appetite, and visual disturbances[2].

Vitamin E

Eight different substances—classified as tocopherols and tocotrienols—with vitamin E activity have been identified. Alpha-tocopherol is the most potent of these. The vitamin is found in all cell membranes. It is hypothesized that vitamin E functions in the body as an antioxidant preventing destructive nonenzymic oxidation of polyunsaturated fatty acids. Its role as an antioxidant that might possibly retard aging is discussed in Chapter 1.

There is evidence that vitamin E may act as a cofactor in the cytochrome system of the electron transport chain and may play a role in the synthesis of heme. In animals, deficiency states of vitamin E interfere with reproduction and cause muscle degeneration. Comparable disorders in humans have never been linked to a deficiency of the vitamin.

Hemolytic anemia in infants, in which the red blood cells are easily destroyed, has been related to vitamin E deficiency caused by the use of commercial formulas low in the vitamin. In adults, deficiency caused by impaired intestinal absorption results in a shortened red blood cell lifespan.

The use of vitamin E supplements for numerous conditions ranging from heart disease and sterility to poor athletic performance have been studied. Results are inconclusive. Daily doses of 300 mg (300 T.E.)* of vitamin E have been reported to alleviate idiopathic nocturnal leg cramps, and larger doses of 1,200 mg (1,200 T.E.) have been used for relief of intermittent claudication (leg cramps), caused by inadequate blood supply to an extremity[5]. Recently a study reported on the value of 600 mg a day of vitamin E as

*α Tocopheral Equivalents: 1 mg d$-\alpha-$tocopherol$=1 \alpha$ T.E.

an analgesic useful in treatment of osteoarthritis[6]. Until the role of vitamin E in human metabolism is more completely elucidated, it will continue to be tested as a remedy for many disorders.

The RDA of vitamin E for adults is 8 T.E. for females and 10 T.E. for males. The average intakes of vitamin E have been estimated to range between 2.6 to 15.4 mg. This suggests that some people may be ingesting less than optimum levels. This may also be true among the elderly, who may use only small amounts of vegetable oils, which are the best dietary source of this vitamin, and who may also have disorders which interfere with fat absorption, which would reduce the amount of vitamin E available to the body.

Animal foods are poor sources of vitamin E, except for eggs and liver which contain moderate amounts. The richest sources are vegetable oils. Green leafy vegetables contain moderate amounts. It is generally accepted that increased amounts of polyunsaturated fats in the diet increase one's need for vitamin E. While vegetable oils are rich in polyunsaturated fatty acids, studies have shown that the polyunsaturated vegetable oils also contain sufficient amounts of vitamin E to meet the increased need caused by their ingestion. The mineral selenium has been shown to replace vitamin E in some but not all of its functions when given to animals deficient in this vitamin.

Vitamin E is not very toxic. However, it has been suggested that an unbalanced ratio between vitamin E and vitamin K may lead to impairment of blood coagulation mechanisms[7]. There have been other reports of headache, dizziness, nausea, and vitamin A antagonism due to larger doses of the vitamin. The latter is interesting because vitamin E is known to have a sparing effect on vitamin A which may be the result of its antioxidant effect. Because of this antagonism and the findings that plasma levels of tocophlerol increase to the same level following intakes of 100 to 800 mg daily, there is no reason to ingest more than 150 mg of this vitamin daily[8]. Elderly persons should be encouraged to consume vitamin E-rich foods to ensure sufficient intake.

Vitamin K

Vitamin K is necessary for the liver's synthesis of prothrombin, a coagulant protein of the blood. The vitamin regulates the synthesis of other clotting factors as well. In vitamin K deficiency, the time that it takes for blood to clot is prolonged—i.e., prothrombin time is increased.

Vitamin K is found in green leafy vegetables and in beef liver. Most other animal foods are poor sources. It has been estimated that one-half of the body's supply of vitamin K is produced in the intestines by bacteria normally present there and the other half is obtained by diet. For this reason, a primary deficiency (a serious reduction in supply) of this vitamin has not been described in adults. Newborn babies, because of their sterile intestinal tract and the fact that both breast milk and cow's milk are poor sources of the vitamin, may require a supplement of vitamin K.

Deficiencies in adults occur because of malabsorption of fats or in cases of biliary obstruction. (Bile salts are needed for the absorption of all fat-soluble vitamins, including vitamin K). Antibiotic therapy, which kills intestinal bacteria, and prolonged use of salicylates or mineral oil may also produce deficiency states. In severe liver disease, prothrombin synthesis may be impossible even with an adequate supply of vitamin K.

Many of the above mentioned disorders can occur in elderly persons who may also use anticoagulant drugs (coumarin derivatives) which indirectly interfere with (i.e., antagonize) the normal metabolism of vitamin K. This antagonism is dose-dependent and is affected by the concentration of vitamin K in the plasma. Overdose with these anticoagulent drugs is treated with vitamin K; persons on anticoagulant therapy may be asked to limit their intake of foods rich in vitamin K.

The estimated safe and adequate dietary intake of vitamin K, as stated in the 1980 RDA, is 70–140 mcg. It is estimated that the ordinary mixed diet provides approximately 400 mcg, which is more than adequate to supply the dietary requirements for the vitamin. A synthetic form of vitamin K (menadione or K_3) has been removed from over-the-counter drug preparations because it is toxic. Moreover, it has been found that only a small part of it (1 percent or less) is converted in the body to the active vitamin.

WATER-SOLUBLE VITAMINS

Vitamin C

Vitamin C (ascorbic acid) has a variety of functions in the body. One of these is the hydroxylation of proline to hydroxyproline, which makes up about 13 percent of collagen, the body's most abundant protein, and the maintenance of which is important in blood vessel and capillary integrity. It is presumed that vitamin C has an important function in the formation of collagen needed for wound healing; it is known that ascorbic acid migrates to the site of a wound. It is also known that stress, fevers, and infections tend to deplete the body's stores of vitamin C. It is for these reasons that daily supplements of 100–300 mg of ascorbic acid are recommended before and after surgery.

Because of its role in the hydroxylation reaction, vitamin C may be important in the detoxification of certain poisons in the body. Vitamin C is a strong antioxidant and protects other nutrients such as vitamins E and A and polyunsaturated fatty acids from oxidation. The conversion of the inactive form of the B vitamin folic acid to its active form, folinic acid, requires vitamin C. Iron absorption is facilitated by the presence of vitamin C.

The use of vitamin C in the prevention and treatment of the common cold is controversial. Many individuals seem convinced that ingesting large amounts of ascorbic acid helps them avoid catching colds. Some studies suggest that although vitamin C does not lower the incidence of colds, it does, by an antihistaminelike effect, reduce cold symptoms. Conservative opinion holds that it is not wise to dose oneself with large amounts of vitamin C for only the small benefit of reducing the symptoms of an occasional cold. Excessive intakes of vitamin C (8 mg or more daily) may cause formation of oxalate stones in the renal tract. Vitamin C also is known to interfere with the activity of heparin and the dicoumoral anticoagulants[9]. Other studies show that habitual overdose of vitamin C may result in its own accelerated metabolism and excretion that may cause symptoms of deficiency if a large intake is suddenly reduced[8].

There is some contradictory evidence about the deleterious effect of vitamin C on vitamin B_{12}. Although the effect is uncertain, it has been suggested that persons with a low intake of vitamin B_{12}—such as strict vegetarians—may become deficient in B_{12} if they take large doses of vitamin C[10].

A recent study suggests that episodes of fever blisters, *herpes labialis*, can be reduced in time and severity by supplements of ascorbic acid and bioflavinoids[11].

Severe deficiency of vitamin C causes scurvy, a disease characterized by weakness, swollen joints, spongy and bleeding gums, loose teeth, and impaired wound healing. It can be prevented by intakes of only 10 mg of the vitamin daily. The RDA for vitamin C is

60 mg daily. Good sources are citrus fruits, strawberries, cantaloupe, tomatoes, broccoli, rose hips, and acerola berry. Potatoes are a source of moderate amounts of the vitamin, and if they are eaten in large amounts may be a significant source. Vitamin C is easily destroyed by heat and also is soluble in water so that cooking reduces the vitamin C content of potatoes and other foods.

Although one does not ordinarily refer to storage of water-soluble vitamins like C, a well-nourished adult can exist for five to eight months before depleting the body sufficiently of C so that wound healing would be compromised. Vitamin C undernutrition may occur in the elderly as a result of a poor diet which excludes necessary foods over a long period of time.

Some studies have found lowered leucocyte levels of ascorbic acid in the elderly that can be increased with vitamin C supplements. Males tend to have lower leucocyte vitamin C levels than females[12]. Thus it is believed that men have greater requirements for C than do females.

Some researchers have found low plasma ascorbic levels to be associated with an increased rate of morbidity. The survival rate of geriatric patients admitted to a hospital was found to be associated with the vitamin C level in their blood[13].

The elderly do not absorb vitamin C as well as do younger people. On the same diet, elderly people had lower blood levels of several vitamins (C, thiamine, B_{12}, pantothenic acid) than did younger people. Several studies suggest that higher-than-normal intakes of vitamin C appear to reduce the aches and pains that the elderly are prone to, to lower mortality when the aged are ill, and to increase their longevity. Some evidence of greater needs of the elderly for C comes from a study that found that elderly subjects who had low levels of C in the body failed to reach the same tissue level as younger people even after four and one-half months supplementation of 50 mg of the vitamin daily[14].

Thiamine, or Vitamin B₁

Thiamine functions in the form of thiamine pyrophosphate (TPP) as a coenzyme in energy metabolism. It activates the enzymes for decarboxylation of certain metabolites, and thus is needed for the metabolism of carbohydrates, proteins, and fats. In states of thiamine deficiency, the levels of pyruvic and lactic acids increase in the blood and tissues.

The RDA of thiamine for those over fifty-one years is 1.2 mg for males and 1.0 mg for females. For younger people the recommended daily thiamine intake is a function of caloric intake—0.5 mg per 1,000 Calories. The suggested allowance for the elderly takes into account the fact that in the aged, gastric secretions (especially those lacking hydrochloric acid) tend to inactivate thiamine. Additionally, the intestinal flora characteristic of the elderly may bind ingested thiamine. Thus the elderly are apt to develop thiamine deficiency[1].

Thiamine, like the other B vitamins and vitamin C, is water-soluble and thus easily excreted from the body. The use of diuretics may increase the excretion of thiamine[1]. Therefore, daily intake of the vitamin is important. Thiamine is found in many foods, but few foods are good sources. Whole grain or enriched breads and cereals are major sources in the diet because large quantities of these foods are eaten. Dry yeast is a good source of all the B vitamins. Pork has more thiamine than other meats. *Alliin,* a substance found in onion oil and garlic oil, combines with thiamine to form *alliithiamine,* a form which permits the vitamin to be readily absorbed. Thiaminase, present in some varieties of uncooked fish, may decrease the thiamine content of food eaten with it. Tannin, found in tea, has anti-thiamine activity. This action can be reduced by the presence of ascorbic acid[15]; however, elderly persons who subsist on marginal diets and consume large amounts of tea may develop thiamine deficiency.

Age, consumption of alcohol (which contains none of the thiamine of the grains from which it is made), barbiturates, fever, malignant disease, and parenteral administration of glucose solutions increases one's need for thiamine. A high dietary intake of carbohydrate (frequently found in the elderly) increases the need for thiamine, while protein and fat are considered to be thiamine sparers.

Beri-beri, a disease caused by thiamine deficiency, is found in the United States almost only in alcoholics. Two forms of beri-beri have been described—the dry form, in which there is tissue wasting, and the wet form, in which there is edema and an accumulation of fluid in the heart.

In the past, thiamine was used as a tonic to increase the appetite. Its value for this is unsubstantiated. However, administration of both B-complex vitamins and ascorbic acid to a group of forty elderly people who had been ingesting deficient diets did result in improved mental and physical health.

Riboflavin, or Vitamin B₂

Riboflavin functions as part of the flavoprotein coenzymes which are necessary for the capture of energy from carbohydrates, fats, and proteins via electron transport and other enzyme systems.

Usually, riboflavin deficiency occurs along with a lack of other B vitamins. Though a deficiency of riboflavin alone does not lead to a specific disease, cellular growth cannot continue in the absence of this vitamin. Cracks at the angles of the mouth, vascularization of the cornea, inflammation of the tongue, and seborrheic dermatitis around the nose and scrotum are symptoms of riboflavin deficiency. It is believed that an alteration of microflora in the intestine may interfere with utilization of the vitamin.

The Recommended Dietary Allowance for riboflavin is based on caloric intake—0.6 mg/1,000 calories for people of all ages. For adults fifty-one years of age and older this is 1.4 mg for men and 1.2 mg for women.

Meats, milk, eggs, and green vegetables are the best sources of riboflavin. Enriched cereals and grains contain riboflavin in lesser amounts. If milk is not a part of one's diet, riboflavin intake is likely to be low. Riboflavin is stable to heat but can be lost by leaching into cooking water or by exposure to light, which destroys it.

As with other water-soluble vitamins, little riboflavin is stored in the body, so it must be a regular part of the diet. Excess amounts are excreted in urine and there is no known toxicity from riboflavin.

Tetracycline, probenecid, and thiazide diuretics increase the urinary excretion of thiamine. Therapy with testosterone increases the need for riboflavin, as does bodily injury because riboflavin is utilized in the cellular growth associated with wound healing.

Niacin

Niacin is a component of the respiratory coenzymes nicotinamide adenosine dinucleotide (NAD) and nicotinamide adenosine dinucleotide phosphate (NADP). These function as hydrogen acceptors in cellular respiration and in the metabolism of carbohydrate, fat, and protein.

Pellagra is the disease state due to severe niacin deficiency. It is characterized by a symmetrical skin discoloration and rash, inflammation of mouth, tongue, and intestine, and mental confusion as well as depression. A moderate deficiency of niacin may be manifest solely by hypermotility of the gut. Pellagra is no longer commonly found in the United States though it can occur as a result of alcoholism or severely restricted diets.

The amino acid tryptophan can be converted to niacin in the body. A dietary intake of 60 mg of tryptophan can give rise to 1 mg of niacin so that in defining recommended allowances both 1 mg of niacin and 60 mg of tryptophan are considered to be one niacin equivalent.

The RDA for niacin is 6.6 mg/1,000 Calories; for individuals aged fifty-one years and older, the daily allowance is 12 mg for females and 16 mg for males. Animal proteins like milk, eggs, and meat contain about 1.4 percent of tryptophan while vegetable protein has about 1 percent tryptophan. Animal products are better than vegetable products as sources of niacin not only because they contain preformed niacin but because of their tryptophan content.

Whole grain and enriched breads and cereals are good sources of niacin, as are peanut butter, other legumes, and yeast. In many cereals, the niacin is bound to certain cellular components and thus is unabsorbable. Large amounts of the vitamin may be lost in cooking water and drippings from cooked meat.

The acid form of niacin (nicotinic acid) causes vasodilation with burning, flushing, and tingling around the face, neck, and hands. Nicotinic acid has been used to lower plasma lipid levels, but prolonged use produces side effects which include cardiac arrhythmias and gastrointestinal problems. Niacin has been reported effective in helping some cases of mental confusion in the elderly.

Pyridoxine, or Vitamin B$_6$

Vitamin B$_6$ refers to three chemically, metabolically, and functionally related compounds—pyridoxine, pyridoxal, and pyridoxamine. In the body, all of these are converted to pyridoxal phosphate.

Vitamin B$_6$ in its coenzyme form (pyridoxal phosphate) is involved in over sixty enzyme systems. For the most part it is associated with nitrogen metabolism. It participates in decarboxylation (a degradation that forms carbon dioxide), transamination (transfer of amino group from one acid to another), and condensation reactions. Vitamin B$_6$ is necessary for conversion of tryptophan to niacin.

Although dermatitis, poor growth, and fatty livers are among deficiency symptoms observed in animals, there are no distinctive signs of B_6 deficiency in humans. Depression, irritability, a loss of sense of responsibility, and other symptoms, however, have been reported in adult subjects fed diets deficient in B_6. High intakes of protein hasten the onset of the deficiency. Some individuals have been described with anemia that is refractory to iron, folic acid, and vitamin B_{12}, but which responds to doses of 2.5 mg or more of vitamin B_6 daily.

Serum glutamic–oxaloacetic acid transaminase (SGOT) is an enzyme system that requires pyridoxal phosphate for its activity. The elderly have lower levels of this enzyme than do younger individuals and this is taken as evidence for decreased serum pyridoxal phosphate levels in the aged. Vitamin B_6 may not be well-absorbed by the elderly, and intestinal synthesis of this vitamin (as well as that of folic acid and vitamin B_{12}) may be reduced due to lowered intestinal acidity and decreases in intestinal mucus secretion.

The RDA of the vitamin for all adults is 2.2 mg a day for males, 2.0 mg for females. The best dietary sources of vitamin B_6 are pork, wheat germ, organ meats, and whole grain cereals. Cooking causes a considerable loss of the vitamin. Pyridoxine supplements are given along with the antitubercular drug *isoniazid* (INH) because this drug reduces the availability of the vitamin, which may result in neurological problems. The antibiotic *chloramphenicol,* the chelating agent *penicillamine,* and some diuretics increase one's need for vitamin B_6. The interaction of levodopa and vitamin B_6 is discussed in Chapter 8. Note that the toxicity of vitamin B_6 is very low.

Folacin

The newer term folate is used to cover all the substances which give rise to folacin in the body. Folacin functions in the transfer of methyl groups, single carbon units needed for the synthesis of a wide variety of compounds including purines and pyrimidines (components of DNA). Much of folacin's function is closely linked to the function of vitamins C, B_6, and B_{12}. As its names implies, folacin is found in green leafy vegetables, and also in liver, meat, orange juice, legumes, yeast, and whole grains. Folacin is easily destroyed by heat, and losses in cooking may be as high as 100 percent.

The deficiency of folacin causes megaloblastic anemia, with abnormal blood cell production similar to the pernicious anemia caused by a deficiency of vitamin B_{12} (see page 83). If an anemia is caused by a B_{12} deficiency, this blood condition improves upon administration of large doses of folacin. However, the neurological symptoms characteristic of pernicious anemia are not improved, and may be worsened, by folacin administration. For this reason, the Food and Drug Administration limits the amount of folic acid (folacin) permitted in nonprescription vitamin supplements to 400 mcg (0.4 mg), which is the RDA of folacin for all adults and which is not a large enough amount to mask the blood dyscrasia of pernicious anemia. Since there is an interdependence of vitamins B_{12}, B_6, C, and folic acid, the anemia found in a deficiency of any of these is similar to that found in other deficiencies and may respond to treatment with one or several of these.

There is some evidence that the influence of bacteria in intestinal blind loops may contribute to reduced folacin absorption. A low iron intake may result in decreased absorption of folic acid as well as of vitamin B_{12}.

While the elderly do not often have megaloblastic anemia as a result of folacin deficiency, studies show that low serum folacin levels in the aged may be correlated with organic brain syndrome. One study concluded that the elderly do not absorb folate from most foods in adequate amounts but do absorb folate as it is found in yeast[16].

Folate deficiency, common in those over age 70, can cause progressively increased folate malabsorption. That is to say, the malabsorption of folate, caused perhaps by a decrease in mucosal secretion of conjugase necessary to convert folates to a form which can be absorbed, may hinder cellular metabolism so as to induce changes in the epithelial structure and enzyme secretion of the small intestine, which may lead to a decreased ability to absorb folate[16].

A folic acid antagonist, *methotrexate*, is a highly toxic substance used in the treatment of leukemia and the skin disorder psoriasis. It acts to induce a deficiency of active forms of folate, which is necessary for the activity of methotrexate. Ingestion of large amounts of folate during methotrexate treatment may hinder its effectiveness.

Cobalamin, or Vitamin B_{12}

Vitamin B_{12}, the anti-pernicious anemia factor, is also known as cobalamin because it contains the mineral cobalt. Vitamin B_{12} is necessary for the synthesis of DNA and a deficiency state results in the formation of red blood cells that are larger than normal (megaloblastic anemia). The vitamin has another role in the maintenance of myelin in nervous tissue. B_{12} also catalyzes the release of folacin from its conjugated form as it is found in foods. The RDA for vitamin B_{12} is 3 mcg for adults. Sources are animal products such as seafood, meat, eggs, and milk. Vegetable products such as soy milk contain B_{12} only if fortified with it.

Since vitamin B_{12} is found only in animal tissues, strict vegetarians who eat no animal products may develop a deficiency. However, the deficiency usually takes a long time to develop, as very little is needed (1 mcg daily prevents symptoms) and there may be large stores of the vitamin in the liver. It may also be possible that sufficient B_{12} may be obtained from mold or other contaminants in vegetable foodstuffs, as well as from bacteria living in the intestine.

In order to absorb B_{12}, the *intrinsic factor*—a glycoprotein secreted by the parietal cells of the stomach—is needed so that the intrinsic factor–B_{12} complex can be absorbed by the intestine. In the elderly, abnormal bacterial growth in the intestine decreases the amount of B_{12} absorbed as bacteria utilize the vitamin for their own growth. Additionally, if the intrinsic factor is absent, the vitamin must be injected in order to enter the bloodstream. Hydroxycobalamin is preferred to cyanocobalamin as it is retained longer in the body and thus can be injected less often. Sorbitol has also been found to increase absorption of vitamin B_{12} in elderly people with depressed gastric secretion.

Absorption of B_{12} is reduced in the elderly and they show reduced serum levels of the vitamin with increasing age. A study of thirty-five subjects aged sixty-five to ninety who complained of fatigue found that the symptoms of fatigue disappeared in 89 percent of the subjects when given a B_{12} supplement[13]. Substitution of a placebo for the vitamin resulted in a return of the fatigue.

Disorientation and confusion in the elderly have been attributed to a deficiency of B_{12} in some instances. Other workers have found that some elderly persons with neurological symptoms but no anemia responded to treatment with vitamin B_{12}.

Pantothenic Acid

Pantothenic acid is part of coenzyme A, which is important in many steps of intermediary metabolism. It is involved in the metabolism of carbohydrate, protein, and fat.

Pantothenic acid (as its name implies) is widely distributed in foods, particularly eggs, liver, yeast, and whole grains. The estimated safe and adequate daily intake of this vitamin is 4 to 7 mg. As the average American diet is estimated to provide 5 to 10 mg of pantothenic acid daily, deficiencies rarely, if ever, occur.

Rats show deficiency of pantothenic acid by the greying of fur. Pantothenic acid will not prevent greying hair in humans, although this claim is often made for it by vitamin hucksters.

Choline

Choline, inositol, biotin, and lipoic acid are substances that are sometimes grouped with water-soluble vitamins, although their designation as vitamins is uncertain. Choline can be synthesized in the body but probably not in amounts sufficient to maintain good health. In the body, choline supplies labile methyl groups for the synthesis of essential substances; it is a precursor of acetylcholine, a substance which transmits nerve impulses at synapses. Choline is also a structural component of the phospholipids lecithin and sphingomyelin. It has been used to treat fatty livers resulting from alcoholism and severe protein deficiency.

In 1975, it was reported that choline from food is taken up directly by the brain from circulating blood and is used almost at once to help the brain make acetylcholine. Choline has been studied in the treatment of Alzheimer's disease, which is believed to be the most common cause of dementia in persons over age forty-five. It is estimated that 15 percent of persons over age sixty-five have severe memory problems stemming from this disorder. Choline supplements were found to slow the usual progress of this disease when initiated in its early stages[17].

Choline is found in egg yolks, meat, legumes, and wheat germ. The commercial form of lecithin, a choline-containing compound used as an emulsifier in chocolate candy, salad dressings, and other processed foods, may contain very little choline.

MINERALS

There are approximately twenty-two minerals presently known to be essential in the diet of humans for the maintenance of good health. These have been grouped as macronutrient minerals and micronutrient (trace) minerals according to the amount of each needed in the diet. The macrominerals have a dietary requirement of 100 mg or more daily, while the microminerals are required in the diet in much smaller amounts. Microminerals are also known as trace minerals because early workers were not able to measure their concentrations precisely with the analytical methods then available and so referred to these minerals as occurring in traces. The name is still used, although their concentrations can now be measured precisely.

Trace minerals are receiving increasing recognition as essentials in the diet, as evidenced by changes in the RDA. The seventh edition of the Recommended Dietary Allowances, published in 1968, included only two trace elements, iron and iodine, in the table. Concrete recommendations for fluorine were given in the text. In 1974, the eighth revision of the RDA added zinc to the table[18]. The ninth edition of the RDA, 1980, for the first time provides estimated safe and adequate daily dietary intakes for copper, manganese, flouride, chromium, selenium, and molybdenum as well as for the electrolytes sodium, potassium, and chloride. To ensure adequate intake, it is necessary to obtain an accurate measurement of the level of these trace minerals in foodstuffs. It is most likely that the mineral content of unprocessed food reflects the soil mineral content of the region in which it is produced; therefore the mineral content of food is variable.

Minerals serve a variety of functions in the body. To illustrate the scope of their activity, an abbreviated list of mineral functions follows. Sodium, potassium, calcium, phosphorus, and chlorine help control water and electrolyte balance; zinc, manganese and molybdenum function as activators for enzyme-catalyzed reactions; calcium and phosphorus are components of skeletal tissue; iodine, iron, cobalt, and chlorine are components of essential body compounds; sodium and potassium function in the transmission of nerve impulses; muscle contractility and relaxation depend on calcium and magnesium. Needless to say, in the body, minerals work in concert and are essential for a myriad of functions.

It has been said that a mineral deficiency is less likely to arise from a dietary lack than from factors which interfere with a mineral's absorption. This concept should be examined in light of the increased tendency for our diet to include convenience foods which are processed, partitioned, or fabricated, and because of the increased use of sweet, carbonated, and alcoholic beverages.

Partitioning of grain reduces its mineral, vitamin, and fiber content. Partitioning sugar produces a product practically devoid of anything but calories, and partitioning butter from milk removes calcium which may affect the potentially harmful effect of the fat and cholesterol it contains. (A study has shown that when healthy elderly females were given calcium supplementation, their bone density improved and serum cholesterol levels were decreased.) Fabricated or engineered foods such as soybean meat analogs, meal replacement snacks, cakes, and carbonated beverages further reduce the amount of nutrients, including trace minerals, in the food supply. In the manufacture of these foods, an attempt is not made to include completely the nutrients found in whole foods.

At the present time, a complete list of all necessary nutrients cannot even be drawn up. For example vanadium, nickel, silicon, and tin have been shown to be necessary elements for animal health but are not yet known to be essential for human health. An experiment in which animals were raised on chemically pure diets containing optimal amounts of all nutrients known or suspected to be necessary for health showed that there are some as yet unknown factors that are needed to maintain good health, because the animals involved in the study became sick and did not grow[19].

The 1980 RDA recognizes the importance of many minerals. We are not sure of the body's need for other minerals such as arsenic, vanadium, and silicon. Excesses of the mineral cadmium, not believed necessary for life, have been implicated as a cause of hypertension. Both excesses and deficiencies of minerals are undesirable. There may be a very small margin between the amount of a mineral that is needed for good health and the amount which is toxic. Therefore, use of mineral supplements should be approached with caution.

The body usually conserves minerals and also regulates their absorption so that mineral balance is maintained. Mechanisms for this include renal and biliary excretion and controlled absorption from the intestine. Large amounts of trace minerals can be lost in sweat. Persons who live in hot climates may need to compensate for this loss by ingesting larger amounts of iron, copper, zinc, and other minerals. Lead, tin, and nickel are also lost in sweat, which may prevent the undesirable buildup of these in the body.

Macronutrients

Calcium   The total calcium content of an adult's body is generally two to three pounds. It comprises about 2 percent of body weight. Of this amount, 99 percent is in the bones and teeth, with only 1 percent in muscle and extracellular fluid. The amount of calcium in blood serum (10 mg/100 ml) is held constant by the actions of the thyroid gland, parathyroid gland, and kidney, with the bone acting as a reserve source of this mineral so that the serum level is not dependent on dietary intake.

The absorption rate of calcium ranges from 10 to 40 percent of that ingested. The amount absorbed tends to correspond to the amount needed by the body. The acidic environment of the duodenum facilitates calcium absorption by rendering it more water-soluble, as does the presence of ascorbic acid. Calcium absorption is also enhanced by the presence of lactose. Phosphorus intake also affects calcium absorption, with greatest absorption occurring with calcium:phosphate ratios of 1:1 or 1:1.5.

Calcium absorption is decreased by a deficiency of vitamin D, as well as by a high concentration of fatty acids in the intestine, which can form insoluble soaps with calcium. Oxalic and phytic acids, found in vegetables such as spinach and legumes, may also form insoluble complexes with calcium and hinder its absorption. Generalized intestinal malabsorption syndromes, which are common in the elderly, may also reduce the absorption of calcium.

Besides its function as a structural component of bones and teeth, calcium is needed for blood clotting, activation of many enzymes, and for normal neuromuscular function.

The Recommended Dietary Allowance for calcium is 800 mg (1 quart of milk contains 1,000 mg, or 1 gm), but surveys show that many adults receive only one half that amount[20]. It is generally accepted that long term dietary insufficiency of calcium is a factor in the etiology of osteoporosis. This disease is estimated to affect at least 10 percent of the American population over age fifty, and is a factor in the estimated six million spontaneous fractures occurring annually in the United States in persons over forty-five. Osteoporosis, also called osteopenia, is a disease involving a decrease in total bone mass without a change in the chemical composition; that is, there remains a normal calcium:protein ratio. This reduction in mass permits fractures of the vertebra, hip, and femoral neck to occur even with little or no trauma.

A slight imbalance in calcium absorbed relative to what is lost (in digestive juices, feces, and sweat, and to demands of pregnancy and lactation in women) sustained over a long period of time can cause radiographically demonstrable osteoporosis. Osteoporosis can be radiographically diagnosed when about 30 percent of the bone mineral has been lost, though a fracture may have occurred by this time[21]. Studies show that once a vertebral fracture has

occurred, osteoporosis can be slowed down but not reversed. This indicates that preventive therapy for osteoporosis should begin in
youth. While some factors other than nutrition (hormonal, inactivity) are involved in the etiology of osteoporosis[21], nutritional intervention seems to be of value in preventive therapy. Although the
Recommended Dietary Allowance for calcium is 800 mg per day for
adults, some experts believe that this is only a minimum figure for
the prevention of osteoporosis. Intake of over one gram (1,000 mg)
results in maximum calcium absorption. Unless 1 quart of milk (or
the equivalent of cheese) is consumed daily, it is difficult to ingest 1
gm of calcium without supplementation. Calcium is also supplied by
green leafy vegetables, legumes, nuts, and whole grains. However,
milk is the major source and has the highest content of any food.
Skimmed milk fortified with dry milk solids has a higher calcium
content than does whole milk which is not similarly fortified.

A study of females aged seventy-nine to eighty-eight showed
that a daily supplement of 750 mg of calcium and 375 I.U. of vitamin D not only stopped bone loss but resulted in an increase in bone
density of up to 12 percent. The pattern of change varied, but, on
the whole, little or no improvement was observed during the first
six to nine months. This indicates that dietary supplementation
may have to be maintained for long periods before the desired
results are evident[22].

It has been hypothesized that bone dissolution often occurs in
order to buffer the acid load caused by a diet high in meat. In order
to test this idea, one study compared the bone density of vegetarians with others who ate animal and plant foods (omnivores). The
two groups were matched for age and sex. It was found that the
bone density of vegetarians showed a significantly lower decrease
with age than did the bone density of omnivores. Furthermore, this
decrease in bone density in vegetarians did not continue after age
sixty-nine as it did with the omnivores. These results suggest that
vegetarians are less likely to develop osteoporosis in old age[23].

An interesting fact which has emerged from the studies on
osteoporosis is that periodontal disease can be an early manifesta-
tion of osteoporosis. It can occur five to ten years before there has
been significant bone loss in other parts of the skeleton. This early
demineralization is reversible by dietary calcium supplements and
may provide an important means of early detection of osteoporosis[24].

Most renal stones are calcium compounds. When there is immobilization or bed rest for long periods of time, bones decalcify and
this raises the amount of calcium that must be excreted in the urine.

For this reason, when an individual is immobilized for a long period of time, dietary calcium should be maintained at adequate levels but should not exceed usual daily allowances. If a patient has a history of renal stones, calcium intake should be reduced at such a time. As the elderly are often confined to bed or wheelchair, the monitoring of calcium intake is essential to prevent the complication of renal stones.

Phosphorus   Phosphorus is a major constituent of all plant and animal cells, where it plays a vital role in cell functioning. It is thus present in all natural foods. Foods rich in calcium and protein are generally also good sources of phosphorus. The RDA for phosphorus is 800 mg a day for adults. Phosphorus is also a frequent additive in processed and fabricated foods. Present–day diets, which are high in meats and soft drinks (beef consumption is up 72 percent and soft drink consumption up 157 percent since 1910), provide large amounts of phosphorus. Foods that are high in phosphorus and low in calcium lower the calcium:phosphorus ratio from its optimum level of 1:1 and may be a predisposing factor in osteoporosis unless calcium supplements are used.

Recently, animal studies have shown that increased dietary phosphorus may confer protection against dental decay in children and might improve bone structure as well. Increasing phosphorus in the diets of the elderly poses a problem, however. Phosphorus is readily absorbed (over 70 percent) and its level in the body is regulated primarily by urinary excretion. Because of the reduction of renal function with age, the kidney may be less able to handle the excretion of large amounts of phosphorus. Elevated blood levels of phosphorus are commonly found in renal disease. Thus, low-phosphorus, low-protein diets are used to alleviate stress in the kidney in these situations.

Adults frequently use antacids to relieve digestive upset. The prolonged use of high levels of nonabsorbable antacids (aluminum hydroxide) may deplete the body of phosphorus by hindering its ability to be absorbed, thus causing weakness, loss of appetite, and bone demineralization. This is treated by discontinuing the use of antacids and increasing phosphorus intake.

Magnesium   All body tissue contains small amounts of magnesium. It is an essential part of enzyme systems responsible for the transfer of energy. The RDA for magnesium is 300 mg and 350 mg for women and men respectively. Most foods, especially milk and vegetables, contain magnesium (magnesium is part of chlorophyll), and 45 percent of the dietary supply is absorbed. Magnesium deficiency is rarely found in individuals unless there are some complicating factors.

Impaired absorption or excessive excretion may cause a deficiency state. Loss of gastrointestinal fluids from prolonged diarrhea or vomiting and increased renal excretion, which occurs in chronic renal disease and in drug-induced diuresis, can all lead to magnesium deficiency. Chronic alcoholism causes increased magnesium excretion and the usual malnutrition found in alcoholism results in a decreased intake of all nutrients including magnesium. Parenteral feedings often contain little or no magnesium; therefore, their prolonged use may also lead to a magnesium deficiency.

The elderly may experience many of these conditions and so are likely candidates for deficiencies or marginal deficiencies. Clinical signs of magnesium deficiency are muscle tremors, personality changes, nausea, and apathy.

It has been suggested that the magnesium found in hard water is a protective factor against coronary vascular disease. A recent study, however, failed to find any statistically significant difference in serum magnesium levels between those who had suffered myocardial infractions and controls[25].

Sulfur   Sulfur is found in proteins, principally in two sulfur-containing amino acids, methionine and cystine, and these are the chief sources of sulfur in the diet. Some enzymes depend on sulfur for their activity. Thiamin and biotin contain sulfur. Generally, sulphur-containing compounds act to detoxify harmful substances in the body.

Obtaining adequate sulfur in the diet is not a problem. Diets providing sufficient protein should contain adequate sulfur.

Strong Electrolytes

Three macrominerals are strong electrolytes: sodium, potassium, and chlorine. All three play an important role in muscle activity, in maintaining water and acid–base balance in the body, in nerve impulse transmission, and in maintaining the proper aqueous environment for enzymatic reactions. Most diets include large quantities of these electrolytes, and recently excessive sodium ingestion has become a matter of concern (see Chapter 7).

Potassium   Potassium is found in many foods and is easily absorbed. Therefore, primary deficiency of this nutrient is believed unlikely. However, older persons living at home have lower intakes of potassium than do younger adults. Investigators hypothesize that there is extensive subclinical nutritional potassium deficiency which could easily be corrected by nutrition education. Dietary potassium intake has been found to correlate directly with muscle strength. Thus, low potassium intake may be a factor in muscle weakness in the elderly.

Potassium functions in fluid and electrolyte balance and in acid–base balance. It functions with sodium to regulate neuromuscular excitability and stimulation. Even small variations in serum potassium values cause changes in heart rhythm.

Low serum levels of potassium can be caused by prolonged diarrhea, renal disease, diabetic acidosis, and certain diuretic drugs. Recently, the use of predigested protein diets for weight reduction resulted in some fatalities attributed to inadequate potassium levels. Elevated serum levels of potassium may occur as a result of renal failure or severe dehydration. Both low serum values (hypokalemia) and high serum values (hyperkalemia) require medical treatment.

The estimated safe and adequate daily intake for potassium is 1.875–5.625 mg for adults. Potassium is widely distributed in milk, meats, fruits, and vegetables, with dietary intake of oranges, tomatoes, and bananas commonly recommended as means of increasing potassium intake.

It is believed that a high intake of dietary potassium increases the body's tolerance to the hypertensive effects of sodium[26].

Sodium   Sodium is normally ingested in the form of sodium chloride (common table salt). The normal intake is approximately 10–15 gm of salt daily. This value, however, has been determined by habit, not need. The estimated safe and adequate daily intake of sodium is 1100–3300 mg (table salt is 40 percent sodium, 60 percent chloride). Of the sodium ingested, 90 percent is excreted in the urine; additional sodium is lost in the stool and in sweat. In healthy adults, sodium intake and output are balanced.

Sodium functions in fluid and electrolyte balance and in acid–base balance. It also facilitates the passage of glucose and potassium through cell membranes. In addition, sodium ions serve as transmitters of neural impulses.

In cases of kidney or heart failure, sodium may be retained and thus dietary restrictions must be imposed. There are different levels of sodium restriction: mild, moderate, and severe. These sodium restricted diets will be described in Chapter 7.

In other situations, sodium may be lost because of kidney damage or adrenal insufficiency. Losses of sodium in body fluids may occur as a result of continued vomiting, diarrhea, or drainage from open wounds. This can lead to dehydration and resultant shock or even death.

There is currently concern that high sodium intake beginning in infancy and continued throughout life may affect the incidence of hypertension. Animal experiments have shown that rats with a predisposition develop hypertension only when maintained on diets containing high levels of sodium comparable to those levels we consume habitually. In view of this, there have been recommendations in the "Dietary Goals for the United States" that sodium intake be reduced for all people, including those in good health[27]. However, aged individuals who have been prescribed diets severely restricted in sodium and who live in hot climates may develop muscle cramps from sodium deficiency. In these situations, an increased intake of sodium may be advised.

Chloride   The principal role of chloride is to regulate the osmotic pressure and water content of the body. It is also a component of hydrochloric acid in the stomach, a coenzyme for digestive amylase, part of the buffer system which maintains acid–base balance in the body, and important in the transmission of nerve impulses. Large losses of chloride from vomiting and diarrhea can cause a disturbance in acid–base balance. The estimated safe and adequate daily intake of chloride is 1700–5100 mg for adults. The major dietary source of chloride is in sodium chloride (common table salt).

Microminerals

Iron   The body of the average adult may contain less than 5 grams of iron (1 teaspoon), but this small amount performs vital functions in cellular respiration and is essential to hemoglobin's oxygen-carrying capacity.

Usually, only about 5–10 percent of dietary iron is absorbed, but in deficiency conditions, this percentage increases to 10–20 percent. Most iron is absorbed in the acidic environment of the upper portion of the small intestine. Ascorbic acid forms a soluble complex with iron and aids in its absorption, as does adequate dietary calcium which binds phosphates, oxylates, and phytates which can combine with iron and inhibit its absorption. Absorption of iron may be hindered by gastrectomy, malabsorption syndromes, or severe infection. EDTA (ethylenediamine tetraacetic acid), an antioxidant widely used in processed foods such as soft drinks, beer, mayonnaise, and salad dressing, combines with iron and reduces its absorption[28].

Iron deficiency and its resultant nutritional anemia are common among the low income elderly living on poor diets[29]. Although iron deficiency is the most common form of nutritional anemia, deficiencies of folic acid, vitamin B_{12}, and other nutrients can cause anemia as well. The problem of anemia in the elderly will be described more fully in Chapter 7.

The Recommended Dietary Allowance for both males and females over fifty-one is 10 mg of iron daily. The recommendation for females represents a reduction from the 18 mg advised for premenopausal women.

The iron found in meat and whole grain is absorbed better than that in eggs and vegetables or fortified bread. In fact, meat eaten at the same time enhances the absorption of iron from other foods[30]. However, relatively little iron is absorbed at any time in the diet. On the other hand, under usual conditions little iron is lost in urine and sweat. Moreover, the iron in hemoglobin is usually recycled into new hemoglobin. Despite this, the ingestion of iron-rich foods such as meat, whole grain and fortified cereals, dried peas and beans, eggs, or iron supplements are necessary to prevent iron deficiency.

Because iron supplements irritate the gastric mucosa, they are often manufactured *enteric-coated.* In this case the iron is not exposed until it has passed the upper portion of the small intestine, though that is where iron absorption occurs most readily.

Recently the possibility of iron fortification of milk and doubling the amount of iron added to flour and cereal in enrichment was considered. It was opposed by those who feel that excessive iron intake from these sources might be harmful for a small segment of the population who have hemochromatosis, which permits an abnormal, harmful accumulation of iron in the body[31]. Such an iron overload might also become a problem in alcoholics, who also have increased iron stores.

Iodine   The 10 to 20 mg of iodine in the adult body is found primarily in the thyroid gland where it is essential for proper functioning of the gland. It is a component of hormones produced by this gland, thyroxine and triiodothyronine. Iodine deficiency leads to an enlargement of the thyroid gland, known as goiter. Intakes of 50–75 mcg daily prevent this type of goiter.

The iodine content of farm products depends on the amount of iodine in the soil. Thus, the use of iodized salt has been recommended as protection against iodine deficiency. The use of salt-restricted diets by many elderly individuals has presented some problems in providing the recommended levels of iodine daily. The Recommended Dietary Allowance is 150 mcg for adults.

Recently it has been proposed that we may, in fact, be receiving more than enough iodine adventitiously, as iodine-containing solutions are used for sanitizing equipment used on farms, in dairies, and in mass food preparation. Iodine is also supplied in iodine-containing dough conditioners and oxidizing agents used in making bread and in coloring agents. Additionally, the burning of fossil fuels increases the iodine levels in the air and this iodine is also absorbed into the body. An increased incidence of toxic goiters (from excessive iodine intake) has been reported in some countries[32]. Therefore, the use of iodized salt may be discouraged because we receive sufficient iodine from the above-mentioned sources and from our food supply which is produced from a variety of soils in different parts of the country.

Zinc   Zinc is a constituent of at least thirty enzyme systems and is a component of insulin. Clinical signs of deficiency in humans are retarded growth and retarded sexual maturation. More recently, zinc deficiency has been cited as a factor in decreased taste and smell sensitivity[33]. This is of importance in the elderly, who may have reduced appetite for several reasons, including a diminished number of functional organoleptic (taste and odor) receptors.

Marginal intakes of zinc may be occurring as an increasing proportion of the diet is comprised of refined and processed foods. Phytates in bran may form insoluble complexes with zinc and further reduce the amount available. Additionally, blood loss may cause zinc deficiency.

The 1974 revision of the Recommended Dietary Allowances suggested an intake of 15 mg of zinc daily[34]. (The recommendation is the same for the 1980 RDA.) A study of elderly participants in a congregant feeding program showed that daily intake of all nutrients listed in the RDA approximated the suggested level except for zinc. Fifty-nine percent of the subjects consumed less than two-thirds of the allowance for zinc[35]. Studies show that some hospital diets contain only 11 mg zinc/2,700 Calories. Thus, older people with poor diets, chronic wounds, and illness may be especially vulnerable to zinc deficiency. Low plasma zinc levels have been found in individuals with alcoholic cirrhosis of the liver, myocardial infarcts, and pulmonary infections[36].

The best food sources of zinc are red meats, seafood, and eggs—that is to say, animal products in general[37]. Thus, diets based on vegetable protein, including meat analogs, are likely to offer only marginal intakes of zinc.

Evidence is accumulating that suggests that cadmium may play a role in hypertension, a condition that is prevalent in the elderly. High zinc intakes may protect against the effect of excess levels of cadmium in the body. Sources of cadmium are air, water, seafood, and refined grains. As cadmium remains in endosperm (where it is bound to protein) when grains are refined, and zinc is removed in the germ and bran, refined grains tend to have cadmium but no zinc. To obtain an adequate balance between zinc and cadmium, one needs to be sure to include zinc–containing foods in the diet to compensate for the cadmium obtained from refined grain products.

There are conflicting reports regarding the effect of zinc supplements on the rate of wound healing. It is known that a high local zinc concentration is required for rapid tissue regeneration and repair and also that high urinary losses of zinc occur following trauma from surgery, accident, or extensive burns. Impaired wound healing treated with 660 mg zinc sulfate, given in three divided doses daily for several weeks, caused no apparent side effects. However, high levels of zinc supplements continued for several months can lead to other mineral imbalances. Copper deficiency, evidenced by hypocupremia, leukopenia, and anemia, was found in a patient treated with ten times the RDA of zinc for a prolonged period. Similar results have been reported in others[38]. High zinc intakes interfere with metabolism and absorption of copper. It appears to be more reasonable to treat apparent deficiencies of zinc by supplements of no more than two or three times the RDA. Such intakes have been shown sufficient to alleviate dwarfism and hypogonadism caused by zinc deficiency. If higher levels are indicated because of abnormalities in the gastrointestinal tract, serum copper levels should be carefully monitored.

Oral zinc supplements given to the elderly have been shown to increase the rate of wound healing, improve taste acuity, and also increase blood flow to extremities where circulation was poor[36].

Some authorities feel that the amount of zinc in supplements may be inadequate. More research is needed to clarify this.

Fluorine   When consumed in drinking water that contains 1 part per million (1 mg/liter of water), fluorine is reported to protect teeth from decay. It has been suggested that this effect is due to fluorine's strengthening of tooth structure by way of limiting the solubility of enamel. If the practice of fluoridating water were to become universal, we might not have the problem of endentulous elderly.

Sodium fluoride in doses from 50 to 150 mg/day has been investigated as a treatment for osteoporosis. There is disagreement regarding the efficacy of this treatment. Some fear the toxic effects of fluorine and believe its favorable effects are negligible.

One and a half to four mg of fluorine daily is the estimated safe and adequate intake for adults. Excessive fluorine intake (more than 20 mg per day) continued for more than ten years can cause fluorosis—calcification of ligaments in the neck and vertebrae, and an increased density of the skeleton which leads to increased bone fragility and mottled or defective tooth enamel[2]. Deficiencies of calcium, vitamin C, or protein increase one's susceptibility to fluorosis. Anti-fluoridation groups claim an association between fluoridated water and allergic reactions, also between fluoridated water and higher incidences of cancer. These associations have not been supported by subsequent independent reviews.

All foods contain trace amounts of fluorine, with seafood and tea especially rich sources. A cup of tea contributes 0.1-0.2 mg fluoride. Therefore, the elderly tea drinker may be getting an appreciable amount of fluoride daily from this source.

Copper   Copper is involved, along with iron, in the synthesis of hemoglobin. Copper is also a constituent of, and essential to, the function of several enzyme systems. Copper intake is adequate for most individuals, as copper is widely distributed in foods. Deficiencies have been reported in conditions of malabsorption, in kidney disease, and in individuals maintained on parenteral nutrition for prolonged periods. A recent hypothesis is that a deficiency of copper along with a high ratio of zinc to copper in the diet may cause elevated blood cholesterol levels.

Wilson's Disease is an inborn error of metabolism in which abnormal amounts of copper accumulate in the body, resulting in cirrhosis of the liver and neurological symptoms. This disease is an example of copper toxicity. Copper toxicity, apart from this disorder, is seldom found because extremely high levels of copper need to accumulate before symptoms are seen.

The safe, adequate daily intake of copper is 2–3 mg daily for adults. The average American diet provides insufficient amounts. Foods with the highest copper content are dry yeast, oysters, lobster, and liver, with whole grains, poultry, fish, nuts, and seeds providing moderate amounts. Copper water pipes, especially in soft water areas, add copper to drinking water.

Manganese　　Manganese plays a role in bone formation, brain function, and reproduction. It is also a component of several enzyme systems. Its deficiency can be produced in laboratory animals but it has not been described in man. Tea is a rich source, as are whole grain cereals, legumes, and leafy vegetables. The safe and adequate daily intake of this mineral is 2.5–5.0 mg for adults.

Cobalt　　Cobalt is a constituent of vitamin B_{12} and four cobamide enzymes. Fish, meat, whole grains, and fat are good sources of cobalt. Several years ago, beer containing cobalt, which was added to improve its foaming qualities, caused severe cardiac problems and death in a number of heavy beer drinkers. It appears that high cobalt intakes along with high alcohol intakes and low protein or thiamine intakes are necessary for the cardiac problems to appear. A satisfactory explanation of the biochemical basis of the syndrome has not been put forth[39].

Molybdenum　　Molybdenum is considered an essential nutrient because it is an activator of xanthine oxidase and other enzymes. It is found in highest concentration in legumes and meats. The safe and adequate daily intake for this mineral is 0.15–0.5 mg daily for adults.

Chromium　　Chromium functions in glucose and fat metabolism. It has been shown to improve glucose tolerance in some diabetics. Middle-aged and older people with maturity onset diabetes and intakes of 50 mcg of chromium daily showed improved glucose tolerance when given a chromium supplement of 150 mcg a day. Chromium is neither a hypoglycemic agent nor a substitute for insulin but probably corrects only that part of the diabetic condition caused by chromium deficiency.

Chromium supplements were found to reduce serum cholesterol in some elderly individuals. The safe and adequate daily intake is 0.05–0.2 mg for adults. Impaired glucose metabolism has been shown to cause increased excretion of chromium. Chromium exists in foods in different forms which vary in stability, potency, and absorption from the gastrointestinal tract. The trivalent form of chromium which normally occurs in foods is not as toxic as are the chromates used industrially. Chromium is found in whole grains, liver, egg yolk, dry yeast, and potatoes with the skin. Chromium, along with other minerals, is often lost in food processing so that whole wheat flour supplies four times as much chromium as does white flour. It is estimated that a 2,500 kcal diet provides 0.06 mg of chromium. With the lower caloric intakes characteristic of many elderly, chromium consumption is often below the lowest suggested intake.

Selenium   Selenium is found in all body cells with the highest concentration being present in the kidney. Selenium apparently functions with vitamin E in the enzyme glutathione peroxidase. Some selenium deficiency states in animals also respond to vitamin E supplements. However, it is now believed that selenium is an essential element for man with a role beyond that of a substitute for vitamin E[40]. The safe and adequate daily intake of selenium is 0.05–0.2 mg. Protein foods are the best known sources of selenium, with fish, meat, eggs, and whole grains the best dietary sources. The amount of selenium present in foods depends on the amount in the soil in the region the food is produced. Selenium, like other minerals, is soluble in water and may be discarded in cooking water.

NUTRIENT
SUPPLEMENTATION

In 1969, a study of the health practices and opinions of a representative sample of adults in the United States found that 86 percent of the people polled agreed that those who eat balanced meals can get enough vitamins in their regular food. Nearly three-fourths of the same individuals also agreed that feeling tired and run-down indicates a need for more vitamins[41]. This apparent contradiction in beliefs is underscored by the quantities of nutrient supplements that are sold in the United States.

The more than 600 million dollars that is spent yearly by the approximately 35 million people who self-prescribe nutrient supplements is an indication that many believe these supplements to be beneficial or even necessary to good health. The elderly, as a group, because they tend to have many health concerns, are particularly vulnerable to suggestions that nutrient supplements are valuable for the maintenance of health and to forestall the undesirable effects of aging. Taking supplements is perceived as doing something positive. The supplements are always considered helpful, never harmful. This is because the elderly (as well as younger people) for the most part learn about nutrition and health from advertisements in the popular media.

In the 1965 Household Food Consumption Survey discussed in Chapter 3, it was found that 34 percent of the adults aged seventy-five years or older who were polled indicated that they had taken a vitamin or mineral pill, capsule, oil, or other supplement in the preceding twenty-four hours. The type of preparations taken was not described. Another survey in 1957 of Social Security recipients living in Rochester, New York, showed that 37 percent of the households reported using supplements. These were primarily multivitamins with very few containing iron or calcium. An interesting finding was that those households in which the diets were adequate, as indicated by meeting two-thirds of the RDA, were more likely to take supplements than those with poorer diets. Supplements were most popular among single elderly women and two-woman households[42].

More recent information about the use of nutrient supplements by the elderly will be available when the data collected in the 1977–78 Household Food Consumption Survey is tabulated. However, it would seem that the use of supplements—nutrients and other substances considered to be of nutritional significance such as bioflavinoids (see Chapter 9)—is more widespread now than ten or more years ago. Nutrition and diet concerns are given wide coverage in books, newspaper and magazine articles, and on television and radio. Frequently, a single nutrient such as vitamin C or E or, more recently, the mineral zinc is touted as being beneficial for numerous conditions which plague the elderly, such as loss of taste, arthritis, and the like. It is no wonder that the aged use supplements which they are led to believe will help them cope with the increasing effects of aging in their bodies.

A varied, well-chosen diet of 1,800 to 2,000 Calories can provide all needed nutrients, but the elderly, particularly low income elderly, are apt to consume inadequate diets. Additionally, nearly all elderly persons are subject in some degree to interference with absorption, storage, and utilization of nutrients. Other physical, psychological, and social factors operate to place the elderly at nutritional risk (see Figure 10–1). Therefore, while it is true that it is possible for a normal individual to obtain all the nutrients necessary for good health from food, the elderly may not be able to do so.

Nutrient supplementation is indicated when deficiency status can be clearly demonstrated by biochemical tests and clinical signs. Their use is debatable in the absence of clearcut signs of deficiency, and these signs themselves are not definitive. Clinical signs of deficiency are often nonspecific and may take many years to develop. Tissue stores must be depleted before enzyme function is reduced, which then leads to nonspecific clinical signs or symptoms such as loss of appetite and irritability, and finally to more specific anatomical lesions. The time span between deficient intake of a nutrient and clearcut overt symptoms may be two years or longer[43]. It is unusual for an individual to manifest deficiency symptoms of a single nutrient; more often it is a multiple deficiency.

There have been few studies to evaluate the use of nutrient supplements in the aged. Some of those published have been criticized because of poor design, inadequate description, and lack of controls[44]. There are several studies which seem to support the value of nutrient supplementation, particularly in deficient elderly individuals.

An indication that higher vitamin intakes may benefit the elderly was found in a study done in California in the late 1940s and early 1950s. When mortality data were compared with nutrient intakes, it was concluded that there was an inverse relationship between mortality and intake of vitamin A, niacin, and ascorbic acid. Those with highest intakes of vitamin A (800 or more I.U. daily) had a mortality rate of 4.3 percent compared to a mortality rate of 13.9 percent for those whose intakes of vitamin A were less than 500 I.U. daily. The reduction in mortality with increased intakes of niacin was not as pronounced. For vitamin C, however, there was a mortality rate of 18.5 percent among those who ingested less than 50 mg of vitamin C daily as compared to a rate of 3.9 percent for those subjects ingesting 50 to 100 mg daily[45].

Another study describes 200 older women who complained of fatigue, backache, persistent headache, and joint pains, among other things. These symptoms improved when supplements were given. Before supplementation, these people were found to be ingesting, on the average, only 40 percent of the 1957 RDA for vitamins A and C. The mortality rate among these subjects was found to be related to nutrient intake, with the mortality rate higher for those who reported intakes of less than 40 percent of the RDA for one or more nutrients[45]. This indicates that elderly persons on restricted diets may have vague, nonspecific complaints which respond to increased vitamin intake. This increased intake can be achieved both by improving the quality of the diet and by supplementation of specific vitamins as needed.

In a carefully controlled study of eighty chronically ill, hospitalized elderly patients, 95 percent of whom had some nutritional deficiency (90 percent having low levels of thiamine or ascorbic acid), one-half of the subjects received a vitamin supplement daily for one year. The supplement contained 15 mg thiamine, 15 mg riboflavin, 50 mg nicotinamide, 10 mg pyridoxine, and 200 mg of vitamin C. The other half of the group was given an identical placebo. The supplemented group showed a striking improvement in general physical and mental condition, including improved color of skin and mucus membranes; while in the placebo group, conditions did not improve and in many cases worsened. The improvements took as long as one year to occur. When the supplement was discontinued, there was a dramatic reappearance of signs of nutritional deficiency within six to nine months[45]. This again supports the thesis that supplementation can be of value to deficient individuals.

The question of whether or not to recommend nutrient supplements across the board to all elderly has not been answered definitively. On the basis of studies showing only 5-10 percent of the elderly to have deficient states, and then only of certain vitamins, Barrows and Beauchene concluded that, "along with complete lack of information on the effect of continued long-term vitamin therapy in older people it seems unwise to propose mass vitamin and other nutrient supplements to the aged at this time and therapy should be administered on the merits of individual cases"[46]. On the other side of the coin, Whanger writes, "Realistically, a diet that has less than 2,000 Calories is likely to be deficient in vitamins. . . . I tend to use multi-vitamin preparations rather liberally in treating elderly patients. The potential benefit outweighs considerably any remotely possible complications of their use"[1].

While the advisability of routine nutrient supplements for all elderly is debatable, *the advisability of high doses or therapeutic intakes is clearly unwarranted in the absence of specific medical indications for their use.*

A potentially dangerous level of intake has been defined as a megadose, which is an amount ten times the RDA for that nutrient. Thus a megadose of vitamin C would be 600 mg or more daily. Vitamin C and many other vitamins function in the body as coenzymes that, along with protein, form enzymes which facilitate metabolic reactions. Vitamins ingested in amounts greater than can be utilized in this function can either be excreted, stored, or act in some non-vitamin function. Some of these non-vitamin functions may be harmful. Problems specific to excessive intake of various nutrients have been described for the individual nutrients earlier in this chapter.

Because excessive vitamin intake can be dangerous, use of vitamins should be carefully monitored. If it has been decided that a single RDA level dose of vitamins and minerals is a good idea to ensure dietary adequacy of the nutrients found in the supplement at a small cost, then a single dose daily is all that should be taken. It would seem desirable to take a vitamin-mineral preparation, as the likelihood of mineral deficiencies is as great as that of vitamin deficiencies. Additional doses should *not* be used to replace missed meals. Nor should additional doses be taken if the individual is not feeling up to par or if the weather seems threatening. Vitamin pills, like other medications, should be counted out daily or weekly by the individual or the person caring for him, so that a forgetful person will not take an additional tablet in the mistaken belief that it is the only one taken. Containers with seven compartments are available for use in apportioning the weekly supply of medication needed. This can help a forgetful person comply with appropriate medication dosage.

If supplements have been purchased in containers with child-proof lids, they may also be "elderly-proof" and should be repacked into a suitable container so that the contents are readily accessible to those whose manipulative movements are impaired.

It is important that the individual who is taking a nutrient supplement be cautioned not to rely on the supplement to balance an otherwise poor diet. *The basis of good health rests on an adequate diet containing a variety of foods supplying sufficient amounts of calories and essential nutrients.*

CITED REFERENCES

1. Whanger, A. D. 1973. Vitamins and vigor at sixty five plus. *Postgrad. Medicine* 53:167.
2. National Nutrition Consortium, Inc. 1978. *Vitamin-mineral safety, toxicity and misuse.* Report of the Committee on Safety, Toxicity and Misuse of Vitamins and Trace Minerals, Chicago: The American Dietetic Association.
3. Corless, D., et al. 1975. Vitamin D status in long-stay geriatric patients. *The Lancet* 1:4044.
4. Anwar, M. 1978. Nutritional hypovitaminosis-D and the genesis of osteomalacia in the elderly. *J. Amer. Geriatrics Soc.* 26(7):309.
5. *Vitamin E, a scientific status summary by the Institute of Food Technologists.* 1977. Expert Panel on Food Safety and Nutrition and the Committee on Public Information. *Nutrition Review* 35(2):57.
6. Machtey, I., and Ouaknine, L. 1978. Tocopherol in osteoarthritis: A controlled pilot study. *J. Amer. Geriatric Soc.* 26(7):328.
7. Hypervitaminosis E and coagulation. 1975. *Nutrition Reviews* 33(9):269.
8. DiPalma, J. R., and Ritchie, D. M. 1977. Vitamin toxicity. *Ann. Rev. Pharmacol. Toxicol.* 17:133.
9. Vitamin C toxicity. 1976. *Nutrition Reviews* 34(8):236.
10. Hathcock, J. N. 1976. Nutrition: Toxicology and pharmacology. *Nutrition Reviews* 34(3):65.
11. Accelerated remission of episodes of Herpes Labialis in response to a bioflavinoid-ascorbate supplement. 1978. *Nutrition Reviews* 36(10):300.
12. Bender, A. E. 1971. Nutrition of the elderly. *Royal Society of Health J.* 91(3):115.
13. Schlenker, E. D., et al. 1973. Nutrition and health of older people. *Amer. J. Clinical Nutrition* 26:1111.
14. Riccitelli, M. L. 1972. Vitamin C therapy in geriatric practice. *J. Amer. Geriatric Soc.* 20(1):34.

15. Rungruangsak, K., et al. 1977. Chemical interactions between thiamine and tannic acid I. Kinetics, oxygen dependence and inhibition by ascorbic acid. *Amer. J. Clinical Nutrition* 30:1680.

16. Baker, H.; Jaslow, S. P.; and Frank, O. 1978. Severe impairment of dietary folate utilization in the elderly. *J. Amer. Geriatrics Soc.* 26(5):218.

17. Schmeck, H. M., Jr. January 9, 1979. Memory loss curbed by chemical in foods. *New York Times* Section C-Science Times, p. 1.

18. Munro, H. 1979. The 1970 RDA's. Speech read April 23, 1979, at Memorial Sloan Kettering Cancer Center, New York.

19. Mertz, W. 1977. Dietary changes pose unknown health dangers. *CNI Weekly Report* 7(44):4.

20. Albanese, A. A. 1976. Nutrition and health of the elderly. *Nutrition News* 39(2):5.

21. Jowsey, J. 1977. Osteoporosis: Dealing with a crippling bone disease of the elderly. *Geriatrics* 32:41.

22. Albanese, A. A. 1978. Calcium nutrition in the elderly. *Postgrad. Medicine* 63(3):167.

23. Ellis, F. R.; Holesh, S.; and Ellis, J. W. 1972. Incidence of osteoporosis in vegetarians and omnivores. *Amer. J. Clinical Nutrition* 25:555.

24. Institute of Food Technologists' Expert Panel on Food Safety and Nutrition and the Committee of Public Information. 1975. The effects of food processing on nutrition values. *Nutrition Reviews* 30(4):123.

25. Abraham, A. S., et al. 1978. Magnesium levels in patients with chronic ischemic heart disease. *Amer. J. Clinical Nutrition* 31:1400.

26. Meneely, G. R., and Battarbee, H. D. 1976. Sodium and potassium. *Nutrition Reviews* 34(8):225.

27. Select Committee on Nutrition and Human Needs, United States Senate. 1977. *Dietary goals for the United States.* 2nd ed. U.S. Government Printing Office, Washington, D.C.

28. Underwood, E. J. 1978. Trace element imbalances of interest to the dietitian. *J. Amer. Dietetic Assoc.* 72:177.

29. Nutrition of the elderly. 1977. *Dairy Council Digest* 48(1).

30. Underwood, E. J. 1971. *Trace elements in human and animal nutrition.* 3rd ed. New York: Academic Press, Inc.

31. Elwood, P. C. 1977. The enrichment debate. *Nutrition Today* 12(4):18.

32. Mertz, W. 1978. Trace elements. *Contemporary Nutrition,* General Mills Nutrition Department 3(2).

33. Greger, J. L., and Geissler, A. H. 1978. Effect of zinc supplementation on taste acuity of the aged. *Amer. J. Clinical Nutrition* 31:633.

34. *Recommended dietary allowances.* 8th ed. 1974. National Research Council, National Academy of Sciences, Washington, D.C.

35. Greger, J. L., and Sciscoe, B. S. 1977. Zinc nutriture of elderly participants in an urban feeding program. *J. Amer. Dietetic Assoc.* 70:37.

36. Prasad, A. 1977. Nutritional aspects of zinc. *Dietetic Currents* 4(5):27.

37. Haedlein, K. A., and Rasmussen, A. I. 1977. Zinc content of selected foods. *J. Amer. Dietetic Assoc.* 70:610.

38. Sandstead, H. H. 1978. Zinc interference with copper metabolism. *J. Amer. Medical Assoc.* 240(2):2188.

39. National Academy of Sciences. 1973. *Toxicants occurring naturally in foods.* 2nd ed. Washington, D.C.

40. Stadtman, T. C. 1977. Biological function of selenium. *Nutrition Reviews* 35(7):161.

41. Schnieder, H. A., and Hesla, J. T. 1973. The way it is. *Nutrition Reviews* 31(8):233.

42. Horwell, S. C., and Loeb, M. B. 1969. Nutrition and aging. *Gerontologist* 9(3):17.

43. Brin, M. 1978. Vitamin needs of the elderly. *Postgrad. Medicine* 63(3):155.

44. Vitamin supplements for older people. 1970. *Nutrition Reviews* 28(10):260.

45. Mickelsen, O. 1976. The possible role of vitamins in the aging process. In *Nutrition, longevity and aging,* eds. M. Rockstein and M. Sussman. New York: Academic Press, Inc.

46. Barrows, C. H., and Beauchene, R. E. 1970. Aging and nutrition. In *Newer methods of nutritional biochemistry,* vol. 4, ed. A. A. Albanese, p. 163. New York: Academic Press, Inc.

OTHER REFERENCES

Aloia, J., et al. 1977. Combination therapy for osteoporosis. *Metabolism* 26(7):787.

Catalanotto, F. A. 1978. The trace metal zinc and taste. *Amer. J. Clinical Nutrition* 31:1098.

Esposito, S. J.; Vinton, P. W.; and Rapuano, J. A. 1969. Nutrition in the aged. *J. Amer. Geriatrics Soc.* 17:790.

Exton-Smith, N. 1972. Physiological aspects of aging: Relationship to nutrition. *Amer. J. Clinical Nutrition* 25:853.

Harrill, A., and Cervone, N. 1977. Vitamin status of older women. *Amer. J. Clinical Nutrition* 30:431.

Institute of Food Technologists' Expert Panel on Food Safety and Nutrition and the Committee of Public Information. 1975. The effects of food processing on nutrition values. *Nutrition Reviews* 30(4):123.

Kositawattanakul, T., et al. 1977. Chemical interactions and tannic acid, II. Separation of products. *Amer. J. Clinical Nutrition* 30:1686.

Myron, D. R., et al. 1977. Vanadium content of selected foods as determined by flameless atomic absorption spectroscopy. *J. Agric. and Food Chemistry* 25(2):297.

Schwarz, K. 1974. Recent dietary trace element research exemplified by tin, fluorine and silicon. *Federation Proceedings* 33(6):1748.

Taylor, R. J. 1972. *Micronutrients.* Unilever Research Division, Unilever Limited.

Underwood, E. J. 1975. Cobalt. *Nutrition Reviews* 33(3):65.

|||||||||||||||||||||||||||||||||||||||||||| 6

Fiber and Water

A review of dietary essentials requires a discussion of fiber and water, both of which are important components of one's dietary intake. Although they are considered to be nonnutritive substances, fiber and water are both essential in nutrient absorption and intestinal motility. Further, all cells in the body depend on an aqueous medium for their metabolic reactions as well as for maintaining the integrity of their surrounding structures. Fiber, also known as unavailable carbohydrate, or roughage, is currently of great interest because of some indications that it may help prevent the occurrence of certain disease states in the body.

FIBER

Dietary fiber is a generic term that includes plant constituents resistant to digestion by secretions of the human gastrointestinal tract. These are carbohydrate substances such as cellulose, hemicellulose, mucilage, pectin, gum, and lignin (a woody, non-carbohydrate substance found in older plants). One may speak of dietary fiber, or one may speak of crude fiber. The two are not equivalent. Crude fiber is the material remaining after a food sample is subjected to rigorous treatment with acid and alkali[1]. Therefore, the figure for the crude fiber content of a food item is mainly the cellulose and lignin content of the food since the other fibrous components are dissolved by this chemical treatment. However, many of the other fibrous components of dietary fiber would not be digested in the body. Data on fiber content of foods, as it is shown on packages and in food composition tables, indicates crude fiber which is considerably *less* than the total dietary fiber (the nutritionally relevant fiber) in the food. Nine gm of crude fiber may represent 18–90 gm of dietary fiber[1]. Total dietary fiber estimation is expensive and time consuming, which is why crude fiber values are most commonly given[1].

All food of vegetable origin contains fiber in varying amounts. Whole grain cereals are a major source (bran has 9–12 percent crude fiber); dry peas, beans, lentils, and nuts have larger amounts of fiber than fruits and vegetables. Processing food affects its fiber content. Peeling reduces it, while browning or toasting slightly increases a food's fiber content. White bread contains more fiber after it has been toasted (white bread is 2.1 percent fiber; toasted white bread is 3.0 percent fiber)[2].

Low fiber diets have been linked epidemiologically with a variety of diseases and disorders, including diverticulosis, colon and breast cancer, constipation, heart disease, and obesity[3]. These conditions are more prevalent in developed countries where the consumption of fiber has been steadily decreasing. Stools of individuals whose diets are low in fiber are less bulky and have a harder consistency and therefore necessitate straining at the stool. This is believed to be an etiological factor in hiatus hernia, varicose veins, and hemorrhoids. Diverticula disease, which is the most common pathological condition of the large bowel, is believed to affect almost one-half of the population over age sixty. This disorder is believed to be caused as a consequence of increased pressure in the sigmoid colon (S-shaped portion of colon) due to hard dry contents which are difficult to propel.

High fiber diets may have a normalizing effect on diarrhea, if it is not caused by infection, because of fiber's affinity for water. Diverticulosis and constipation are also treated by a high fiber diet because the addition of fiber to the diet increases the size of the stool and softens its consistency as lignin and cellulose absorb water. A ten-week study in the geriatric unit of a hospital showed that elderly patients were able to reduce the necessity for laxatives by as much as 46 percent as a result of moderate additions of fiber to their diet[4]. Recent evidence shows that a person suffering from irritable-bowel syndrome may also benefit from a diet high in wheat fiber[5].

Increased stool size causes greater peristalsis, which decreases the transit time of the stool through the large intestine. This decreased transit time reduces the time in which the large intestine is in contact with carcinogenic substances formed by the action of the colon's bacteria on feces[6]. This is the hypothesis which is used to explain the association of colon cancer and a low fiber diet. The high fiber diet not only reduces transit time, but it may also alter the type of microorganisms present in the colon so that production of carcinogens is inhibited. Also, the increased water content in the colon due to the presence of fiber reduces concentration of these potential carcinogens[7].

A high fiber diet has been utilized to reduce serum cholesterol[8]. Recent evidence reports that it is the pectin component of the fiber rather than the bran which reduces serum cholesterol. This effect is thought to be brought about by a binding of the bile acids, which contain cholesterol, to dietary fiber in the intestine. These bile acids play a role in the digestion of fats. They are secreted into the intestine, where they emulsify fats. The bile acids then are normally reabsorbed and reused by the body. If the bile acid is bound to fiber, its reabsorption is inhibited and the size of the body's bile acid pool is reduced. The body then converts cholesterol to bile acid and thereby reduces the circulating level of cholesterol. The elderly should have adequate liquid intake along with fiber to avoid risk of fecal impaction which can be caused by the combined effect of fiber and the relaxed intestinal muscle tone found in the aged.

Breast cancer has been associated with a high fat, high meat diet. It has been hypothesized that this type of diet increases levels of hormones in breast tissue which predispose individuals to cancer. Because fiber interferes with fat absorption, it may lower the amount of fat in the body available for synthesis of these hormones and thus lessen their concentration in breast tissue[9].

A high fiber diet may also help to prevent or control obesity because the nonnutritive fiber displaces other foods in the diet. Fiber also requires more chewing than other foods, which slows down intake and promotes a feeling of satiety[1]. Additionally, the absorption efficiency of the small intestine is reduced by the presence of fiber so that approximately 92 percent of the calories in the food are available for absorption, compared with a 97 percent availability of calories from foods low in fiber.

This last factor can have an undesirable effect on absorption of important trace nutrients, particularly some minerals[5]. Phytic acid, which is a component of fiber, binds iron, calcium, zinc, and other minerals, preventing their absorption so they are unavailable to the body. This has been documented in studies in which a trace mineral deficiency was found in animals on a high fiber diet. This might especially be a problem in diets characteristic of the elderly, which may be marginal in their mineral content. Mineral supplementation may be advisable for indviduals on a high fiber diet.

Large amounts of bran in the diet have been found to temporarily increase flatulence and abdominal distention[10]. In rare cases, esophageal obstruction was caused by large quantities of bran and other fiber-containing foods eaten dry. It is important to drink plenty of liquid when eating fiber. Additionally, the stomach and intestinal linings can be irritated and damaged from too much fiber in the diet.

At the present time, the status of knowledge about the desirable and undesirable effects of fiber in the diet does not indicate the need for a major change in diets of the total population. Rather it appears that a moderate consumption of fiber is not just beneficial, but contributes to good health.

The elderly can increase fiber in their diet by eating more bread made from whole wheat flour. Food labels must be carefully read to be sure that the bread assumed to be whole grain actually lists whole wheat as the first (major) ingredient. Many dark, rough looking breads available actually are made primarily from enriched white flour, and are colored with burnt sugar and raisin juice. Another way to increase dietary fiber is to eat more whole grain cooked cereals such as oatmeal, barley, and dry ready-to-eat cereals such as bran and shredded wheat. Granola-type cereals are usually too high in fat and sugar to be eaten regularly. Fruits, vegetables, and legumes—rather than pastries and sweets—should be used for meals and snacks.

Many individuals have begun to buy unprocessed bran (the outer layer of the wheat kernel) and add it to soups, cereals, muffins, and baked foods. This is an effective way to introduce fiber, but it should be done with moderation. At first a small amount—one teaspoon—should be added each day. This amount can be increased gradually to a maximum amount of two to three tablespoons per day. Most adults need no more than this amount to prevent constipation[11].

It has recently been reported that insulin-dependent diabetics have significantly lower levels of plasma glucose when fed a diet containing twenty grams of crude fiber when compared with others on an isocaloric diet containing only three grams of crude fiber[12]. There is no adequate explanation for this.

WATER

Water is more critical to survival than food. Lack of water intake will result in death sooner than will lack of food. Water is the medium in which all the body's various metabolic activities take place. It dissolves the vast majority of biologically important molecules and ions and is able to provide a constant, balanced internal environment for the body. Water is an essential structural component of every cell in the body. Its solvent properties allow water to function in digestion, absorption, circulation (blood is 80 percent water), and excretion (urine is 97 percent water). Water also acts to help regulate body temperature as well as lubricate joints and abdominal viscera.

Approximately two-thirds of the body's weight is water. The specific amount of water in the body varies with age and with the amount of body fat present. Elderly persons tend to have less body water present than they did when they were younger[13]. Fat tissue contains little or no water. Thus, an individual with a large amount of body fat might be expected to have a smaller-than-average fraction of his body weight made up of water.

Normally, there is a balance between water intake and water output. One's water intake is that water consumed through food (and some foods have very high water content—even potatoes are 60% water) and drink, as well as the water that is formed metabolically by the oxidation of carbohydrates, fat, and protein. One's water output is that water lost as urine, in the feces, and through the skin and lungs.

The minimum amount of water ingested should cover the total lost each day. A good rule of thumb is that one's liquid intake should be sufficient to produce one quart or more of urine each day. For the average 132-pound individual, aged sixty-five to ninety years, it was found that 1.3 quarts of water intake daily were necessary to maintain water balance[14]. Further, it is believed that approximately 50 percent of this 1.3 quarts can be obtained in one's daily food intake, exclusive of liquids.

Despite the apparent ease with which fluid needs may be met, many elderly become dehydrated. Elderly people may fail to drink the necessary amount of fluid each day for a variety of reasons. Weakness and disability may act to sharply reduce one's intake. Sometimes a sufficient amount of drinkable fluid is simply not conveniently available. In many adult homes and extended care facilities, water is not routinely placed on the table at mealtimes. Even though water is placed at the bedside, the bedridden person may find it difficult or impossible to drink this water without assistance. At other times, elderly persons restrict their fluid intake because they are troubled by nocturia and wish to avoid disturbing their sleep. In this case, the elderly person should be encouraged to drink more fluids earlier in the day so that frequent urination at night is not necessary. The incontinent bedridden person may avoid fluids to lessen embarrassing "accidents." Lastly, some elderly persons are simply not aware of thirst, which normally stimulates one to drink.

Drinking plenty of fluids is beneficial to many body processes. It is useful in washing down partially masticated food. High water intake reduces the amount of osmotic work the kidney must do and may prevent the formation of renal stones. Additionally, water aids in peristalsis and thus drinking plenty of water will combat constipation. Water may also be a source of trace minerals such as zinc, fluorine, and copper. However, water also may be a carrier of potentially harmful substances such as nitrates and cadmium[13]. It is estimated that 5 percent of the communities in the United States have very high nitrate levels in their drinking water[15].

Dehydration can be manifest by sunken eyes, dry tongue, and dry skin. Dehydrated skin is loose and lacks elasticity. When such skin is pinched between thumb and forefinger, it stands up away from underlying tissue. Severe fluid deprivation interferes with many metabolic processes. Dehydration may cause confusion which, in an elderly person, might be mistaken for chronic brain syndrome.

In the past, fluid has been restricted in several situations: cardiac or renal failure, pulmonary edema, and cataract surgery. The trend now, however, is to allow normal fluid consumption along with the use of diuretics. This reduces the possibility of dehydration.

CITED REFERENCES

1. The role of fiber in the diet. 1975. *Dairy Council Digest* 46(1):1.
2. Van Soest, P. J. 1976. The secret my friends is the fiber. *Human Ecology Forum* 6(4):1.
3. Brodribb, A. J. M., and Humphreys, D. M. 1976. Diverticular disease: Three studies. *Brit. Med. J.* 1:424.
4. Bass, L. More fiber—less constipation. 1977. *Amer. J. Nursing* 77(2):254.
5. Kelsay, J. L. 1978. A review of research on effects of fiber intake on man. *Amer. J. of Clin. Nutrition* 31:142.
6. Van Soest, P. J., and McQueen, R. W. 1973. The chemistry and estimation of fiber. *Pro. Nutrition Soc.* 32:123.
7. Mendeloff, A. I. 1975. Dietary fiber. *Nutrition Reviews* 33(11):321.
8. Leveille, G. A. 1976. Dietary fiber. *Food and Nutrition News* 47(3):1.
9. Hill, P., and Wynder, E. 1976. Diet and prolactin release. *Lancet* 2:806.
10. Connell, A. M. 1978. Fiber and gastrointestinal functions in nutrition in disease. Ohio: Ross Laboratories.
11. Kramer, P. 1975. The importance of dietary fiber in gastrointestinal disorders. *G.I. Tract* 5(3):4.
12. Diabetes and dietary fiber. 1978. *Nutrition Reviews* 36(9):273.
13. Davidson, S., et al. 1975. *Human nutrition and dietetics.* London: Churchill Livingstone.
14. Albanese, A. A. 1976. Nutrition and health of the elderly. *Nutrition News* 39(2):5.
15. Ibrahim, M. A., and Christman, R. F. 1977. Drinking water and carcinogenesis: The dilemmas. *Amer. J. Public Health* 67(8): 719.

OTHER REFERENCES

Recommended Dietary Allowances. 8th ed. 1974. National Research Council, National Academy of Sciences, Washington, D.C.

Watkin, D. M. 1973. Nutrition for the aging and the aged. In *Modern nutrition in health and disease,* eds. R. S. Goodhart and M. E. Shils, p. 681. Philadelphia: Lea and Febiger.

7

Nutrition and Health Problems

As would be expected, the elderly are more likely to be affected with illness—primarily chronic conditions and physical impairment—than are younger people. After age sixty-five, few persons are free of chronic illness or impairment. About 72 percent of those aged forty-five to sixty-four years have one or more chronic health problems. At age sixty-five and over, the percentage having chronic illness increases to 86 percent, with many individuals having several chronic impairments. About 50 percent of people in this age group report some limitation of normal activity due to chronic health problems[1].

Therefore, the major health care problem of the elderly is that of chronic conditions. Arthritis, auditory and visual impairments, hypertension, and heart conditions are the most prevalent of these. Each of these can affect the nutrition of the elderly. All have nutritional implications, while hypertension and heart conditions require nutritional intervention. The major causes of death, accounting for 70 percent of the deaths of people over age forty-five, are heart disease, cancer, and cerebrovascular disease (primarily strokes)[1]. These have nutritional implications, as do two other major causes of death in the elderly, arteriosclerosis and diabetes. The nutritional implications of some of these aforementioned diseases will be considered in this chapter, along with several others which afflict the elderly and therefore are of concern to those who work with them. It

116

should be kept in mind, however, that, based on our present understanding, dietary intervention in health problems of old age is practiced more to maintain the individual in a stable condition than to ameliorate any long-standing health problem.

CARDIOVASCULAR DISEASE

Cardiovascular diseases are those diseases affecting the heart and blood vessels, primarily the arteries. These diseases comprise two of the three major causes of death in the United States. Many elderly are affected by one or more of the cardiovascular diseases, including hypertension, atherosclerosis, congestive heart failure, angina pectoris, and arteriosclerosis. It is believed that diet probably plays a role in the etiology of these disorders, and certainly has a role in their treatment. Modifications in the type and amount of fat and carbohydrate eaten are the primary dietary changes that have been recommended for both the prevention and treatment of several of these diseases.

There is an increased risk of developing cardiovascular disease with increasing age. The risk factors most commonly correlated with the susceptibility of populations to coronary heart disease are elevated serum cholesterol levels, high blood pressure, and excessive cigarette smoking. Several other risk factors associated with the incidence of cardiovascular disease include genetic predisposition, lack of physical activity, emotional stress, personality type, other lipid abnormalities, diabetes mellitus, obesity, and gout. Several of these risk factors are responsive to dietary intervention[2].

High levels of dietary fat and elevated serum lipid levels have been associated with atherosclerosis (deposits of fat-containing plaques on the arterial walls), which is the pathological basis for cardiovascular disease; however, no cause-and-effect relationship between the two has been proven.

Hyperlipidemia refers to an elevation of one or more of the lipids in the blood. This generally refers to increased levels of cholesterol or triglycerides. There are actually three major fats or lipids in the blood—cholesterol, triglycerides, and phospholipids. They are carried bound to protein which enables the insoluble lipids to be transported easily. These combinations of lipids and protein, called lipoproteins, vary as to the amounts of lipids (cholesterol, triglycerides, phospholipids) and protein they contain. The chylomicrons are primarily triglycerides with small amounts of protein, phospho-lipid, and cholesterol. Low density lipoproteins and very low density lipoproteins contain mostly lipids and lesser amounts of protein, while high density lipoproteins are about one-half protein and one-half lipid. Levels of these lipoproteins, as well as triglycerides and cholesterol, can be measured in the blood to determine those individuals with values higher than what is considered normal. It is believed that measurements of lipoproteins are better indicators of lipid abnormalities than analysis of blood lipid levels alone. Choles-terol and triglyceride measurements are nonspecific, while the determination of which lipoproteins are elevated provides direction in the medical management of the conditions. On the basis of these concentrations, an individual may be classified into one of the six types of hyperlipoproteinemia that have been identified. The differ-ent types are treated with different drugs and dietary modifica-tions[3]. The dietary modifications involve manipulation of the amount of fat (saturated and polyunsaturated), cholesterol, carbo-hydrate, protein, and alcohol ingested. General modifications are outlined in Figure 7-1. Complete diet regimens appropriate for the various hyperlipoproteinemias are available in most diet manuals. A list of recommended diet manuals can be found in Figure 7-2.

The American Heart Association has made some recommenda-tions about diets that may help to protect the individual from devel-oping cardiovascular disease. These are:

1. Adjustment of the caloric content of the diet to achieve and maintain optimal weight.

2. Reduction of the total fat content of the diet to no more than 30–35 percent of the total calories, restriction of satu-rated fat to less than 10 percent of total calories, and inclu-sion of polyunsaturated fat to comprise up to 10 percent of the calories (remaining percentage of calories as monoun-saturated fat).

3. Restriction of dietary cholesterol to approximately 300 mg per day.

4. Limitation of concentrated "empty" calories (i.e., simple sugars), which provide only calories without vitamins and other essential nutrients.

5. Prudent use of salt until its role in hypertension is better defined[4].

The Senate Select Committee on Nutrition in the revised Di-etary Goals (1977) underscored these recommendations and went

Type	Diet
I	
increased chylomicrons, triglycerides, cholesterol (may be normal) *normal* VLDL and LDL	Fat restricted to less than 35% of calories, cholesterol not restricted, protein and carbohydrate not limited, alcohol not recommended.
IIA	
increased cholesterol and LDL *normal* triglycerides and VLDL	Limited saturated fat, increased polyunsaturated fat, calories not restricted, cholesterol less than 300 mg, protein and carbohydrate not limited, alcohol permitted in limited amounts.
IIB or III	
increased cholesterol, triglycerides, LDL, and VLDL	Fat is 40% of calories (substitute polyunsaturated fats for saturated fats), calories restricted to reduce weight to ideal, cholesterol less than 300 mg, protein 20% of calories, sugar and concentrated sweets restricted, alcohol limited to 2 oz. whiskey.*
IV	
increased VLDL, triglycerides *normal or increased* LDL, cholesterol	Fat not limited (substitute polyunsaturated for saturated fat), calories restricted to reduce weight to ideal, cholesterol 300–500 mg, protein not limited, carbohydrate 40% of calories, sucrose and concentrated sweets restricted, alcohol limited to 2 oz. whiskey.*
V	
increased chylomicrons, VLDL, cholesterol, triglycerides, *normal or increased* LDL	Fat is 30% of calories (substitute polyunsaturated fats for saturated fats), calories restricted to reduce weight to ideal, cholesterol 300–500 mg, protein 20% of calories, sugar and concentrated sweets limited, alcohol not recommended.

*3 ounces sweet wine, 5 ounces dry wine or 10 ounces beer

FIGURE 7-1　　Dietary modifications for treatment of the six types of hyperlipoproteinemia.

Diet Manual
Diet Therapy Committee, Louisville
  District
Kentucky Dietetic Assoc.
order from: Nancy W. Ratfiff
            300 Chestsey Ct.
            Louisville, Ky. 40243

Diet Manual
Massachusetts General Hospital
Boston, Mass. 02114
1971

Diet Manual
Nashville District Dietetic Assoc.
P.O. Box 37219
Nashville, Tenn.
1979

Diet Manual
New Jersey Dept. of Health
Trenton, N.J.
1975

Diet Manual
Southern California Region
Kaiser Permanente Medical Care
  Program
Kaiser Foundation Hospitals
Los Angeles, Calif.
1973

Diet Manual Utilizing a Vegetarian
  Diet Plan
Seventh Day Adventist Dietetic
  Assoc.
P.O. Box 75
Loma Linda, Calif. 92354
1975

Long Island Diet Manual, 3rd Ed.
Long Island Dietetic Assoc.
P.O. Box 27
Syosset, N.Y. 11791
1978

Mayo Clinic Diet Manual
Committee on Dietetics of the
  Mayo Clinic
W.B. Saunders Co., Philadelphia,
  Pa.
1971

FIGURE 7–2   A selection of recommended diet manuals.

---

beyond them to recommend a greater reduction of total calories from fat to 30 percent and to specify that salt be restricted to 5 gm daily. The Dietary Goals include the recommendation that the consumption of complex carbohydrate and "naturally-occurring sugars" (sugars as they occur in natural foods, not refined) be increased from about 28 percent of the caloric intake to 48 percent while consumption of refined sugars be reduced by 45 percent[5].

Questions are often asked about the necessity, or indeed the advisability, of recommending dietary changes for elderly individuals in order to modify blood lipids which may be factors in the etiology of cardiovascular disease. It is obviously of less value to urge dietary changes for an aged individual in good health than for a younger person. For the aged person who suffers from atherosclerotic disease, the value of the diet changes are debatable because it is uncertain at what point the changes in the arteries become irreversable. It is believed that this point may vary from person to person. Despite the uncertainty, it is a general practice to recommend low fat and cholesterol diets to many elderly. However, many other dietary factors and even the interaction between dietary components may influence blood lipid levels. Dietary protein, carbohydrate, and fiber have been shown to affect blood lipid levels, as do dietary fats.

With elderly people, hyperlipidemia is not as important a risk factor as it is in the young. Also, cardiovascular disease has multiple causes only one of which is diet, and all factors are best dealt with in middle years or even earlier.

HYPERTENSION

Hypertension (high blood pressure) or elevated systolic or diastolic arterial pressure is found in persons of all ages. It has been estimated to affect 20 percent of the total population in the United States. It is, however, more prevalent in the elderly than in younger persons[6]. In men over seventy years of age, the incidence of hypertension has been estimated to range between 40 percent and 65 percent. Hypertension causes increased cardiovascular morbidity and mortality. The risk is as great in older persons as in the young, in women as well as men. The cause of the elevation in blood pressure is, in about two-thirds of all cases, unknown. These cases of hypertension are termed "essential" or idiopathic. In other situations, the cause of hypertension is secondary to renal and endocrine disorders. In these cases the causative disorder must be treated as well as the symptom. In cases of unknown etiology only the high blood pressure symptom is treated.

Healthy young adults have arterial pressure readings of about 120 mm Hg for the systolic (given as the upper figure in the reading) and 80 mm Hg for the diastolic. For most people there is an increase in these readings with age, but the increase is variable. There is a possible physiological need for higher pressure to compensate for decreased cardiac output that might otherwise result in inadequate perfusion of the brain, kidneys, and heart. Additionally, one's weight and other conditions at the time of examination affect the blood pressure readings. For these reasons, it is hard to define precisely what blood pressure levels in an elderly individual constitute hypertension that requires treatment. Many practitioners agree that any pressures over 160 mm Hg systolic and 95 mm Hg diastolic (160/95) should be treated regardless of age[6]. Others consider any readings below 215 mm Hg systolic and 110 mm Hg diastolic acceptable for those aged eighty and over, so long as there are no other symptoms such as left ventricular hypertrophy[7].

Nutritional factors involved in the treatment of hypertension are weight control and sodium restriction[8]. Weight loss of two to three pounds per week in the overweight individual often may result in a significant fall in blood pressure. Reduction of dietary sodium accomplished by restricting salt intake (often along with use of diuretics that enhance sodium excretion) also contributes to a reduction in blood pressure level[6]. Recently, generous fluid intakes have been found helpful in enhancing sodium excretion by the body. The elderly often must be encouraged to consume adequate fluids. Overtreatment of mild hypertension in the elderly may result in hypotension and inadequate blood supply to the brain, causing confusion which may not be recognized as due simply to low blood pressure.

Sodium-restricted diets are indicated in a variety of disorders afflicting the elderly and others, such as hypertension, cardiovascular disease, some renal diseases, and cirrhosis of the liver with edema. Diets may be planned containing various amounts of sodium. Four levels of sodium restriction are used commonly. The level is prescribed by the physician after evaluating the patient.

Mild Sodium Restriction

Intake of 2–3 gm of sodium per day is also referred to as the "no salt shaker diet" because, although small amounts of salt may be used in cooking, no salt is added at the table. Additionally, all prepared and processed foods in which salt has been added as a preservative or flavoring are excluded. These include all salted and smoked meats and fish such as bacon, ham, bologna and other luncheon meats, anchovies, salt cod, and condiments such as seasoned salt, bouillion cubes, catsup, pickles, olives, soy sauce, and Worcestershire sauce. Salted snacks such as chips, nuts, popcorn, and pretzels may not be eaten. Some ordinarily salty foods such as cheese and peanut butter are now readily available (and tasty) in low sodium versions, and these should be used in place of the usual salty types.

Moderate Sodium Restriction

This involves ingesting only 1,000 mg of sodium per day. In addition to those foods eliminated in the Mild Sodium-Restricted Diet, no salt is used in cooking. There is also a limited intake of those vegetables that are high in sodium, such as beets, carrots, celery, kale, white turnips, dandelion, mustard and beet greens, spinach, and Swiss chard. Regular canned vegetables, vegetable juices, soups, meat, and fish may not be used. There are several varieties of canned soups, vegetables, and tuna processed without added salt and these are allowed. All commercially prepared baked products, other than those labeled low sodium, should not be eaten. Because meat, milk, and milk products like yogurt are high in natural sodium, their use is limited as well.

Strict and Severe Sodium Restriction

These involve limiting salt intake to 500 mg and 250 mg per day, respectively. These diets are difficult to implement and are not appropriate for home use. For the 500 mg allowance, milk is limited to two cups daily, meat to 5 ounces daily, and eggs to one daily. This is in addition to all restrictions outlined in the preceding sections on the less restricted diets. Additionally, frozen peas, lima beans, and fish are excluded because salt is used in processing them. All other products containing any salt or sodium compounds such as the preservatives sodium benzoate or sodium propionate are eliminated. All baked goods, including bread, must be of the low sodium variety[9].

For the severe restriction of only 250 mg of sodium daily, low sodium or dialyzed milk is used, meat intake is reduced to two to four ounces daily, and eggs to three a week. If the local water supply contains more than 10 mg of sodium per 100 cc (most municipal water supplies contain less than this amount), only distilled water should be used. Hardness or softness of water does not affect sodium content, but if water is softened by some methods in which the calcium and magnesium, which are responsible for the hardness of the water, are replaced by sodium, the water may be unsuitable for use by persons following a restricted sodium diet.

It is important for the individual following a diet restricted in sodium to be aware of sodium levels of medications such as antacids, saline cathartics, and even toothpaste. Some foods which are not usually considered salty, such as ice cream, may contain appreciable amounts of salt and other sodium-containing substances.

A study of the usefulness of potassium-containing salt substitutes to replace the potassium lost in diuretic therapy found them to be uniform from sample to sample of each brand as well as among different brands. They are less expensive than prescription potassium supplements which may also be unpleasant to take. Thus, the potassium-containing salt substitutes might serve a dual function: seasoning food and combating the hypokalemia that may result from diuretic therapy[10]. The salt substitutes should be used with caution and under a physician's supervision. Potassium salt substitutes are not appropriate for those individuals with impaired renal functions.

MALDIGESTION AND MALABSORPTION

The gastrointestinal tract prepares foods for digestion, digests foods, and selectively absorbs the products of digestion. The gastrointestinal tract also contains several organs that secrete substances necessary for the digestive process. The various digestive juices —saliva, gastric juice, pancreatic juice, and intestinal juice—are all fundamentally solutions of enzymes. Bile, produced in the liver and secreted by the gall bladder, is an exception as this fat emulsifier contains no enzymes. Enzymes, which are protein substances, may require nonprotein substances or cofactors for activity. These cofactors may be either metal ions or organic molecules (coenzymes), many of which are vitamins. Finally, the gastrointestinal tract is an excretory organ through which by-products of ingested materials, secretions, and sloughed-off cells are eliminated.

The gastrointestinal tract is a tube twenty-five to thirty feet long in adults. The human body has accurately been described as a "tube within a tube," to describe the relationship between the gastrointestinal tract and the rest of the body. Ingested food is processed within this tube to convert it to the size and composition suitable for absorption by the intestine. Food within the gastrointestinal tract is considered to be outside the body since it has not yet been absorbed into the body proper. Under normal circumstances, an average of 98 percent of dietary carbohydrate, 95 percent of dietary fat, and 92 percent of dietary protein is digested and absorbed.

The elderly, however, are subject to varying degrees of maldigestion and malabsorption. These conditions can be caused by lack of hydrochloric acid, enzymes, or bile salts; bacterial overgrowth in the small intestine; reduction in the number of functioning intestinal villi, which reduces the absorptive capacity of the small intestine; infections, tropical sprue, enteritis, or parasitic infestation; localized surgery; removal of part or all of the stomach or small intestine, as well as by the effects of certain drugs[11].

Hydrochloric acid secretion may gradually diminish with age. This reduction in acid reduces the absorption of iron and also can permit the proliferation of bacteria in the stomach, as maintenance of a pH less than 4 is necessary for gastric secretions to have bacteriacidal effect.

Pancreatic insufficiency can result from pancreatitis, cancer of the pancreas, resection of the pancreas, and cystic fibrosis (in children and young adults). This insufficiency may necessitate the oral administration of the pancreatic enzymes needed for digestion. These pancreatic enzyme supplements are usually given before each meal, although they have been shown to be more effective if they are given at six to twelve regular intervals throughout the day.

Insufficient secretion of bile acid salts, caused by liver disease, cystic duct obstruction, or bacterial overgrowth, may result in steatorrhea (excessive fat in stools)[12]. This condition reduces the absorption of fat-soluble vitamins A, D, and K and calcium. Medium-chain triglycerides (MCT), composed of fatty acids wth six to ten carbons, are frequently administered for this condition and for a number of other malabsorption disorders, including pancreatic insufficiency, sprue and gastrectomy. About one-third of the MCT ingested can be absorbed without the presence of bile salts.

Bacterial overgrowth in portions of the small intestine is caused mainly by stasis—the slowing or stopping of the movement of intestinal contents down the gastrointestinal tract. This bacterial overgrowth interferes with the absorption of fat, iron, folic acid, and vitamin B_{12}. Antibiotics are useful to combat the overgrowth, and nutrient supplements are used to overcome deficiencies.

Adult celiac disease is an important cause of malabsorption in temperate climates. Tropical sprue is found in areas suggested by its name, and can be treated with a gluten-free diet. This excludes all cereal grains except rice and corn.

Disaccharidase deficiency, the most common of which is lactase deficiency (discussed in Chapter 4), is another cause of malabsorption. In such a case, only small amounts of lactose are tolerated without symptoms.

Acute infection can cause transient but severe malabsorption, as does parasite infestation. Some parasites have been shown to cause atrophy of the intestinal villi.

Intestinal angina is found in older persons with atherosclerosis. Insufficient blood supply to the gastrointestinal tract results in cramping pain after eating. The afflicted person may lose weight because of fear of eating. Small, frequent meals may help somewhat.

Surgical alterations of the gastrointestinal tract, naturally, affect digestion and absorption. For example, a total gastrectomy results in poor digestion of fat and protein, as the digestive juices of the stomach are no longer secreted into the gastrointestinal tract. There is also a lack of the intrinsic factor which is secreted by the stomach and is necessary for the absorption of vitamin B_{12}. Thus, parenteral administration of vitamin B_{12} is needed after gastrectomy. Additionally, iron is not well absorbed after gastrectomy so that iron supplements may be needed. The dumping syndrome, with its symptoms of flushing, sweating, and lightheadedness, results from rapid entry of the gastric contents into the jejunum of the small intestine. Treatment of this problem includes small, frequent meals, rest after eating, avoiding liquids with meals, and decreasing sugar intake.

In ileal resection, disease, or bypass there is malabsorption of vitamin B_{12} and bile salts. Vitamin B_{12} is given parenterally, and *cholestyramine,* a resin which binds bile salts, is used to help the diarrhea caused by the osmotic effect of the unabsorbed bile salts.

Drug use also contributes to digestive problems and malabsorption. Elderly people use laxatives with much greater frequency than younger adults. Excessive use of cathartics and mineral oil (lubricant) can result in decreased transit time and impaired absorption of fat and fat-soluble vitamins. Excessive use of alcohol interferes with fat absorption as well as with the absorption of vitamin A, thiamine, vitamin B_{12}, and folate. *Neomycin* and *tetracyline* also cause specific malabsorptions. Nutrient–drug interactions will be discussed in Chapter 8.

Some other diseases and disorders commonly found in the elderly interfere with normal digestion and absorption, including congestive heart failure, vascular insufficiency, endocrine problems such as diabetes, and radiation injury to the gastrointestinal tract[13]. Skin disorders such as psoriasis and eczema are associated with malabsorption of fat, vitamin B_{12}, and folate.

Correction of the underlying cause for maldigestion and malabsorption is not always possible. For this reason, vitamin, mineral, and calorie supplements are used in a program of nutritional management. Chemically defined formulas which are predigested are useful when digestion is severely impaired. Total parenteral nutrition (TPN) is used to provide complete nutrition when a patient cannot be fed enterally. The diet is administered as a hypertonic solution through a major body vein. The use of TPN necessitates careful and continued monitoring of a wide variety of biochemical and physiological parameters.

Conditions of the Gastrointestinal Tract

Several conditions of the gastrointestinal tract are more commonly found in the elderly than in younger people. A discussion of these follows.

Hiatus Hernia   This protrusion of the stomach upward through the esophageal opening of the diaphragm occurs in about 69 percent of those aged seventy and over[14]. Hiatus hernia may be due to muscle weakness, straining at the stool, wearing clothes that are tight around the waist, and other conditions which cause increased intraabdominal pressure. Some individuals are unaware of this condition while others experience symptoms including bleeding and ulceration of the esophagus. Hiatus hernia is treated by weight reduction, small, frequent, bland meals, antacid use, avoiding constricting clothes, and sleeping with head and shoulders raised.

Diverticulosis   Small distended sacs (diverticulae) in the colon are found in 40 percent of those over seventy years of age[15]. Diverticulosis usually causes no symptoms, but a portion of those afflicted develop diverticulitis, an inflammation of a diverticulum. This is treated by bed rest, liquid diet, antibiotics, antispasmotics, and sedatives. Complications of diverticulitis, such as perforation, may necessitate surgery.

It is believed that consumption of a low fiber diet predisposes one to diverticulosis as this disorder is more commonly found in those who consume primarily refined and processed foods (see Chapter 6). High fiber diets are proposed as a possible preventive measure to avoid diverticulosis. Additionally, when the inflammation of diverticulitis is controlled, moderate amounts of fiber are introduced to the diet to avoid recurrence of the inflammation.

Cholelithiasis   This condition indicates the presence of gallstones, which is common in the elderly. It is estimated that 12 million women and 4 million men in the United States have gallstones, one-half of whom have no symptoms. Those who have diabetes and intestinal disorders interfering with bile absorptions, as well as individuals who take estrogens for menopausal symptoms and clofibrate (a drug used to reduce serum cholesterol) are at increased risk of developing gallstones. They have been found in 38 percent of patients aged seventy to eighty who have autopsies[15]. If there is not any obstruction or inflammation of the gallbladder, the gallstones are asymptomatic. Many individuals who do not tolerate fatty foods believe that gallstones are the cause. However, intolerance to fats is not necessarily a symptom of cholelithiasis.

Constipation   This is a frequent problem in the elderly and is very common among the bedridden. Many elderly were taught that a daily bowel movement was necessary to prevent accumulation of "poisons" in the body. Some healthy people may have a bowel movement only once every two or three days while others may have movements daily or even two to three times a day. The term constipation should be reserved for prolonged retention of feces with infrequent and difficult passage of dry, hard stools[16].

Constipation can be caused by a variety of factors, including lack of fiber and fluid intake, decreased intestinal muscle tone, ignoring of the normal urge to defecate, laxative abuse, prolonged bedrest, insufficient food intake, medical problems such as tumors or spasms, and certain medications—tranquilizers, sedatives, and antacids. Laxative abuse is a particular problem in the elderly. One study showed that individuals over age seventy used laxatives twice as frequently as those aged forty to fifty years. The first step in restoring normal bowel functions in severe constipation is to eliminate all laxatives. (Initially, enemas may be used to induce bowel evacuation until responsiveness of the rectum is reestablished.) Then, a regular time each day for a bowel movement should be established, usually after breakfast. A hearty breakfast which includes foods high in fiber such as whole grain breads or cereals should be eaten daily. Bran can be helpful in moderate amounts —that is, no more than three tablespoons a day with generous fluid intake. Too much dry bran can itself cause an impaction.

Six or more glasses of liquid daily will help keep the feces from becoming dry and hard. A glass of prune juice, which has laxative effect, may make up part of this intake. Some elderly persons drink a glass of warm water and lemon juice upon arising each day and find that this is helpful.

Exercise is important to regular bowel movements. Walking and an appropriate exercise program should be a part of an elderly person's daily routine. A person dependent on laxatives must make an effort to substitute better health habits to regain regular, normal bowel elimination.

Intestinal Gas   A common complaint of many individuals, intestinal gas especially plagues the elderly. Gas in the gastrointestinal tract may be formed by the fermentation of food residues by intestinal microflora or may simply be swallowed air (aerophagia, common in smokers who inhale), or gases which diffuse into the gastrointestinal tract from the blood.

Certain foods such as beans, cabbage, cucumbers, and radishes are generally believed to be "gassy" and are avoided by many people[17]. It has been said that gas is produced by the individual, not the food. Be that as it may, some persons do not expel the gas as easily as do others. This may be due to the fact that their intestinal motility is compromised. Unexpelled gas is that which is responsible for gas pains.

The most effective way for the individual to eliminate intestinal gas is to selectively eliminate foods from the diet in order to discover which foods are most "gassy" for that individual and then substitute nutritional equivalents for these in the diet. If no offensive foods are found, then simply eating and drinking more slowly in an effort to swallow less air will usually ameliorate the situation.

CANCER

"Diseases of the heart" far outrank any other cause of death among persons sixty-five and over. Malignant neoplasms (cancer) rank second. Twenty percent of all American men die of cancer. The most common malignant tumors occur in the lung, breast, and large bowel[18]. The overall incidence of cancer tends to increase with age. However, a recent study has shown that the incidence of cancer of the stomach, lung, esophagus, liver, and pancreas tends to decline after age eighty-five in men and after age seventy-five in women[19].

Nutritional support of cancer patients plays a vital role in therapy. It can help shorten a patient's hospital stay, increase the effectiveness of cancer therapy, and, in some cases, increase the length of his or her life[18].

Nutritional support for the cancer patient can be *supportive, adjunctive,* or *definitive*[20]. Supportive nutrition therapy is designed to maintain or improve nutrition of the patient prior to some more definite therapy. This type of nutritional support might be used prior to surgery. Adjunctive nutrition therapy is based on the concept that improving nutritional status will contribute to the efficacy of the primary modality of treatment. For example, if a patient is in a state of good nutrition, higher doses of radiation or chemotherapeutic agents may be used.

It is well known that the response to oncologic treatment and the tolerance of that treatment by the patient depends in part upon the nutritional status of the patient[21]. When definitive nutrition therapy is employed, the therapy is the primary cancer treatment. For example, a severely debilitated patient may not be able to tolerate other types of cancer therapy. The malnourished cancer victim is a poor risk for chemotherapy because the chance for help is minimal while the side effects of the therapy will be severe. Until the patient's nutritional status is improved, in most cases, other forms of treatment are avoided.

Feeding the cancer patient is a challenge that must be met if therapy is to be successful[22]. The cancer patient is often anorexic (lacking appetite)[23], and this anorexia will lead to malnutrition and ultimate failure of therapy unless it is treated. In some cases the patient feels "full" after eating a very small amount. His taste sensations may be altered, making some foods unpalatable, and swallowing may be difficult due to a decreased saliva production. Psychological deterrents such as depression may also cause anorexia and must be handled[24].

During radiation therapy, the patient may suffer "mouth blindness"[22]. This is an alteration or a complete loss of taste sensations. The bitter sensation is often magnified, making the patient acutely sensitive to the amino acid bitterness in meats. This is a serious problem since most cancer patients should be receiving about 100 grams of protein daily[18]. It has been observed that non-meat protein sources (eggs, cheese, and milk) are better accepted. Poultry and fish may also be less offensive to the patient than red meat. Cold protein food may be better tolerated, and the use of soy sauce, salt, fruit sauces, and wine sauces may make items more palatable[28].

The cancer patient's sweet threshold tends to increase and sweetened food may be readily accepted, though within a narrow range of sweetness[22]. For example, instead of using one teaspoon of sugar in a bowl of cereal the patient may now prefer five teaspoons of sugar per bowl. If six teaspoons are added, however, the patient will find the additional sweetness intolerable and nauseating. Sugar substitutes should be avoided since they are sweeter than sugar and tend to leave an aftertaste. Each sweetened food should be prepared so that it meets the individual patient's preference for sweetness. This can be accomplished by modifying the food at the time of service, adding extra sugar or diluting items like pudding with milk to reduce sweetness. The taste sensations for salty and sour food frequently remain normal. Therefore, high calorie snack foods such as peanuts, peanut butter, crackers, and pretzels can be used. These foods also stimulate fluid intake and if calories are added to fluids, using several products available from different manufacturers, the daily caloric intake can be further increased[21].

Often cancer patients become acutely aware of smells[22]. Many foods, especially meats, smell rancid and may cause nausea. Uncovering the patient's tray outside his room will help odors to dissipate. Isolating and eliminating offensive items can help prevent rejection of an entire meal. Offensive liquids and soups can be served with covers and sipped through a straw.

Difficulty in swallowing is often the result of decreased salivary flow, a side effect of irradiation of the head and neck. A dry mouth and throat causes great discomfort during eating. The patient should be encouraged to drink more liquids with meals and eat foods moistened with sauces, gravies, and butter so that they can be more easily swallowed[22]. Dentists at the Houston Veterans Administration Hospital have devised a saliva substitute, named VA-Ora Lube that greatly relieves dry mouth problems[25, 26].

Most chemotherapeutic agents cause nausea and vomiting, which interferes with food intake. Stomatitis (inflammation of oral mucosa), diarrhea, and malabsorption of nutrients can also arise to varying degrees in patients. Most treatments tend to be scheduled for late in the day to allow for food to be consumed prior to therapy. The breakfast meal and breakfast foods, such as cold cereal, are well accepted and often the patient will consume half of the day's calories at this time.

Despite all efforts, some patients continue to lose weight and alternate feeding methods may be necessary. These will be discussed briefly on pages 135 to 137. Most patients, however, will remain more confident of their prognosis if they continue to be served conventional foods in a conventional manner.

Colon-Rectal Cancer

The incidence of colon carcinoma or carcinomas of the rectum increases with age[15]. Older patients tend to have a better prognosis than younger patients with carcinoma of the colon. Surgery to remove the malignant growth is usually indicated. If the patient is inoperable because of general debility or other associated disease, procedures can be performed to reduce the obstruction, bleeding, and discharge. Radiation therapy may also provide longterm palliation of an inoperable carcinoma of the rectum.

An ileostomy or colostomy is frequently performed to treat colonic cancer. The intact intestine is brought through the abdominal wall, creating an opening or *stoma* which provides a new route for defecation.

Ileostomy and colostomy patients require a great deal of support and help from the medical staff. They not only must accept having cancer but also must accept this new anatomical condition and its inherent problems and care. The older patient, particularly, needs to be made to realize that his life is not over. After the initial convalescent period, independent living and normal activities can resume. Prompt return to a normal diet is an important indicator of progress and will often help motivate an otherwise depressed patient[27].

Colonic surgery in itself does not cause nutritional problems of clinical significance[28]. Consequently, set dietary rules are not prescribed. Almost all food tolerated before surgery will be tolerated after healing has occurred. The postoperative diet should be balanced and tailored to the individual's preferences and condition. In some patients, vitamin B_{12} absorption is reduced or may be totally absent. Vitamin B_{12} is absorbed in the terminal ileum, and if a large portion of the ileum is removed by surgery, the vitamin must be administered parenterally so that megaloblastic anemia does not develop[27].

Postoperatively, the colostomy patient is generally given clear fluids with a gradual return to a normal diet, beginning with a diet that minimizes residue in the digestive tract. New foods should be introduced one at a time and in small amounts so that offending foods can be easily identified. Any food that causes discomfort should be discontinued and then tried again in a few months when healing is more complete. Gas and odor may be caused by beans, onions, green peppers, turnips, cabbage, beets, antibiotics, and some vitamin-mineral supplements, but the extent of the problem varies among individuals. Blockage may occur if a food bolus gets caught in the ileostomy at the point where it narrows and passes through the abdominal wall. Avoidance of very fibrous vegetables, such as corn, celery, and coconut is advised. These foods, however, are usually tolerated if eaten in small amounts. Loose stools and watery discharge may be triggered by alcohol, raw vegetables, fruits, and highly spiced foods. The extent of the discomfort varies with the quantity eaten and the individual tolerance to the particular food[20].

The patient should be cautioned that restricting fluids will not control diarrhea or watery stools. The patient's water-absorbing capacity has been surgically impaired and he will require one to two quarts of additional fluids each day. The use of additional dietary sodium may also be necessary. The surgery will not change preexisting food intolerances nor cause any new distress from favorite foods. An acceptable diet must be established on an individual basis since every person's gastrointestinal tract responds differently to different stimuli. Practical help for the patient may be obtained from the *United Ostomy Association* (1111 Wilshire Blvd., Los Angeles, Ca. 90017), which has chapters throughout the country[27].

MALNUTRITION

Malnutrition covers a wide spectrum of disease states, ranging from morbid obesity to cachexia due to the loss of significant amounts of lean body mass. The following section will briefly discuss these extremes of malnutrition seen in the geriatric patient.

Undernutrition

Physicians are frequently dealing with patients who are undernourished. Many of these individuals who suffer a significant degree of malnutrition include the elderly who are hospitalized or in a nursing home and elderly patients who have recently been discharged from a hospital. Regardless of the cause (physical, psychological, or both), malnutrition is a serious health problem and aggressive nutritional support is necessary for its treatment.

The debilitation of undernutrition is accompanied by weakness, depression, skin breakdown, poor wound healing, and decreased immune mechanisms. The condition is progressive; an already poor eater becomes increasingly apathetic, lethargic, and irritable, and then eats even less. What develops is a self-reinforcing phenomenon that may result in starvation[29].

Undernourished patients can be loosely grouped into two categories: patients who can't eat and patients who won't eat. The former are patients who cannot feed themselves or whose gastrointestinal tract is not functioning (who are thus unable to digest or absorb food normally)[23]. Patients who won't eat have some factor interfering with their willingness to eat[24]. The elderly person may not eat due to a lack of socialization at meals, prolonged illness, or the effect of drugs which often alter the sense of taste. Depression, common to the aged, classically manifests itself as loss of appetite. The presence of pain, such as from arthritis, significantly interferes with eating. Fear and anxiety may also inhibit one's appetite. Additionally, an unnecessarily stringent or restrictive diet prescription may result in too few foods that are acceptable to the patient, resulting in a severely limited intake.

Many elderly patients rebel through food. In order to get attention they will often make a fuss about their diets or refuse to eat. An elderly person may be angry because he is sick, angry with relatives who deserted him in a nursing home, or angry with a physician who ordered a necessary but painful treatment. The focal point of his anger may become food. In addition, some aged persons refuse to eat because they wish to die. Undernourished patients are difficult to treat and often cause the staff or relatives who look after them to become frustrated and resentful. However, if the alleviation of malnutrition is not integrated into a total treatment program, an undernourished person will continue to have a poor prognosis.

If maintenance of good nutrition is crucial to the patient's recovery, then the caretaker must be able to recognize early signs of nutritional deterioration. The easiest way to detect a problem is to record the patient's weight and keep track of it[30, 31]. When weight loss is obvious, corrective approaches should be instituted. Patients who are grossly overweight or grossly underweight initially, are particularly "at risk," the former because their obesity tends to mask the loss of body protein and the latter because of limited protein reserves in organs of the body.

The easiest corrective approach is to modify the undernourished person's diet and provide regular food. Five hundred calories over the daily need will produce a weight gain of one pound per week[29]. Higher levels of calorie intake may be required for more acute states but it is inadvisable to increase caloric intake too quickly, for some patients are repelled by an overladen plate of food. The additional calories can come from food or from commercial nutrition supplements. These supplements tend to be convenient, reliable, and acceptable to the patient. Some patients may tolerate between-meal snacks; for others, these snacks depress the appetite for the following meal. In this case, a bedtime snack can provide the five hundred extra calories and not interfere with the three daily meals. Foods that can be kept by the bedside to be nibbled on throughout the day or a supplementary liquid formula made accessible at the bedside in an ice bath can account for an appreciable caloric intake by the end of the day[23].

It is not necessary to provide excessive amounts of protein to undernourished patients. A daily protein intake of 100 gm has been recommended. Other authorities feel that normal quantities (41–56 gm) are all that is needed, provided the patient consumes all the protein and that there are enough calories to prevent the body from utilizing undue amounts of the protein as a source of energy[24, 30].

When supplementation with food is not applicable, the patient may receive a tube feeding or special feeding that can be administered orally. These products are available commercially prepared as complete feedings or as supplements that supply specific nutrients. Currently, there are many such products available on the market and the physician, working in conjunction with the dietitian, can select the type most appropriate for the particular patient. Each patient must receive a good balance of nutrients in proportion to his caloric requirements. The patient must be carefully monitored. When weight is not maintained or the patient is not in nitrogen balance, his intake should be increased[32]. Many elderly people (particularly non-Caucasian elderly) are deficient in the enzyme lactase which splits lactose in milk. The resulting lactose intolerance may be of particular importance if the patient is to receive a tube feeding, as many of these feedings contain large amounts of milk and lactose. If lactose intolerance is diagnosed or suspected, commercially available alternative tube feedings, containing neither lactose nor milk, should be given to the patient.

Feeding through a nasogastric tube or a tube emptying directly into the stomach or small intestine is appropriate for a patient who cannot be fed orally but whose gastrointestinal tract is functioning enough for adequate nutrition to be obtained via this route. In some cases, the gastrointestinal tract is nonfunctional and patients must be sustained by parenteral feedings. Traditional intravenous feedings of glucose and water are inadequate for more than a few days. Patients maintained for more than ten days on simple solutions of glucose and saline are at risk for undernutrition[31]. Even when these feedings are fortified with vitamins and minerals and supplemented with intravenous amino acids they are not adequate to sustain body weight or prevent tissue breakdown. When a patient is still unable to eat after ten to fourteen days of peripheral intravenous therapy, *total parenteral nutrition* (TPN) should be considered[31].

TPN is a method of feeding by which a concentrated solution is administered through a catheter inserted into the superior vena cava. The entering solution is rapidly diluted by the large volume of blood in this large vein. Unlike intravenous glucose, which provides 400 to 600 calories per day, TPN can supply 5,000 or more calories per day—enough energy to ensure anabolism. Supplying calories appreciably in excess of the normal requirement is called intravenous *hyperalimentation*[20].

TPN may be used to maintain nutritional status, as well as to rehabilitate a severely undernourished patient. By providing all nutrients intravenously, positive nitrogen balance can be achieved and sustained for indefinite periods. This method of feeding has been particularly beneficial to cancer patients. Repletion of nutritional status allows for a more positive response to oncological treatment.

Total parenteral nutrition administered to a patient aged sixty-five and over may result in the onset of hyperosmolar nonketotic hyperglycemia[33]. This usually results from a too rapid infusion of the hypertonic solution. The patient becomes weak, listless, and finally comatose, suffering from osmotic diuresis, dehydration, central nervous system irritability and convulsions. This syndrome is preventable with careful clinical observation and laboratory monitoring.

Whether the patient is receiving parenteral nutrition through a peripheral or a central vein, it is important that these feedings are not abruptly discontinued. After prolonged intravenous feedings, there may be a degree of disuse malabsorption in the gastrointestinal tract[23]. The patient should be taken from the intravenous feeding by a graduated series of diets culminating in total oral feeding with a normal diet. This gradual transition prevents protein and calorie consumption from falling off, thereby ensuring that body protein will not be catabolized.

Any person on TPN needs careful biochemical and physiological monitoring. Periodic determinations of urinary glucose, urine specific gravity, urine acetone, serum electrolytes, blood urea nitrogen (BUN), blood glucose, calcium, phosphorous, serum protein, prothrombin time, blood ammonia, magnesium, and blood counts help avoid complications[32].

Obesity

Statistical evidence for humans indicates that overweight in adults is associated with a shortened lifespan. The percentage of overweight individuals continues to increase, and a 1973 survey showed 71 percent of women and 84 percent of men over fifty were obese, that is, 25 percent over desirable weight for men and 30 percent over desirable weight for women. Most men reach their peak weight between the ages of thirty-five and forty-four while women peak between age fifty-five and sixty-four[34].

Obesity has been suggested as a predisposing factor in cardiovascular disease, hypertension, atherosclerosis, hernia, gall bladder disease, diabetes, liver disease, and hyperuricemia. Excessive weight is an additional risk factor in surgery. When the surgery is elective, the patient's overweight condition may be the deciding factor in whether or not to perform the operation. Obesity further complicates the treatment of arthritis and Parkinson's disease[35, 36].

This evidence appears to support the advisability of weight reduction therapy in all older obese individuals. An aggressive weight reduction program, however, may not always be beneficial and in some cases may actually be detrimental.

Animal feeding experiments indicate that when a strict program of food restriction is imposed on mature rats, it results in a reduction of lifespan. With less stringent food restriction, life expectancy is increased. This research shows an inverse relationship between length of life and level of caloric restriction in mature rats. For the older rat, both overnutrition and excessive restriction exert a detrimental influence on life expectancy. It has been proposed, therefore, that elderly humans not subject themselves to stringent weight-loss regimens, and consider a slight increase in weight with age to be acceptable[37].

Epidemiological data on humans is in keeping with some of these findings. The elderly are somehow buffered from the consequences of a poor diet; neither undernutrition nor obesity have the noxious effects that would be anticipated in younger persons. In both cases, but most particularly in obesity, the treatment program should not be overly vigorous. Obesity in the over-65 age group may in fact carry with it few negative side effects. In a longitudinal study of several diseases in 3,142 elderly poor aged sixty-five to seventy-four, obesity did not increase the risk of death. In fact, the fattest groups had the lowest total mortality rate and the lowest cardiovascular renal disease, and stroke mortality rates. Bedridden, obese, elderly patients suffer from decubitus ulcers far less often than their leaner counterparts.

In some cases, weight reduction may be necessary to promote successful treatment of a primary condition, such as diabetes or arthritis where excessive weight can be a complicating factor[35]. In these cases, a weight loss program should be planned over a long period of time with a graduated schedule of caloric restriction. This slow, steady weight loss plan is more advantageous than the stress of abrupt caloric restriction imposed by a more stringent plan. Animal studies have shown a high mortality rate when older, heavier animals lost a considerable proportion of body mass in a short period of time. Length of life of these older, heavier animals, however, could be extended when the restriction of food intake was less severe[37]. Elderly humans may be found to behave similarly.

Opportunities for improvement of the dietary status in the overweight elderly do exist and should not be overlooked. Improvement of inadequate diets and correction of serious nutritional deficiency is warranted and will add to the individual's quality of life. However, the effect of these improvements on morbidity and mortality are speculative at this time.

DIABETES

Diabetes mellitus is a chronic metabolic disease characterized by a deficiency in the production or utilization of the pancreatic hormone insulin. The usual clinical symptoms of polyuria, polydipsia, polyphagia, and weight loss are not usually symptoms in the aged or middle aged person who is found to be diabetic. The discovery of diabetes is usually a result of an examination for some other problem. As with cardiovascular disease, the incidence of diabetes increases with age. It rises steadily from childhood to a peak at age sixty-five to seventy-four. Five percent (or 1.2 million) of those over age sixty-five have diabetes and are under treatment. There are believed to be many more undetected cases. Elderly women and those aged individuals who are overweight are more likely to develop diabetes.

The disorder is generally considered as falling into one of two types—juvenile-onset or maturity-onset. The juvenile or growth-onset form occurs in those under age forty. It is characterized by rapid onset and is ketosis-prone. This type is generally controlled by insulin. The latter type, often called insulin-independent, is usually slow in onset, resistant to the development of ketosis, and may be controlled by weight loss and diet alone. This is not true for all cases as some 30 percent of elderly diabetics require insulin for adequate control and others are treated with oral hypoglycemic agents.

Diagnosis of diabetes in the elderly is based on laboratory criteria for glucose tolerance. The norms have been determined from studies of healthy young people. Accordingly they may not be appropriately used for elderly persons, as a progressive decline in glucose tolerance has been found to be part of the aging process. Studies show that at least 50 percent of those over age sixty show abnormal blood glucose responses to oral glucose tests. In spite of this, for the ambulatory, healthy, elderly patient, it is blood glucose levels of above 130 mg per 100 cc of whole venous blood and above 150 mg per 100 cc of plasma that are considered diagnostic evidence of diabetes[38].

The elderly diabetic is susceptible to many complications of the disorder involving large and small blood vessels, peripheral veins, the central nervous system, and the autonomic nervous system. Kidney and eye disorders are common, with kidney infections frequently found. Cataracts, retinopathy, and glaucoma are the chief eye problems. Diabetic retinopathy is a leading cause of blindness among elderly persons [39]. Control of the clinical symptoms of diabetes through diet, insulin, or other hypoglycemic agents does not protect against the occurrence of these longterm complications. Even though the elderly with maturity-onset diabetes have not had the disease over the major part of their lifespan, an asymptomatic form of the disorder may have been present for many years. Accordingly, they are subject to longterm complications such as blood vessel degeneration which can lead to premature cardiovascular disease and a decreased life expectancy[40].

The most important aspect of dietary treatment of maturity-onset diabetes is reduction of weight until ideal weight (or even slightly below ideal weight) is reached. The desirable weight for a diabetic is 10 percent less than ideal weight. Larger fat cells are more insulin-resistant than smaller fat cells, so much higher levels of insulin are needed for glucose metabolism in an obese individual. The loss of weight often results in an improvement or correction of the condition as well as reducing other risk factors for cardiovascular disease such as hypertension and hyperlipidemia. Accordingly, many elderly persons can control their diabetes with a simple loss of weight (if necessary) and continued use of a balanced diet without sweets. Restriction in type and amount of fat used may be indicated to maintain optimum weight and to reduce the development of vascular problems. (Nearly 75 percent of diabetic deaths in the United States are from vascular disease.) Such a diet would be of value to the elderly nondiabetic as well.

In the past, approximately 30 percent of those with maturity-onset diabetes were treated with oral hypoglycemic agents when dietary control alone was found to be ineffective. There is some indication that longterm use of these oral hypoglycemic agents is associated with increased mortality from cardiovascular disease. At the present time the Food and Drug Administration is suggesting that the labeling on all oral hypoglycemic agents be changed to indicate that their use should be reserved for those times when dietary restrictions or dietary restrictions plus insulin have failed to control the hyperglycemia. Accordingly, it is recommended that most cases of diabetes in the elderly be treated by diet alone.

About 30 percent of maturity-onset diabetics require insulin along with dietary control. There may be problems when the elderly individual must inject his own insulin. Measurement and injection of insulin require mental alertness and manipulative skill. Poor eyesight may cause many errors in measurement; forgetfulness may result in missed or duplicated doses[41]. These problems may make insulin use undesirable for a person who is likely to have difficulty managing the medication. A slightly higher blood glucose level may be acceptable in older persons as this may overcome the problems of getting glucose into body cells. Also, hypoglycemia is more dangerous in older persons than in those younger. Special devices are available for the insulin-dependent, visually handicapped diabetic. A listing of these can be obtained from the New York Association for the Blind, New York City, New York.

Different types of dietary control are used with diabetics. The *unmeasured* or *"free"* diet used with some young juvenile-onset diabetics matches caloric intake to energy needs. The *weighed diet* which calls for weighing of all food, is rigid and permits little flexibility. It is usually not carefully followed.

The *measured diet* is considered the best choice for the majority of maturity-onset diabetics who are obese and thus require a fixed caloric intake. Dietary needs for calories, carbohydrate, protein, and fat for the elderly individual are determined. Total caloric needs may be derived by multiplying body weight in kilograms by 25 Calories (Kcal). The carbohydrate allowance is usually between 45 and 55 percent of total calories[42]. In the past, carbohydrate restriction was the cornerstone of diabetic treatment in the belief that excessive carbohydrate intake would aggravate the condition. However, in areas of the world where diabetics habitually consume diets that contain 60–70 percent of the calories as carbohydrate, principally starch, longterm complications are less frequent and control is maintained as well as with more restricted carbohydrate intakes. Several studies seem to support the concept that diabetics do best when consuming diets relatively higher in carbohydrate and lower in fats[43]. Protein intake should make up about 15 percent of the calories with fat as the remaining 30 to 35 percent. Restriction of cholesterol and saturated fat is often recommended.

When the energy and nutrient requirements have been established, these amounts are divided into *exchanges*. The exchanges group foods according to their carbohydrate, protein, and fat content. There are six exchange food groups: milk, vegetables, fruit, bread (includes cereal and starchy vegetables), meat, and fat. All exchanges within one group contain about the same number of calories. An individual is allowed to eat a specified number of food exchanges from each group every day. The use of the term *exchange* confuses some individuals who believe that they can exchange a food in one group for a food in another group. Exchanges are made only *within* an individual food group, not among the various groups. It is obvious that one ounce of a food such as applesauce listed under the fruit exchanges is not a substitute for one ounce of meat found in the meat exchanges. The use of fructose in the diabetic diet was discussed in Chapter 4. One-tenth-ounce package of fructose is equal in calories to one teaspoon of sugar, and is thus equal to one-fourth of a fruit exchange.

The Diabetic Exchange Lists generally used for diet planning for the diabetic were revised in 1976. The revisions make it easier for individuals to choose those foods useful in fat-restricted diets. The revised lists are found in Appendix 5.

The diabetic need not buy special "diabetic" foods to meet his needs. Fruits canned in water instead of syrup are needed by diabetics but these can usually be found in a well-stocked supermarket. Fruits canned in unsweetened fruit juice can be used but the juice must be counted toward the fruit servings allowed for the day. Beverages artificially sweetened with saccharin may be used, as may candy and baked goods containing sorbitol (an alcohol of glucose) as a sweetener. Sorbitol is a source of calories but since it is absorbed slowly and does not require insulin for its metabolism it is useful for diabetics. The calories in sorbitol, however, must be counted as part of the daily intake and excessive sorbitol consumption may cause diarrhea.

The diabetic individual who undergoes surgery has temporary stresses imposed which require careful management. If the surgery is not an emergency, the patient should be hospitalized for three days before the operation so that diabetic control can be assured. If an emergency condition exists, surgery can usually be undertaken.

As of July, 1980, there will be federal regulations governing the labeling of any food represented for use in the diet of a diabetic. The label must include complete nutrition labeling and the statement: "Diabetics: This product may be useful in your diet on the advice of a physician. This food is not a reduced calorie food."

ANEMIA

Anemia is a reduction below normal levels of erythrocytes, hemoglobin, or hematocrit.

Physical signs of anemia in the elderly are headaches, lightheadedness, angina pectoris, pallor of mucus membranes and fingernails, tachycardia, functional systolic murmurs, and cardiac dilations. Severe anemia in the elderly can also lead to congestive heart failure[45].

Anemia can be caused by the chronic hemorrhaging associated with hemorrhoids, hiatus hernias, cancer, diverticulitis, peptic ulcers, or alimentary bleeding due to aspirin. Cases of anemia have reportedly been caused by intestinal polyps, ulcerative colitis, defects in cardiac valves, and parasites in the intestine. Anemia can also be caused by disorders of the gastrointestinal tract that lead to impaired absorption of the B_{12}-intrinsic factor complex as well as by genetic defects resulting in decreased intrinsic factor production.

A variety of nutrients is needed for the production of erythrocytes: iron, folic acid, B_{12}, protein, pyridoxine, ascorbic acid, copper, and maybe also vitamin E. A deficiency of any of these can cause anemia. A deficiency in iron intake leads to hypochromic–microcytic anemia, characterized by a paleness of the blood and the presence of very small red blood cells. A deficiency of either folate or vitamin B_{12} leads to megaloblastic anemia, characterized by enlarged red blood cells of irregular shape and increased color.

Anemia is generally diagnosed by a hemoglobin value of less than 12 gm/100 ml. However, the measurement of hemoglobin concentration alone does not distinguish between types of anemia. A value of below thirty for the mean corpuscular hemoglobin concentration (MCHC, which is the hemoglobin value divided by the hematocrit value) indicates hypochromic anemia and a need for increased iron intake. Also, a value of over 95 cubic micrometers for mean corpuscular volume (MCV) indicates that the red blood cells are larger than normal, which suggests a deficiency of either folic acid or Vitamin B_{12}[46].

Iron deficiency anemia is the most common type of anemia found in elderly persons[45]. Of 2,700 consecutive admissions to geriatric wards, 6.4 percent had anemia with hemoglobin values below 10 gm. Iron deficiency was present in two-thirds of the cases of anemia while megaloblastic anemia was present in one-half. Thus some patients present with both megaloblastic and iron deficiency anemia[47].

Pernicious anemia is a form of megaloblastic anemia. It is due to an inadequate production in the stomach of intrinsic factor, which is necessary for vitamin B_{12} absorption. The incidence of pernicious anemia is age-related. The frequency increases with age as follows:

1 per million in those people aged six months to one year

1 per 10,000 in those aged 1–10

1 per 5,000 in those aged 30–40

1 per 200 in individuals aged 60–70

This incidence follows the observed pattern of achlorhydria, found in 15 percent of people aged forty–sixty, 25 percent of those aged sixty–seventy, and in 30 percent of those over seventy[44]. Also, there is an increased incidence of pernicious anemia in those people with thyroid disorders or diabetes.

A supply of intrinsic factor is necessary for absorption of vitamin B_{12}. Therefore if intrinsic factor *or* vitamin B_{12} are in short supply, pernicious anemia may result.

In the Ten State Nutrition Survey of low income people (discussed in Chapter 3), low hemoglobin was found to be most prevalent in people over sixty. Following is a discussion of iron, folic acid, and vitamin B_{12} deficiencies, the major causes of anemias in the elderly. It should be remembered that anemia is not a normal concomitant of aging.

Iron

The Recommended Dietary Allowance of iron for both men and women over fifty-one is 10 mg. Ferrous salts are the most readily utilizable source of iron. They are better utilized than ferric compounds. It is known that ascorbic acid and sorbitol enhance absorption of iron, while phytates, phosphates, and antacids bind iron and reduce its absorption.

Hemochromatosis (excessive iron deposits throughout the body) is unlikely with a daily iron intake of 10–20 mg[48]. In hemochomatosis, iron deficiency, and during cobalt treatment, iron absorption is increased. On the other hand, absorption of iron decreases in people with iron overload, malabsorption, malignant diseases, and achlorhydria.

The iron in meat is better absorbed (12–20 percent) than the iron in vegetables (1–7 percent) due to a factor present in meat that is not in vegetables. Thus, diets containing food with little meat impart poor absorbability to supplementary iron no matter what iron compound is used in the supplement. Enteric-coated and delayed-release iron preparations are generally poorly designed. A delay in iron release serves to dump iron in the lower intestine where, because the lower portion is less acidic, absorption capabilities are less than in the upper portion[45].

Three to four tablets of ferrous sulfate (60 mg elemental iron per tablet) or ferrous fumarate (66 mg of iron per tablet) are equivalent to six tablets of ferrous gluconate since it contains only 36 mg of elemental iron per tablet[45]. Iron tablets are best given with or after meals and with snacks at bedtime. Even though there is increased absorption of iron if it is given on an empty stomach, this benefit is outweighed by the problem of gastrointestinal irritation by iron. One patient in ten will show the undesirable side effects of gastric irritation if iron treatment continues four to six months.

Parenteral administration of iron is indicated only if a patient has a malabsorption problem, refuses iron by mouth, or cannot be relied upon to take his own medication.

Folic Acid

A deficiency of folic acid produces megaloblastic anemia. This is seen most often in pregnant women (one-third of all pregnant women in the world exhibit this), but it can occur at any age.

Folic acid is present in many foods. It is readily available in ba-nanas, lima beans, liver, and brewers yeast. Its availability is some-what lower in orange juice, romaine lettuce, egg yolk, cabbage, de-fatted soybeans, and wheat germ[48]. Folate is easily destroyed by extensive cooking, especially of finely-divided foods like rice and beans.

The body's stores of folate last only four months; thus ninety percent of all hard liquor alcoholics, the majority of wine and beer alcoholics, and also one-half of all narcotic addicts suffer from folate deficiency because they ingest relatively little food. Folate defi-ciency is also caused by anticonvulsant drugs that are used to treat epilepsy. Thus, there is a high incidence of folate deficiency in patients with mental disorders. The chronic use of sedatives includ-ing barbiturates and glutethimide can cause folic acid deficiency and resultant megaloblastic anemia. Aspirin intake at levels com-monly used by people with rheumatoid arthritis can also cause low serum folate levels. Gluten-sensitive enteropathy may interfere with absorption of folate and can occur in the elderly even without the characteristic accompaniment of diarrhea.

In the past the FDA did not permit the addition of more than 0.1 mg folic acid in over-the-counter supplements because it could mask the neurological complications of pernicious anemia. How-ever, in 1973, the FDA revised regulations so folic acid could be added to supplements on the basis of the 0.4 mg RDA for adults. For the elderly, dietary supplementation of 0.4 mg daily may be desirable because their absorption of folic acid may be impaired. The usual therapeutic dose of folic acid is 1.0 mg daily (oral or paren-teral).

Vitamin B$_{12}$

Vitamin B$_{12}$ needs intrinsic factor for its absorption. A deficiency of intrinsic factor is always accompanied by achlorhydria, but individ-uals with achlorhydria are not necessarily deficient in intrinsic fac-tor. The presence of achlorhydria or gastric resection calls for sup-plementation of B$_{12}$. The RDA of vitamin B$_{12}$ is 3 mcg (the liver can store 2,000 mcg). Liver, meat, and fish are good sources, and usually a mixed diet supplies 3 mcg daily. A deficiency of the vitamin may be seen among vegans (vegetarians who eat only plant foods).

Pernicious anemia is treated with vitamin B$_{12}$. At first, 1,000 mcg is injected intramuscularly two times a week for two weeks. If neurologic signs are present, more frequent doses are given for several months. Thereafter, 250–1,000 mcg are injected every two months. Hydroxycobalamin is preferred to the cyanocobalamin form of the vitamin as it combines more easily with body protein and is retained three times better than is cyanocobalamin.

Vitamin B_{12} also can be given by mouth with intrinsic factor prepared from the intestinal mucosa of pigs. Large doses of B_{12} (100–1,000 mcg) can be given orally without intrinsic factor. This is the cheapest way to administer the vitamin.

To prevent anemia, the RDA of vitamins and iron as well as sufficient calories and protein is required in the diet. In order to obtain this, a knowledge and understanding of nutrition is required. Such a regimen may be expensive, and for this reason, and because the eating habits of the elderly are erratic, a multivitamin plus iron supplement is considered by some to be a good form of insurance against the development of anemia in the elderly.

ARTHRITIS

Arthritis is the nation's number one crippling disease, and is a common affliction in the elderly, occurring most frequently in the fifth and sixth decade of life. It has been estimated that 20 million people in the United States suffer from arthritis[1]. Because of the chronic pain and disability associated with arthritis, many sufferers fall prey to charlatans who offer quick and easy cures. Millions are spent each year on "cures" that simply do not work.

Arthritis and Common Sense, first published in 1950, has sold over 500,000 copies. The premise of the book, written by Dan Dale Alexander, is that if large quantities of oil are ingested, they will go to the joints and lubricate them[17]. For years the Arthritis Foundation denounced the book and stated that the thesis proposed was entirely incorrect, yet over 25 years after its first publication, it is still sold and Alexander still lectures on his "cure."

Dr. Jarvis, who wrote *Folk Medicine: A Vermont Doctor's Guide to Good Health*, suggested that apple cider vinegar would be curative for arthritis[49]. The scientific community refuted these erroneous claims, but to no avail since a sequel, *Arthritis and Folk Medicine*, was published and still sells today along with apple cider vinegar, in many health food stores in the United States.

Regardless of their current popularity, low-carbohydrate diets, high protein diets, vitamins, minerals, cod liver oil, honey, and vinegar do not help arthritis. Nothing that is eaten will cause arthritis or cause increased joint inflammation (with the exception of some situations with patients having gout). This is not to presume that diet therapy is totally ineffectual in the treatment of arthritic conditions. Arthritis is a chronic condition and as with any chronic condition, nutrition therapy will become an adjunct to the treatment prescribed.

Rheumatoid Arthritis

Rheumatoid arthritis is a systemic disease of connective tissue in which joint inflammation, pain, and stiffness are common. The disease is deforming, disfiguring, and debilitating, and is subject to exacerbations and remissions. The average age of onset is 35 years but its incidence increases with age and may reach 15 percent in females over sixty, according to some population studies. Rheumatoid arthritis is two to three times more prevalent in women than men[50].

Patients with the disease are often underweight. This condition may be further complicated by the fact that the disease may make the process of food preparation and eating terribly difficult and painful. (See chapter 10 for hints to help the handicapped homemaker.)

A nutritious, well-balanced diet is usually prescribed with calories adjusted to maintain weight at a desired level. A high calorie diet is often indicated. Diet instruction is focused on how to improve intake for the maintenance of good health. Early morning and end-of-the-day pain and stiffness may decrease appetite. The largest meal of the day should be planned at lunch with mid-morning and mid-afternoon snacks encouraged to meet the daily caloric need.

Arthritis victims often have a negative nitrogen and calcium balance, muscle atrophy, decalcification of bone, and when the disease is in the active state, decreased carbohydrate metabolism. Anemia, due to hemolysis rather than to iron deficiency, may also be seen. Oral iron supplementation may help some individuals but in others the anemia remains refractory. In an observation of some elderly patients with mild rheumatoid arthritis, supplementing the diet with liver showed a positive effect on hemoglobin levels[50]. Increased consumption of dairy foods along with the use of calcium supplements can help prevent bone decalcification and restore calcium balance. Steroids, used to treat rheumatoid arthritis, may cause bone demineralization, sodium retention, negative nitrogen balance, and edema. For some patients, mild sodium restriction and potassium supplementation may be necessary[9].

Low serum vitamin B_6 levels have been reported in some patients. These lowered levels may be the result of drug therapy or caused by gastric mucosal lesions common to rheumatoid arthritis patients. Supplemental B_6 was given to restore levels, but further supplementation did not change the arthritis condition[51].

Vitamin C deficiency may exist in some arthritis sufferers. Ingestion of large quantities of aspirin (a common occurrence for arthritis sufferers) has been shown to affect ascorbic acid levels in some patients, resulting in cutaneous bruising that subsides upon vitamin C supplementation[51]. Therapeutic doses of aspirin also may cause gastric upset in many patients. This discomfort can be helped by taking the aspirin after meals or with milk.

Osteoarthritis

Osteoarthritis is a very common form of arthritis found in the elderly, particularly in women after menopause[52]. It is a noninflammatory disorder of the movable joints, also known as degenerative or hypertrophic arthritis. There appears to be no single cause; advancing age is the main predisposing factor. The disease may be the result of the cumulative assaults of life on the joints, or it may follow injury or disease of the joints. There is evidence of a familial predisposition to osteoarthritis.

Degenerative joint changes may affect the knees, hips, spine, shoulders, ankles, and fingers. Stiffness and soreness confined to the afflicted joints are the primary symptoms. An overweight condition can exacerbate the disease and cause additional pain by stressing the weight-bearing joints[53].

The goal of nutrition therapy is to reduce the patient to a desired weight or to maintain weight at a desired level. Symptoms often decrease markedly or subside completely after weight loss occurs. The diet most often prescribed is one low in fat, moderate in protein, and moderate in carbohydrate, providing 1,200 to 1,800 Calories daily.

Since weight control is vital to the treatment of osteoarthritis, a group approach called the Pilot Geriatric Arthritis Program was established as an outreach program from the University of Michigan[35]. The primary goal of this pilot program was weight reduction to relieve joint stress and pain in osteoarthritis sufferers. The program emphasized member involvement at group meetings and positive reinforcement by the group and professional staff. After the group structure was established, support staff withdrew and the group continued on its own. This example could be a model for establishing programs of this type where there is a need. The arthritis/weight reduction program may even become an ongoing supportive service in a geriatric feeding program.

The osteoarthritis sufferer may rely on aspirin for pain relief, and in severe cases of pain, steroids may be used. Refer to the section on rheumatoid arthritis for the dietary implications of the use of these drugs.

In a small group of older patients with osteoarthritis, a daily dose of 600 mg of vitamin E was administered[54]. Fifty-two percent of the patients reported "marked improvement" after ten days of vitamin E therapy. Although the sample used was small, the results were favorable and indicate the need for further study on the analgesic effect of vitamin E in osteoarthritis.

Gout

Gout is an inborn error of purine metabolism in which an excess of uric acid appears in the blood. Individuals with gout have difficulty eliminating uric acid, an end product of purine metabolism, formed in the breakdown of nucleoproteins. Deposits of sodium urate, as *tophi*, occur in the small joints and surrounding soft tissue. In chronic gout, tophi are often also found in the helix of the ear. Familial hyperuricemia is far more prevalent in males than females. Males exhibit characteristics of the condition after age thirty-five. The small percentage of women who have gout usually do' not exhibit symptoms until after menopause[50].

Gout resembles arthritis since its major symptom is joint pain. Attacks are frequently manifest as sudden pain in the large toe radiating up the leg. Control of the serum uric acid level is imperative. If levels are allowed to rise to 9.0 mg percent or more (3–7 mg percent is normal range) there is an 83 percent chance that the patient will develop acute gouty arthritis which may lead to joint destruction and severe crippling. Gout will usually run a mild course if treated appropriately[50].

Specific foods have been implicated in the development of hyperuricemia. Overeating should be discouraged, as should a diet high in fat. The use of alcohol will not induce an attack; however, lactic acid, which appears during ethanol metabolism, disrupts the metabolism of uric acid and results in renal retention of urate. Overindulgence or moderate chronic use of alcohol is not advisable[55].

Fasting can precipitate a gouty attack and should never be attempted by someone who has gout. Since many sufferers of gout are overweight, and weight loss will assist in management, the dieting plan should be formulated so that weight loss is slow and gradual. A sudden weight reduction with the development of ketonemia is acknowledged as a precipitating factor of acute attacks[55].

Diuretic therapy may also induce gouty attacks. A gouty condition may surface for the first time as a result of therapeutically increased fluid excretion when hypertensive cardiovascular disease becomes suspect.

With the use of drugs such as allopurinol, which effectively regulate serum uric acid levels, dietary treatment is now less vital than it once was[50]. However, weight control or reduction, as mentioned, is advantageous. The diet planned should be varied and well balanced, with high carbohydrate, low fat, and moderate protein. A high carbohydrate diet has a tendency to increase uric acid excretion. A high fat consumption retards excretion and may induce acute attacks in some individuals. With drug therapy, a moderate protein intake has little or no effect on the body's uric acid pool. Foods of high purine content (such as anchovies, meat extracts, gravy, heart, herring, kidney, liver, mincemeat, mussels, scallops, baker's and brewer's yeast) may be excluded. Caffeine, theophylline, and theobromine found in coffee, tea, and cocoa are metabolized to methylurates but are not deposited as gouty tophi. Thus these beverages need not be avoided[55].

In cases of severe or advanced gout, a restriction of purines to 100–150 mg per day may be indicated. (A normal diet contains between 600–1000 mg per day.) Dietary protein should be limited to 3 ounces per day and should come from plant and dairy sources predominately. A reliable diet therapy text will group food according to purine content and should be referred to when planning a diet.

During an acute attack, a diet similar to that planned for advanced gout would be used, including high carbohydrate, low fat, and low protein. Fluids should be increased, up to three liters per day, to aid in the excretion of uric acid and to minimize the formation of renal calculi. Increased fluid intake is usually indicated between attacks; two and one-half to three quarts per day is recommended[50].

PARKINSON'S DISEASE

The onset of Parkinson's disease is difficult to assess since early symptoms may be subtle and overlooked. The patient often does not seek medical help until a dramatic symptom, such as a tremor, occurs. Consequently, many patients may have a mild form of the condition three to six years before diagnosis.

Parkinsonism occurs most frequently in late middle age. There are an estimated 200,000 cases in the United States, with 40,000 new cases arising each year[36]. The disease is an incurable, progressive, degenerative condition involving the central nervous system. It is characterized by slowness of movement (bradykinesia), rigidity and difficulty initiating movement (akinesia), and tremor of the extremities. In later stages of the disease, postural reflexes are affected and the patient has difficulty keeping balanced and turning while standing[56]. These symptoms are further aggravated by obesity and therefore loss of weight may help a person with the disease to regain motor function.

The slowness, rigidity, and tremor evidenced in Parkinson's disease creates feeding problems. Most patients suffer from poor grasp, poor hand-mouth coordination, a moderate inability to suck or close their lips, and limited ability to bite, chew, and swallow[36].

Mealtimes are laborious and greatly prolonged due to bradykinesia. The patient often has difficulty feeding himself. However, every effort should be made to permit him to continue to eat independently[56]. Utensils with built-up or loop handles, spouted cups, dishes with plate guards or rims, and other feeding devices may be employed[57]. (See Chapter 10 for more information on self-feeding and food preparation for the person with incoordination.) A relative or caretaker can minimize frustration by presenting a meal in which the meat has already been cut, the bread buttered, and the beverage poured. Using a spoon to "scoop" vegetables may be necessary. A bib should never be used unless absolutely necessary, as this serves only to emphasize the patient's inability to cope and adds to his embarrassment. Weight loss may result from rushing the patient, as he may indicate he is through with his meal long before he is actually satisfied. As chewing and swallowing become increasingly difficult a semisoft, soft, and finally a liquid diet may be required. A regular diet, however, should be continued until dysphagia is present[56].

Constipation is a frequent complaint of sufferers of Parkinson's disease. This is due in part to a lack of saliva to moisten food, inactivity, and the use of drugs that may decrease gastrointestinal motility and salivation. Stool softeners and an increase in dietary fiber and the consumption of four to six glasses of fluid a day is the best treatment. Insufficient fluid intake is common since a tremor may make drinking from a cup extremely difficult. Fluids should be offered frequently and daily intake monitored carefully.

In the 1960s, oral levodopa was given to sufferers of Parkinsonism and effected dramatic relief of symptoms. Levodopa is the metabolic precursor of dopamine, a substance found in decreased amounts in the brains of afflicted individuals. Dopamine, when administered clinically, does not cross the blood–brain barrier. Levodopa does cross and is then converted to dopamine by the action of the enzyme dopa-decarboxylase[59].

The action of levodopa is compromised by pyridoxine (vitamin B_6); therefore, patients on levodopa therapy needed to limit their intake of B_6 by eliminating from their diets foods high in this vitamin, as well as multivitamin supplements containing B_6[58]. Currently, most patients are given carbidopa/levodopa (*Sinemet*) as the primary antiparkinsonism agent. This newer medication has fewer side effects than levodopa, and pyridoxine does not interfere with its action[59].

DECUBITUS ULCERS

Decubitus ulcers—also called bed sores or pressure sores—describe an area that, as a result of pressure, may be reddened, with or without blistered or broken skin, and with or without necrosis of tissue. The incidence of this skin breakdown increases with age, and is almost exclusively the result of prolonged immobilization. Pressure sores are the most accurate name for these ulcers as they occur as a result of prolonged pressure which interferes with the blood supply to the affected skin. The amount of pressure and the time needed to produce the ulcer varies with the condition of the patient. Changes in the subcutaneous tissue—congestion of capillaries and reddening of skin—can occur after only two hours of pressure on an area caused by immobilization of an individual[60].

Many factors such as improper bedding, unmade beds, radiation therapy, barbiturate sensitivity (which can cause blisters), skin condition, and sensory loss are involved in the etiology of pressure sores. A discussion of these factors is beyond the scope of this book. A review of the nutritional considerations in the etiology and treatment of decubitus ulcers follows.

Both obesity and underweight increase one's susceptibility to pressure sores. Obesity does so because adipose tissue is poorly vascularized so that it is more vulnerable than other tissue to breaking down if subjected to sustained pressure or force. On the other hand, small amounts of fat tend to cushion the body against pressure and have a protective function, and it is believed that obesity after age seventy-five may be helpful in protecting against injury from pressure[61]. In the same manner, active muscle provides a flat, weight-bearing surface which prevents bony joints from sticking out against the body surface and cutting off its blood supply, while wasted muscle, often present in a severely underweight person, provides an inadequate cushion for bones.

Anemia (reduced hemoglobin values) results in a lowered oxygen content of tissues which enhances tissue necrosis in areas subject to pressure[62]. (As discussed earlier in this chapter, anemia is not a normal part of aging.) If hemoglobin levels are less than 13 gm per 100 ml, iron supplements are called for. However, oral iron supplements may be of little help if an open pressure sore is already present. In that case, direct transfusions may be necessary. This is because infection may be present, red blood cell formation is inhibited, and the blood cell lifespan is shortened in individuals with chronic infection. Additionally, blood is lost from the dressing on the ulcers as well, though this amount generally is minor[60].

A study of patients with pressure sores found over 45 percent to be anemic (as judged by a hemoglobin of less than 12 gm for females and less than 14 gm for males), compared to an incidence of 26 percent with anemia in a control population. An interesting finding of this study was that 50 percent of those with pressure sores had been maintained on tube feedings[63]. This suggests that nutritional deficits may be an important predisposing factor. It is important to keep in mind that deficiencies of nutrients besides iron (such as protein, folate, vitamin B_{12}, vitamin C, riboflavin) may cause anemia.

Hyperglycemia, elevated blood sugar level, as found in uncontrolled diabetics, increases the likelihood of tissue necrosis if there is skin damage because the abundant sugar makes the damaged skin a more suitable medium for bacteria growth. Atherosclerosis reduces blood supply to the tissues, which may predispose a person to pressure sores[64].

Dehydration with its concomitant dry, fragile, inelastic skin is another factor in the etiology of decubiti. Frequent fluid intake should be encouraged in patients who are immobilized, whether or not they have pressure sores. When possible, liquids provided should be those with caloric value.

The problem of adequate fluid intake is considered fully in Chapter 6; however it should be noted here that a high protein diet may contribute to dehydration because of the increased water excretion necessary to eliminate the end products of protein metabolism. On the other hand, a protein-deficient diet with resultant negative nitrogen balance (see Chapter 4) predisposes an individual to edema, which decreases elasticity and resiliency of skin. Edema also slows down the rate of diffusion of oxygen and metabolites from the capillaries to the cells as the rate of diffusion decreases in proportion to the distance from the capillary to the cell.

It should be emphasized that none of these factors—negative nitrogen balance, anemia, hyperglycemia, atherosclerosis, obesity, underweight—will cause pressure sores in the absence of persistent pressure. Moreover, persistent pressure will eventually cause a pressure sore to arise even in a healthy individual.

The rate of wound healing, including healing of pressure sores, is a biological constant. It may be depressed by physiological and environmental factors, but correction of these factors can only restore the normal rate of healing, it cannot increase it above the normal rate. If the nutritional state of an individual is good, a high protein diet supplemented with other nutrients will not increase the rate of healing. However, if the individual's nutritional state is poor, a retarded rate of healing can be improved by nutritional intervention. Several nutrients are particularly involved in wound healing.

Protein

In 1943, it was observed that healing of pressure sores was delayed during the feeding of a high calorie, low protein diet and that healing began within four days of changing to a high protein diet.

The daily loss of nitrogen in the body due to wear and tear is 3 gm, which is the amount in approximately 20 gm of protein. Trauma such as burns, fever, infection, and emotional stress may increase this nitrogen loss considerably[65]. Additional losses may result if protein-containing pus or exudate drain away from the body. A loss of a significant amount of body protein results in a reduced synthesis of tissue and blood protein, leucocytes, enzymes, hormones, and antibodies with consequent delay in healing and enhanced susceptibility to infection.

The total plasma protein level in individuals averages 6.8 gm per 100 ml, including 4.3 gm of albumin, 2.2 gm of globulin, and 0.3 gm of fibrinogen. In patients with pressures sores the plasma protein level falls, but usually to no lower than 5.5 gm per 100 ml[60]. This may occur because there is a reduction of total plasma volume with prolonged bed rest that occurs more rapidly than would a decline in plasma proteins due to poor nutrition. Thus, even though a bedridden person is in negative nitrogen balance, plasma protein levels may be adequate because of the reduced plasma volume associated with stress and prolonged recumbancy and because the body attempts to maintain homeostasis of serum protein at the expense of tissue protein[66].

A high protein diet is not sufficient to promote good health in an individual with bed sores. There must be sufficient calories plus essential vitamins and minerals in addition to generous amounts of protein. At least 2,500 Calories is necessary as a minimum amount to prevent the use of dietary proteins for energy. Usually a diet containing 2,500 to 3,000 or more Calories is used with 150–200 gm of protein (2–3 gm of protein for each kilogram of body weight). Eggnogs, milkshakes, and high protein–calorie supplements can be utilized to increase protein intake. Protein hydrolysates are useful if there is maldigestion of protein[67].

Vitamins

A high protein, high calorie diet increases the need for thiamine, niacin, pyridoxine, riboflavin, and pantothenic acid. A well-chosen diet will contain sufficient amounts of these nutrients. If their supply is in doubt, supplements should be used.

Ascorbic acid is needed for normal collagen formation, and minimal body stores of ascorbic acid are needed to promote wound healing. Vitamin C deficiency interferes with normal tissue integrity. Guinea pigs with scurvy were found to develop more severe hemorrhagic lesions in a shorter time after pressure than did normal animals[68]. Many conditions cause a depletion of the body's stores of ascorbic acid. Stresses such as hospitalization, wounds, burns, bacterial infections, as well as the use of common drugs such as aspirin, barbiturates, paraldehyde, diphenylhydantoin, and ether, even cigarette smoking, all increase the need for ascorbic acid. However, deficiency must be quite severe before wound healing is affected.

Body tissues are saturated by intakes of 60 to 100 mg of vitamin C per day. Doses above that amount have been found to have little further benefit. In spite of this, it is common practice in some hospitals to give 100 to 300 mg of ascorbic acid daily to surgical patients to ensure that wound healing is not compromised.

Vitamin E, an antioxidant, may reduce the amount of peroxides generated in a wound (which inhibit fibroblast development and, hence, inhibit wound healing). The supply of vitamin K may be reduced by the use of antibiotics since approximately one-half of the supply of this vitamin normally comes from intestinal microbial synthesis. Therefore, both vitamins E and K need to be maintained at adequate levels in a patient being treated for infected pressure sores.

Minerals

Many hospital diets, particularly bland diets (those with little fiber), may contain less than optimal levels of zinc[69]. Chronic alcoholics have greatly increased zinc excretion even when serum zinc levels are low, as do severe burn patients[70]. Loss of appetite may accompany low zinc levels in the body. Therapy with 25 to 50 mg of zinc not only supplies the zinc needed for cell formation in wound healing but also may improve a patient's appetite so that food intake begins to reach the high levels of calories and vitamins needed for recovery from pressure sores[71]. Sufficient copper intake must be ensured when increasing intakes of zinc to avoid possible mineral imbalance (see Chapter 5).

Magnesium intakes have been found deficient in institutionalized populations. Low serum levels of magnesium have been found in alcoholics, diabetics, and those with malabsorption. Magnesium is needed for protein synthesis and its deficiency in animals has been shown to impair immune responses[72]. Magnesium supplements of 250 mg along with 25 mg of zinc, 100 I.U. of vitamin E, 500 mg of vitamin C, and 15 mg of copper have been mixed with liquid protein–calorie supplements and used as an extra snack (cocktail) for patients with decubitus ulcers to ensure sufficient vitamin and mineral intakes for wound healing in the affected individuals.

CITED REFERENCES

1. Shanas, E., and Maddox, G. L. 1977. Aging, health and organization of health resources. In *Handbook of psychology of aging*, eds. J. E. Birren and K. W. Schaie. New York: Van Nostrand Reinhold Co.
2. Walker, W. J. 1976. Success story: The program against major cardiovascular risk factors. *Geriatrics* 31:97.
3. Thiele, V. F. 1976. *Clinical nutrition.* St. Louis: C. V. Mosby Co.
4. Wright, I. S., et al. 1970. Report of inter-society commission for heart disease resources. *Circulation* 42:53.
5. Select Committee on Nutrition and Human Needs, United States Senate. 1977. *Dietary goal for the United States.* 2nd ed.
6. Chrysant, S. G.; Frolich, E. D.; and Popper, S. 1976. Why hypertension is so prevalent in the elderly—and how to treat it. *Geriatrics* 31:101.
7. Schwab, M., Sr. 1973. Caring for the aged. *Amer. J. of Nursing* 73(12):2049.
8. Gordon, E. S. 1974. Dietary problems in hypertension. *Geriatrics* 29:139.
9. Pennington, J. 1978. *Nutritional diet therapy.* California: Bull Publishing Co.
10. Sopko, J. A., and Freeman, R. M. 1977. Salt substitutes as a source of potassium. *J. Amer. Medical Assoc.* 238(7):608.
11. Balacki, John A., and Dobbins, William O. 1974. Maldigestion and malabsorption, making up for lost nutrients. *Geriatrics* 29:157.
12. Sleisenger, M. H. Diseases of malabsorption. 1975. In *Textbook of medicine,* eds. P. B. Beeson and W. McDermott, p. 1217. Philadelphia: W. A. Saunders.
13. Holt, P. R. 1977. *Malabsorption.* Columbus, Ohio: Ross Laboratories.
14. Berman, P. M., and Kirsner, J. B. 1972. The aging gut, I. Diseases of the esophagus, small intestine and appendix. *Geriatrics* 27(3):84.

15. Berman, P. M., and Kirsner, J. B. 1972. The aging gut, II. Diseases of the colon, pancreas, liver and gallbladder, functional bowel disease and iatrogenic disease. *Geriatrics* 27(4):117.
16. *Nurse's aid to understanding constipation.* 1971. Virginia: C. B. Fleet Co., Inc.
17. Levitt, M. D. 1972. Intestinal gas production. *J. Amer. Dietetic Assoc.* 60(6):487.
18. Shils, M. E. 1976. Nutritional problems in cancer patients. *Nutrition in Disease.* Ross Laboratories.
19. Ishu, T., et al. 1979. Cancer in the aged: An autopsy study of 940 cancer patients. *J. Am. Geriatrics Society* 27(7):307.
20. Shils, M. E. 1978. Parenteral feeding of the cancer patient. *Nutrition and the M.D.* 4(11):1.
21. Nutrition in the cancer patient. 1976. *Dialogues in Nutrition* 1(4).
22. Whitworth, F. M. 1978. Consultation: Feeding the cancer patient. *Nursing* 78:87.
23. The patient who can't eat. 1976. *Dialogues in Nutrition* 1(2).
24. The patient who won't eat. 1976. *Dialogues in Nutrition* 1(1).
25. Dental sequelas of radiation. 1978. *Nutrition and the M.D.* 5(13):1.
26. Shannon, I. L.; Trodahl, J. N.; and Starcke, E. N. 1978. Remineralization of enamel by a saliva substitute designed for use by irradiated patients. *Cancer* 41:1746.
27. Dietary management of the ostomy patient. 1978. *Nutrition and the M.D.* 4(7):2.
28. Laerence, W. 1977. Nutrition consequences of surgical resection of the gastrointestinal tract for cancer. *Cancer Research* 37(7):2379.
29. The patient who can't gain weight. 1978. *Nutrition and the M.D.* 4(3):4.
30. Butterworth, C. E. 1974. The skeleton in the hospital closet. *Nutrition Today* 9(2):4.
31. Butterworth, C. E., and Blackburn, G. L. 1975. Hospital malnutrition. *Nutrition Today* 10(2):8.
32. *Insights into parenteral nutrition.* 1977. Deerfield, Illinois: Travenal Laboratories.
33. Organ, C. H., and Finn, M. P. 1977. The importance of nutritional support for the geriatric surgical patient. *Geriatrics* 32:77.
34. Men reach peak weight by 44, women take 20 years longer. 1978. *Newsday* p. 8A, column 2.

35. Templeton, C. L.; Petty, B. J.; and Harter, J. L. 1978. Weight control—a group approach for arthritic clients. *J. Nutrition Education* 10:33.

36. Weiner, J. W. 1973. Parkinson's Disease—A clinical review with special emphasis on dietary problems. *Amer. Dietetic Assoc.* Cassette-A-Month, CAM-7.

37. Ross, M. H. 1972. Length of life and calorie intake. *Amer. J. of Clin. Nutrition* 25:834.

38. Sussman, K. E. 1973. Diagnostic dilemmas. In *The older diabetic patient*, p. 17. UpJohn Co.

39. Thomas, K. P. 1976. Diabetes mellitus in elderly persons. *Nursing Clinics of North America* 2(1):157.

40. Kent, S. 1978. Reevaluating the dietary treatment of diabetes. *Geriatrics* 33:99.

41. Danowski, T. S. 1973. Therapy: Avoiding the pitfalls. In *The older diabetic patient*, p. 24. UpJohn Co.

42. Hillman, R. W. 1974. Sensible eating for older diabetics. *Geriatrics* 29:123.

43. Bierman, E. L., et al. 1971. Principles of nutrition and dietary recommendations for patients with diabetes mellitus. *Diabetes* 20:633.

44. Herbert, V. 1975. Megaloblastic anemias. In *Textbook of medicine*, vol. 2, eds. P. B. Beeson and W. McDermott, p. 1404. Philadelphia: W. B. Saunders Co.

45. Lewis, R. 1976. Anemia—a common but never a normal concomitant of aging. *Geriatrics* 31:53.

46. Brain, M. C. 1975. The anemias. In *Textbook of medicine*, vol. 2, eds. P. B. Beeson and W. McDermott, p. 1399. Phildadelphia: W. B. Saunders Co.

47. Evans, D. 1971. Haematological aspects of iron deficiency in the elderly. *Gerontological Clinica* 13:12.

48. Jukes, T. H., and Borsook, H. 1974. Nutritional management of the anemic geriatric patient. *Geriatrics* 29:147.

49. Deutsch, R. M. 1977. *The new nuts among the berries*. Palo Alto, California: Bull Publishing Co.

50. Bayles, T. B. 1973. Nutrition in diseases of the bones and joints. In *Modern nutrition in health and disease*, eds. R. S. Goodhart and M. E. Shils. Philadelphia: Lea and Febiger.

51. Krause, M. V., and Mahan, L. K. 1979. *Food, nutrition and diet therapy*. Nutritional Care for Patients with Diseases of the Musculoskeleton System. Philadelphia: W. B. Saunders Co.

52. Arthritis, the basic facts. 1976. The Arthritis Foundation, New York, New York.
53. Burnside, I. M. 1976. *Nursing and the aged.* New York: McGraw-Hill Book Co.
54. Machtey, I., and Quaknine, L. 1978. Tocopherol in osteoarthritis: A controlled pilot study. *J. Amer. Geriatrics Soc.* 26(7):328.
55. Boykin, L. S. 1976. Iron deficiency anemia in post-menopausal women. *J. of Amer. Geriatrics Soc.* 24:558.
56. Robinson, M. B. 1974. Levodopa and Parkinsonism. *Amer. J. of Nursing* 74(4):656.
57. Mitchell, H. S., et al. 1976. *Nutrition in health and disease, handicapping problems, self-feeding, chewing, swallowing.* New York: J. B. Lippincott Co.
58. Paddison, R. M., and Paulson, G. June 15, 1971. Levodopa therapy: Why wait? *Patient Care* p. 90.
59. Loebl, S.; Spratto, G.; and Wit, A. 1977. *The nurse's drug handbook.* New York: John Wiley and Sons.
60. Bailey, B. N. 1967. *Bedsores.* London: Edward Arnold, Ltd.
61. Bedsore: Prevention and care of decubitus ulcers. 1974. *Nursing Update* 5(2):3.
62. Pinel, C. 1976. Pressure sores. *Nursing Times* 72(5):172.
63. Michocki, R. J., and Lamy, P. P. 1976. The problem of pressure sores in a nursing home population: Statistical data. *J. of the Amer. Geriatrics Soc.* 24(7):323.
64. Etiology of decubitus ulcers. 1975. *Nursing Clinics of North America.* Philadelphia: W. B. Saunders Co.
65. Love, R. 1972. Nutrition in the burned patient. *J. of Mississippi State Medical Assoc.* 13(9):391.
66. Localio, S. A.; Chassin, J. L., and Hinton, J. W. 1948. Tissue protein depletion, a factor in wound disruption. *Surgery, Gynecology and Obstetrics* 86:107.
67. Blackburn, G. L., and Bistrian, B. R. 1976. Nutritional care of the injured and/or septic patient. *Surgical Clinics of North America* 56(5):1195.
68. Schwartz, P. L. 1970. Ascorbic acid in wound healing a review. *J. Amer. Dietetic Assoc.* 56(6):497.
69. Greger, J. L. 1977. Dietary intake and nutritional status in regard to zinc of institutionalized aged. *J. of Gerontology* 32(5):549.
70. Sullivan, J. F., and Lankford, H. G. 1965. Zinc and wound healing. *Amer. J. of Clin. Nutrition* 17:57.

71. Cohen, I. K. 1973. Hypogeusia, anorexia and altered zinc metabolism following thermal burn. *J. Amer. Med. Assoc.* 223:914.
72. Zieve, F. J.; Fieude, K. A.; and Zieve, L. 1977. Effects of magnesium deficiency on protein and nucleic acid synthesis in vivo. *J. of Nutrition* 107(2):2178.

OTHER REFERENCES

Berg, N. L.; Williams, S. R.; and Sutherland, B. 1979. Behavior modification in a weight-control program. *Family and Community Health* 1(4):41.

Bray, G. 1978. Highlights from the Second Congress on Obesity. *Nutrition and the M.D.* 6(5):3.

Crenshaw, C. 1973. Intake: Perspectives in clinical nutrition. 2. *Nutritional Support for Burn Patients.* Norwich, New York: Eaton Laboratories.

Diet therapy for the diabetic patient. 1978. *Nutrition and the M.D.* 4(5):1.

Gershoff, S. N., et al. 1977. Studies of the elderly in Boston. 1. The effects of iron fortification of moderately anemic people. *Amer. J. of Clin. Nutrition* 30:226.

Gotto, A. M., and Scott, L. 1973. Dietary aspects of hyperlipidemia. *J. Amer. Dietetic Assoc.* 62:617.

Gotto, A. M.; and Scott, L.; and Manis, E. 1974. Prudent eating after forty. *Geriatrics* 29:109.

Jacobs, A. 1971. The effect of iron deficiency on the tissues. *Gerontological Clinica* 13:61.

Kritchevsky, D. 1978. How aging affects cholesterol metabolism. *Postgrad. Medicine* 63(3):133.

Kupers, E. C. 1974. Feeding the elderly heart. *J. Amer. Geriatrics Soc.* 22(3):97.

Leslin, J. August 25, 1977. Nutrition and diet. *Nursing Mirror* p. 31.

Malnutrition in the hospital. 1977. *Dialogues in Nutrition* 2(2).

Mueller, J. F. 1973. A dietary approach to coronary artery disease. *J. American Dietetic Assoc.* 62:613.

The National Council on the Aging, Inc. 1978. *Fact book on aging.* Washington, D.C.

Nugent, C. A., and Van Haldren, L. L. 1979. Diets and coronary heart disease. *Family and Community Health* 1(4):53.

The older diabetic patient. 1973. Kalamazoo, Michigan: Science and Medicine Publishing Co., Inc. for the Upjohn Co.

Ostfeld, A. M., and Lauder, A. 1972. Nutrition and aging-discussant's perspective. In *Epidemiology of Aging,* National Institute of Aging, National Institute of Health, Bethesda, Maryland.

Rudell, J. H. November 1975. Nutrition and aging of the heart. *J. of the Medical Assoc. of State of Alabama* p. 38.

Selected aspects of geriatric nutrition. 1972. *Dairy Council Digest* 43(2):1.

Siegel, J. S. 1972. Some demographic aspects of aging in the United States. In *Epidemiology of Aging,* National Institute of Aging, National Institute of Health, Bethesda, Maryland.

Stern, P. 1973. APA: Insidious foe of an aging swede. *Amer. J. of Nursing* 73(1):111.

IIIIIIIIIIIIIIIIIIIIIIIIIIIIIIIIIIIIIIIIIII 8

Drug Interaction, Caffeine, and Alcohol

Older people comprise 10 percent of the national population, yet they use 22 percent of all prescribed and over-the-counter drugs[1]. These include prescribed sedatives, oral hypoglycemic agents, diuretics, hypnotics, digoxin, and propoxyphene (Darvon), as well as laxatives, aspirin-containing preparations, antacids, and alcohol-containing tonics.

Eighty-five percent of the elderly take prescription drugs and the average elderly person fills over thirteen (new and renewable) prescriptions each year[2]. Further, it has been estimated that the average nursing home patient takes four to seven different drugs each day. Moreover, in 1974, spending by the aged on drugs and drug sundries totaled $2.26 billion, and the average person over sixty-five spends $100 a year for both prescribed and over-the-counter drugs. This is well above the average for all other age groups.

Clearly, the elderly population of this country is receiving a great deal of medication. This is particularly important to note in light of the facts that the elderly are particularly susceptible to drug reactions and also tend to be improperly nourished. Thus they are potentially endangered by particular interactions between drugs and food.

Adverse drug reactions occur seven times more frequently in those over sixty-five than in people aged twenty to twenty-nine.

Twenty-five percent of all patients over the age of eighty have abnormal drug reactions[3]. This may be largely attributable to the effects of aging on the body's ability to handle drugs, be it absorption, distribution, metabolism, or excretion of drugs. The loss of body weight and decrease in body water associated with aging can lead to overdosage with routine amounts of medication. The total circulating plasma albumin—a major carrier of drugs in the circulation—may be reduced in the elderly, especially those with chronic very low protein intakes, and may allow more free (unbound) drug to be in the plasma, causing increased pharmacological effects. Reduced drug-binding protein in the plasma may also effect a competition among various drugs for carrier binding sites. For example, aspirin may replace warfarin (an anticoagulant) on a binding protein and the free excess warfarin may produce an excessive anticoagulant effect[3].

Reduced cardiac output can cause congestion in veins and result in uneven distributions of drugs throughout the body. Also, an increased proportion of body fat may affect the distribution of lipid-soluble drugs throughout the body.

Decreased liver function, with reduced enzyme levels, results in impaired drug detoxification since most drugs are degraded in the liver by specific enzymes[1]. In addition, reduction in kidney function may result in decreased elimination of drugs, and thus may allow for the accumulation of toxic amounts of drugs.

In the following pages, food–drug interactions are to be considered. It is important to distinquish two major types of interaction: that of drugs on the absorption, metabolism, and excretion of food and nutrients, to be considered first; and that of food on the absorption, metabolism, and excretion of drugs, to be considered later in this chapter.

EFFECTS OF DRUGS ON NUTRITION

In addition to the effects of poor diet, stress, chronic or acute disease, poverty, and the myriad of other problems of the elderly that may lead to their being poorly nourished, it is important to note that a great many drugs commonly taken by the elderly may act to cause malnutrition or specific deficiency states. Drugs may act to alter taste perception, alter appetite, suppress nutrient absorption, alter nutrient metabolism in the tissues, and alter nutrient excretion. The following sections will discuss these effects with respect to specific drugs commonly used by the elderly.

Effects on Food Intake

Some drugs are known to specifically alter taste perception in the individual who is taking them. Amphetamines have been reported to increase bitter sensitivity. Benzocaine increases sour sensitivity, and 5–flourouracil (an anticancer agent) alters both bitter and sour sensitivities[4]. Needless to say, altered taste perception may cause changes in food intake.

Some drugs have very unpleasant tastes. These include griseofulvin, (Fulvicin) used for skin problems such as ringworm; clofibrate, used to lower serum cholesterol; and the antibiotic lincomycin (Lincocin). Their unpleasant tastes may act indirectly to suppress appetite.

Appetite can be depressed by ingesting bulking agents such as guar gum and methyl cellulose. These agents absorb water and swell in the stomach, producing a feeling of being full. Amphetamines also depress the appetite.

Any drug that causes inflammation of the upper gastrointestinal tract is apt to cause vomiting, which in turn tends to reduce one's food intake[5]. Digitalis taken at high doses for long periods of time can cause severe wasting due to nausea and decreased food intake even though no gastrointestinal tract inflammation occurs. Cancer chemotherapeutic agents are also known to cause nausea and vomiting and thus reduce food intake.

Moderate-to-large doses of tranquilizers may reduce one's level of consciousness and thus depress food intake. However, smaller doses of tranquilizers offer relief from anxiety and may allow for an increased food intake. Appetite, and hence food intake, can also be increased by insulin, steroids, sulphonylureas, and periactin (Cyproheptadine), an antihistamine that has been used to rehabilitate nutritionally debilitated persons[2].

Effects on Nutrient Absorption and Excretion

Since nutrients are absorbed in the intestine, drugs that alter intestinal motility, bind to certain nutrients, injure the intestine, or block specific nutrient absorption mechanisms generally will alter the intestine's absorptive capabilities[6].

As a rule, all laxatives reduce nutrient absorption because they increase intestinal motility, thus reducing the time that food is in the intestine (i.e., they reduce transit time). Mineral oil, however, retards *gastric* emptying and also reduces the absorption of calcium, phosphorus, and fat-soluble vitamins.

Neomycin, an antibiotic, binds fatty acids and bile acids and decreases the absorption of folic acid and vitamin B_{12}. Some tetracycline antibiotics form complexes with calcium, iron, and magnesium and thereby interfere with the absorption of both the antibiotic and the mineral. Aluminum, a common component of antacids (such as Rolaids), can combine with phosphates in the intestine to prevent their absorption.

Colchicine, used to treat gouty attacks, interferes with cell division and thus injures the intestinal epithelium. The folic acid antagonist methotrexate, used to treat certain types of leukemia as well as psoriasis, also damages gastrointestinal cells, as does the anti-inflammatory analgesic indomethacin, used in the treatment of arthritis. All of these drugs lead to diarrhea which causes a reduction in the amount of nutrients absorbed and also leads to a major loss of fluid and electrolytes.

Diphenylhydantoin (Dilantin), an anticonvulsant, when used for a very long time, depresses the absorption of folic acid and vitamin C. Cholestyramine (Cuemid or Questran) is used to therapeutically block cholesterol absorption and also results in the reduced absorption of fat-soluble vitamins, iron, folic acid, and vitamin B_{12}.

It should be noted that bacteria living in the intestine are an important source of certain vitamins. Therefore, the use of some antibiotics may deplete this source of nutrients by killing these important bacteria.

Some drugs increase the urinary excretion of certain nutrients. In particular, isoniazid (INH), used for treatment of tuberculosis, causes increased urinary excretion of vitamin B_6. Therefore, additional supplements of pyridoxine usually are routinely given along with isoniazid[7]. Thiazide diuretics cause potassium depletion due to excessive loss of this nutrient in the urine. There also exist potassium sparing diuretics; these should not be used in patients with impaired renal function as hyperkalemia (excessive potassium in the blood) would result. When aluminum in antacids blocks phosphate absorption, calcium is excreted by the kidneys in an effort to balance the mineral content of the blood. Thus, the use of antacids can cause osteomalacia in as little as three weeks' time.

DRUG AND NUTRIENT INTERACTIONS IN THE TISSUES

Several drugs interfere with the metabolism and tissue levels of vitamins. In some cases, supplementation of the vitamins affected will prevent any deleterious effects of vitamin deficiency. However, the hindrance of vitamin metabolism by some drugs appears to be essential to their therapeutic value, and with these drugs, the administration of vitamin supplements can compromise their effectiveness. Moreover, in some instances, ingestion of certain nutrients even in normal quantities can cause adverse reactions from drugs that may be extremely harmful.

The antibiotic tetracycline causes a decrease in the ascorbic acid content of leukocytes. In the elderly, such a fall in the leukocyte ascorbic acid level is accompanied by an increased urinary excretion of ascorbic acid.

Isoniazid inhibits the normal metabolism of vitamin B_6 (pyridoxine), and a supplement of 50 mg of pyridoxine is given daily to prevent deficiency symptoms.

Levodopa (L-dopa), used in the treatment of Parkinson's disease, interferes with the normal metabolism of pyridoxine so that there is an increased requirement for this vitamin. However, if the vitamin is taken in large amounts, the levodopa-induced improvement of the disease symptoms is eliminated. It should be noted that carbidopa/levodopa (Sinemet), also used in the treatment of Parkinson's disease, is not affected by pyridoxine. (See Chapter 7.)

The anticonvulsants diphenylhydantoin (Dilantin) and phenobarbitol (Eskobarb), when taken over a long period of time, cause deficiencies of folic acid and of vitamins D and K. However, high doses of folic acid decrease the effectiveness of these anticonvulsant agents. Similarly, the anticoagulants dihydroxycoumarin (Dicoumaral) and warfarin are vitamin K antagonists and interfere with the synthesis of prothrombin and related clotting factors in the liver. Foods high in vitamin K (such as spinach) will interfere with the action of these drugs.

Persons taking monoamine oxidase inhibitors (Parnate, Marplan), used as mood elevators, should be careful not to ingest tyramine-rich foods such as beer, aged cheeses (cheddar, brie, Stilton, Camembert), Chianti wine, chicken livers, figs, licorice, pickled or kippered herrings, cream, and yogurt and should also stay away from caffeine-rich foods such as coffee, tea, and cola drinks. The mood elevators mentioned react strongly with tyramine and caffeine and may cause a wide range of symptoms including headache, hypertension, intracranial hemorrhage, and possibly death. These antidepressants are not widely used at present; however, certain other drugs, such as procarbazine (Matulane), used for Hodgkins Disease, inhibit monamine oxidase[5].

The preceding passages have discussed a variety of ways through which drugs may affect the nutritional status of an individual and have touched upon ways that an individual's diet may affect the action of particular drugs. Following is a more detailed discussion of the effects of diet on drug action, specifically noting instances in which a diet common to an elderly person may affect the absorption, metabolism, and excretion of certain drugs.

DIET AND DRUG ABSORPTION, METABOLISM, AND EXCRETION

When food and drugs are mixed, the absorption of the drug may be enhanced, unaffected, or may be diminished. Griseofulvin, for instance, is absorbed better if it is ingested during a meal that is rich in fat, since such a meal will stimulate the secretion of bile salts into the intestine and these will promote the absorption of the drug. Also, lithium salts and propranolol (Inderal) are both absorbed better when they are taken during a meal. On the other hand, there is delayed absorption of digoxin, aspirin, sulfonilamides, furosemides, probanthine, and lincomycin if food is taken at the same time, particularly if the food has a high fiber content. Moreover, acid-labile drugs such as ampicillin and penicillin G potassium may be totally inactivated if taken at the same time as an acidic food such as cola drinks or citrus juice[8].

Once a drug is absorbed, the duration of its effect is partly determined by the diet of the individual. Patients on high protein, low carbohydrate diets will tend to metabolize (and thus inactivate) most drugs faster than will patients on high carbohydrate, low protein diets. Along these lines, it is known that the charcoaling of beef increases its polycyclic hydrocarbon content and will induce a change in the levels of certain liver enzymes needed to metabolize these compounds. It is also known that an individual with a diet high in charcoaled beef will tend after taking phenacetin-containing compounds to have lowered plasma levels of phenacetin (Aceto-phenetidin), an analgesic and anti-inflammatory drug. The goiterogenic activity of cabbage and brussels sprouts may result in clinical symptoms and an apparent interaction with thyroid-like drugs[9].

It is known that one's diet has an influence on one's urinary pH, and that this may influence the rate of excretion of certain drugs. The effects of acidic drugs tend to be prolonged when one has an acid urine while a basic urine tends to be associated with pro-longed effects of basic drugs such as amphetamines or quinidine (Quinidex, Cardioquin), a cardiac depressant used in treating arrhythmias[10]. Extreme shifts in urinary pH (below 5 or above 8), are hard to achieve through normal diets, but an acid ash diet along with ammonium chloride can serve to acidify the urine while an alk-aline ash diet along with sodium bicarbonate or carbonic anhydride can serve to alkalinize the urine. It should be noted that following a strict vegetarian diet may lead to an alkaline urine. Also, there is a report of a patient who developed quinidine intoxication requiring hospitalization after drinking a quart of orange-grapefruit juice and taking eight antacid tablets daily, which resulted in an alkaline urine and depressed quinidine excretion[10].

A thorough and detailed discussion of the entire spectrum of food–drug interactions is beyond the scope of this text. Yet, an awareness of the types of interactions that may occur is important, as is the realization that many of the interactions may have grave consequences for the patient if appropriate action is not taken. The ten medical problems for which drugs are most often prescribed are: heart conditions, high blood pressure, arthritis, mental and nervous conditions, gastrointestinal diseases, genito-urinary tract infec-tions, diabetes, respiratory tract infections, circulatory diseases, and skin conditions. These are medical problems quite often encoun-tered by the elderly, and when dealing with an elderly individual suffering from a disorder requiring medication, he or she should be informed as to how diet will influence the drug therapy. Moreover, it is important for the professional to be informed of the patient's eat-ing habits, social situation, and health history to ensure that the pa-tient may behave in accordance with an intelligent assessment of his or her condition.

Alcohol and caffeine are both consumed in large quantity by a large proportion of our population. For an illustration of how wide-spread caffeine and alcohol may be in the diets of elderly persons, refer to Tables 8-1 and 8-3, which list the caffeine and alcohol contents of a wide variety of products often ingested. Since both of these agents affect the well-being and nutritional status of the elderly and interact with many drugs commonly taken by the elderly, specific discussions of these interactions are warranted.

CAFFEINE

Since caffeine has pharmacological activity and is present in the diets of essentially all Americans, including the elderly, it is important to be aware of its potential usefulness and danger in the diet. Caffeine is consumed in coffee, tea, cola beverages, cocoa, and in medication (see Table 8-1). It is estimated that in the United States, the average daily per capita intake is 206 mg or the equivalent caffeine present in 2.25 cups of coffee. While most caffeine is consumed in beverages, for some individuals, a highly significant amount comes from over-the-counter caffeine-containing drugs. Only trace amounts are present in chocolate beverages and foods[11].

A pharmacologically active dose of caffeine is defined as 200 mg[11,12] and a large proportion of the elderly population may be receiving at least this amount daily. A wide range of caffeine's effects on humans has been reported in the literature. Following is a discussion of those aspects of caffeine's activity most likely to affect the elderly.

Ingested caffeine is rapidly absorbed from the gastrointestinal tract. Peak plasma levels are reached within one hour and the caffeine quickly diffuses into the central nervous system (CNS) and into other tissues in approximate proportion to the tissue water content. The maximal CNS effects are not reached for two hours but effects may begin within one-half hour after ingestion[13].

The metabolic half-life of caffeine in the plasma and tissues is 3.5 hours. Most ingested caffeine is metabolized and only 3-6 percent is excreted in the urine[13]. Caffeine's mechanism of action is still unclear but its biologic effects are numerous and include diuresis, stimulation of cardiac muscle, and stimulation of the central nervous system. With the ingestion of 200 mg of caffeine, the cerebral cortex is activated; the electroencephalogram (EEG) shows an arousal pattern, and drowsiness and fatigue decrease in the individual[12].

The "stay awake" and "pick-me-up" properties of caffeine can be used to the advantage of the aged. It has been recommended that a morning cup of coffee be used as an energizer. Evidence suggests

Source	Approximate Caffeine per 5 oz cup or 1 tablet
Beverages	
Brewed coffee	80–150 mg*
Instant coffee	60–100 mg*
Decaffeinated coffee	2–4 mg
Brewed black tea	50 mg
Brewed green tea	30 mg
Instant tea	30 mg
Cocoa	5–42 mg
Cola beverage	20 mg**
Prescription medication	
APCs (aspirin, phenacetin, and caffeine)	32 mg
Darvon	32 mg
Migral	50 mg
Nonprescription medication	
Bromoquinine	15 mg
Dristan	30 mg
Sinarest	30 mg
Anacin	32 mg
Bromo Seltzer	32 mg
Cope	32 mg
Excedrin	60 mg
No-Doz	100 mg
Vivarin	200 mg

*Depends on strength of brew
**1 fluid ounce = 4 mg caffeine

TABLE 8-1   Sources and amounts of caffeine in beverages and medications.

that 150–300 mg of caffeine can eliminate fatigue-induced performance, inaccuracies in physical and mental tasks, slow the development of boredom, and *may,* in a rested, interested individual, increase motor and mental efficiency. These effects may be particularly beneficial to the atherosclerotic, brain-impaired individual[12].

While caffeine may be useful in helping the elderly "get going" in the morning, caffeine also has a role in sleep disturbances, which plague many elderly people[14]. Difficulty inducing sleep, frequent nighttime awakenings, and early morning awakenings are common complaints of the aged. In a study of subjects aged fifty to sixty-three, 300 mg of caffeine taken just before retiring decreased sleep time an average of two hours, increased the time required to fall asleep, doubled the number of awakenings, and decreased the amount of deep sleep that occurred. In other studies, doses as low as 150 mg altered sleep patterns. Even heavy coffee drinkers reported sleeping more soundly on placebo nights[13]. Those elderly who continually report difficulty sleeping should be questioned about the amounts and times which they are ingesting caffeine. Metabolic elimination of caffeine requires at least three hours, therefore caffeine ingestion should be limited to times when its activity will not coincide with normal sleep patterns. The elderly should also be alerted to the caffeine content of tea and colas so that they may choose an appropriate alternate nighttime drink.

At high dose levels (approximately 500 mg) caffeine exerts an effect on the autonomic centers of the brain which may cause an increase in heart rate and respiration. The cardiac muscle is strongly stimulated by caffeine. This effect is not always readily apparent because caffeine also stimulates the medullary vagal nuclei which effects a decrease in heart rate. These opposing actions may produce arrhythmias in a small portion of the population[12]. It is prudent to limit caffeine consumption in an elderly patient with any type of heart arrhythmia.

Caffeine consumption must also be considered when evaluating a patient for hypertension. In a recent study, 250 mg of caffeine was shown to increase blood pressure an average of 14/10 mm Hg, enough to cause a false-positive diagnosis of hypertension in a borderline normotensive. The increased blood pressure peaked at one hour after caffeine ingestion but some elevation was still present four hours afterwards[15]. Recent coffee, tea, or cola consumption and consumption habits should be noted when checking the blood pressure of an older patient to be sure that a diagnosis of hypertension is accurate and not temporarily induced by a caffeine load. Known hypertensives should be counseled to avoid abuse of caffeine-containing beverages and medications since caffeine's vasoconstricting effect will further aggravate the existing condition.

Evidence to support the theory that caffeine increases one's risk of myocardial infarction or other cardiovascular disease has not been well documented and further research is suggested[11,16].

However, it has been shown that a dose of caffeine elevates plasma levels of free fatty acids and glucose. One study showed that diabetic patients had higher blood sugar levels after receiving glucose and caffeine than after receiving glucose alone[11]. Caffeine ingestion may need to be considered when counseling elderly diabetics, particularly those who are regulated solely by dietary manipulation.

Nursing home residents are often permitted to drink coffee, tea, or soda throughout the day. An elderly person will drink these beverages with others as part of social activity. This continual caffeine ingestion may possibly interfere with, or potentiate, the effects of some medications. Little literature is available on caffeine-drug interactions. Caffeine can counteract the effect of barbiturates given to induce sleep and also reduce the degree of respiratory depression induced by morphine and codeine. For patients who are mentally ill, caffeine may increase the patients anxiety levels and nullify the effects of medication administered to help calm the patient[13].

Some reports have suggested that the administration of caffeine or caffeine sodium benzoate to patients with senile dementia decreases the incidence of sleep disturbances. Further studies have not supported this hypothesis but have shown an improved sleep pattern in a few patients with senile dementia and no adverse effects from caffeine at single dose levels as high as 228 mg[17].

It is known that caffeine can stimulate gastric secretions in man. This information has suggested the hypothesis that abuse of caffeine contributes to the pathogenesis of peptic ulcer. Management of this condition has routinely included elimination of caffeine from the diet. However, no clear evidence has ever established a cause-and-effect relationship between caffeine ingestion and the onset or exacerbation of a peptic ulcer[13]. Further, it was recently demonstrated that both instant and decaffeinated coffee are more potent stimuli of gastric secretion than doses of caffeine alone. Consequently a patient with a peptic ulcer should avoid all coffee, regular as well as decaffeinated[18].

Caffeine ingestion should be monitored in elderly alcoholics[19]. Both active drinkers and arrested drinkers may be heavy coffee consumers. If a person has impaired hepatic function, continued caffeine ingestion can create additional stress on an already ailing liver[13].

It must be noted in closing that theophylline (a xanthine, similar to caffeine, that is found in tea) is a very effective broncho dilator and has therapeutic use in man. Grandma was right—a few cups of tea will help the cold sufferer breathe more easily[12].

ALCOHOL

Alcoholism refers to a spectrum of problems ranging from deviant drinking behavior to alcohol addiction. Much of this spectrum is synonymous with alcohol abuse, commonly defined as excessive drinking which impairs an individual's social functioning, adversely affects one's health, or both. Often included in the phenomena associated with alcohol abuse are habitual excessive drinking in social situations, drinking to induce sleep during times of insomnia, early morning drinking, and blackouts during heavy alcohol intake. While none of these signs are necessary nor sufficient to establish one as an "alcoholic," alcohol intake that routinely and repeatedly interferes with an individual's social functioning or physical health is definitely dangerous and may be considered to be alcohol abuse[20].

Chronic ingestion of alcohol has many implications for health, socialization, and psychological well-being, most of which are beyond the scope of this text. The following discussion will deal only with nutritional complications from the chronic ingestion of alcohol. However, the reader who copes with the alcoholic patient must recognize that nutritional complications are only one aspect of the alcoholic's problem.

Alcohol (ethanol) yields 7 Calories per gram or about 40 Calories per jigger, 1½ ounces (see Table 8-2). However, alcoholic beverages contain few nutrients besides calories. Thus, chronic ingestion of large amounts of ethanol can lead to malnutrition despite a high calorie intake. Increasing evidence suggests that chronic alcohol ingestion is associated with a hypermetabolic state and that alcohol ingestion may involve a loss rather than a gain in weight[21]. Moreover, ethanol alters the normal absorptive functions of the gastrointestinal tract as well as impairing liver, pancreas, and other body functions. It should be apparent that alcohol abuse poses a major threat to health.

Ethanol requires no digestion and can be absorbed throughout the gastrointestinal tract. Since it is freely soluble in any amount of water, the alcohol content of any given tissue is in direct proportion to the water content of that tissue. Hence, the blood can contain large amounts of alcohol. Alcohol in the blood exerts a depressing effect on the central nervous system resulting in a broad continuum of effects on the functional levels of brain activity. The degree of effect is directly related to the amount of alcohol ingested. Impairment of voluntary motor actions (arm movements, walking, and speech) can result from a blood alcohol content of 10 mg per 100 ml (which is that equivalent of 6 oz of distilled spirits consumed within two hours). A blood concentration of 20 mg per 100 ml (10 oz within two hours) results in staggering and emotional instability. If 22 oz of distilled spirits are drunk during a two hour period, the blood alcohol concentration will be 50 mg per 100 ml, resulting in coma and possible death[22].

Alcohol is toxic to the gastrointestinal tract, pancreas, liver, myocardium, bone marrow, and other tissues[21]. When alcohol is present, the affected tissue cannot utilize or store nutrients in the normal manner. It has been further demonstrated that a good diet cannot prevent the progressive toxic effect of alcohol on body tissues, particularly those of the liver, and, in many instances, the alcoholic is unresponsive to vitamin therapy.

Alcohol interferes with gluconeogensis in the liver. Liver glycogen can be depleted by a seventy-two-hour fast or by ingestion of alcohol with little or no other source of nutrients[23]. This may explain the hypoglycemia (abnormally low blood glucose levels) seen in alcoholics. Hypoglycemic symptoms—weakness, irritability, incoordination, trembling, perspiration, rapid heartbeat, nausea, vomiting, and confusion—may be mistaken as signs of intoxication. In an emergency situation, if signs are misread and a glucose infusion is delayed, the brain may be left with an inadequate supply of glucose, resulting in coma, brain damage, or death[22].

Pancreatitis, associated with abdominal tenderness, distention, and vomiting, can be triggered by binge drinking. Concomitant with these symptoms is the malabsorption of amino acids and fat caused by maldigestion resulting from a decreased production of pancreatic enzymes[23].

Alcohol itself is the direct cause of the liver disease evident in may chronic drinkers. A moderate, but constant, consumption of alcohol causes alterations in the normal metabolic pathways of the liver. When alcohol is present it replaces fat as the preferred energy source of the liver. Oxidation of fat ceases and lipid accumulates in the liver. Continued alcohol use causes lipid deposits to enlarge and liver function becomes depressed due to progressive liver disease; stores of vitamins in the liver are depleted and restoration of these stores is depressed. Prolonged, excessive alcohol abuse may lead to cirrhosis causing permanent structural damage to the liver. How alcohol consumption leads to cirrhosis has not yet been determined. Studies on baboons have suggested that alcohol ingestion can lead to cirrhosis despite an adequate diet, and frequently alcoholic hepatitis is the precursor of cirrhosis[23]. Cirrhosis is the ninth leading cause of death in the United States and a large portion of those who die of cirrhosis are fifty years of age or older[22].

Beverage	Wt.	Approximate Measure	Calories	Protein	Alcohol	CHO	CA
	Gm.			Gm.	Gm.	mg.	
Ale, mild, (8 oz.)	230	1 large glass, 8 oz.	109	1.1	8.9	8.0	30
Ale, mild, (12 oz.)	345	1 bottle, 12 oz.	148	1.7	13.1	12.0	45
Beer, average, (8 oz.)	240	1 large glass, 8 oz.	114	1.4	8.9	10.6	10
Beer, average, (12 oz.)	360	1 bottle, 12 oz.	173	2.2	13.3	15.8	14
Brandy, California	30	1 brandy glass	75	—	10.5	—	—
Brandy, cognac	30	1 brandy glass	75	—	10.5	—	—
Cider, fermented	180	1 glass, 6 oz.	73	—	9.4	1.8	—
Cordials:							
Anisette	20	1 cordial glass	75	—	7.0	7.0	—
Apricot brandy	20	1 cordial glass	65	—	6.0	6.0	—
Benedictine	20	1 cordial glass	70	—	6.6	6.6	—
Creme de menthe	20	1 cordial glass	68	—	6.0	7.0	—
Curacao	20	1 cordial glass	55	—	6.0	4.0	—
Daiquiri	—	1 cocktail	124	0.1	15.1	5.2	4
Eggnog, Christmas type	123	1 punch cup	338	3.9	15.0	18.0	44
Gin, dry	43	1 jigger, 1½ oz.	107	—	15.1	—	—
Gin rickey	—	1 glass	153	Tr.	21.0	1.3	2
Highball	—	1 glass	170	—	24.0	—	—
Manhattan	—	1 cocktail	167	Tr.	19.2	7.9	1
Martini	—	1 cocktail	143	0.1	18.5	0.3	5
Mint julep	—	1 glass	217	—	29.2	2.7	—
Old Fashioned	—	1 glass	183	—	24.0	3.5	—
Planter's Punch	—	1 glass	177	0.1	21.5	7.9	4
Rum	43	1 jigger, 1½ oz.	107	—	15.4	—	—
Rum Sour	—	1 glass	163	0.2	21.0	3.7	4
Tom Collins	—	1 cocktail	182	0.3	21.5	9.0	6
Whiskey, rye	43	1 jigger, 1½ oz.	122	—	17.2	—	—
Whiskey, Scotch	43	1 jigger, 1½ oz.	107	—	15.1	—	—
Wine, California, red	100	1 wine glass	73	0.2	10.0	0.5	—
Wine, California, sauterne	100	1 wine glass	85	0.2	10.5	4.0	—
Wine, champagne, domestic	100	1 wine glass	85	0.2	11.0	3.0	—
Wine, muscatel or port	100	1 wine glass	169	0.2	15.0	14.0	—
Wine, vermouth, French	100	1 wine glass	108	—	15.0	1.0	—
Wine, vermouth, Italian	100	1 wine glass	170	—	18.0	12.0	—

TABLE 8–2   Composition of some common alcoholic beverages.

Source: Turner, D.: Handbook of Diet Therapy. 2nd Ed. Chicago, The University of Chicago Press. Copyright 1952 by the University of Chicago.

			Vitamins					Approx. Excess		
P	FE	A	Thiamine	Riboflavin	Niacin	Ascorbic Acid	D	Acid	Base	Fiber
mg.	mg.	I.U.	mcg.	mcg.	mg.	mg.	I.U.			Gm.
41	0.2	(0)	Tr.	(69)	(0.5)	0	0	—	—	—
62	0.3	(0)	Tr.	(102)	(0.7)	0	0	—	—	—
62	0.0	(0)	Tr.	72	0.5	0	0	—	—	—
94	0.0	(0)	Tr.	108	0.7	0	0	—	—	—
—	—	—	—	—	—	—	—	—	—	—
—	—	—	—	—	—	—	—	—	—	—
—	—	—	—	—	—	—	—	—	—	—
—	—	—	—	—	—	—	—	—	—	—
—	—	—	—	—	—	—	—	—	—	—
—	—	—	—	—	—	—	—	—	—	—
—	—	—	—	—	—	—	—	—	—	—
—	—	—	—	—	—	—	—	—	—	—
3	0.1	—	14	1	Tr.	8	0	—	—	—
74	0.7	84	35	113	Tr.	Tr.	21	2.5	—	—
—	—	—	—	—	—	—	—	—	—	—
1	Tr.	—	7	Tr.	Tr.	4	0	—	—	—
—	—	—	—	—	—	—	—	—	—	—
1	Tr.	35	36	2	Tr.	(0)	0	—	—	—
1	0.1	4	Tr.	Tr.	Tr.	(0)	0	—	—	—
—	—	—	—	—	—	—	—	—	—	—
3	0.1	—	14	1	Tr.	8	0	—	—	—
—	—	—	—	—	—	—	—	—	—	—
4	Tr.	—	20	Tr.	Tr.	14	0	—	—	—
6	Tr.	0	30	Tr.	Tr.	21	0	—	—	—
—	—	—	—	—	—	—	—	—	—	—
—	—	—	—	—	—	—	—	—	—	—
—	—	—	—	—	—	—	—	—	—	—
—	—	—	—	—	—	—	—	—	—	—
—	—	—	—	—	—	—	—	—	—	—
—	—	—	—	—	—	—	—	—	—	—
—	—	—	—	—	—	—	—	—	—	—

TABLE 8-2   Continued

Source: Turner, D.: Handbook of Diet Therapy. 2nd Ed. Chicago, The University of Chicago Press. Copyright 1952 by the University of Chicago.

Alcohol ingestion interferes with the metabolism of minerals. Alcohol can increase the absorption of iron and this excess iron storage can injure the liver. Routine iron supplements are contraindicated in the elderly alcoholic so that the incidence of any further hepatic damage will be minimized[21]. Alcohol increases the urinary excretion of magnesium and this depletion may be responsible for the symptoms of delerium tremens[22]. Decreased zinc absorption along with increased zinc excretion, characteristic of the alcoholic, may exacerbate the decreased taste sensation and lack of appetite common to the elderly resulting in a low food intake[24]. Alcoholism disrupts zinc metabolism and this cannot be corrected by increased zinc intake.

The toxicity of ethanol on the intestinal absorptive mucosa compounds the malnutrition common in the elderly alcohol abuser by causing malabsorption. Taken at moderate levels, alcohol decreases the absorption of sugars, amino acids, calcium, B vitamins, and other nutrients. Malabsorption of vitamins has been associated with both binge drinking and active chronic consumption of alcohol. Deficiencies in thiamine, pyridoxine, and pantothenic acid lead to a variety of neuropathies characterized by progressive muscular weakness and wasting, burning of the skin, and tingling pinprick sensations of the arms and legs. The older a person is when such a deficiency becomes pronounced, the more severe the symptoms and permanent the condition. Along with nutrient malabsorption, the person may suffer the burning pain of gastritis and an increased incidence of diarrhea[22]. Chronic or even intermittent diarrhea poses the possible complication of dehydration to the elderly drinker.

Alcohol and the Elderly

Generally, alcoholism in the elderly is acknowledged in much the same way as is sexuality—for the most part it is ignored. Many physicians are reluctant to designate elderly patients as alcoholic for fear of the effect of social stigma on the patient[25]. Despite this, it has been reported that up to 20 percent of those over age fifty have an alcohol consumption pattern that is problematic. Ten to twenty percent of all nursing home residents are alcoholic, and this distribution extends across all social, racial, economic, and geographic boundaries[25]. However, widowers aged sixty-five and over appear to be the most vulnerable subgroup of this population. It has been suggested that rehabilitation of the elderly alcoholic is more effective than intervention approaches with the younger alcohol abuser. One explanation for this is that elderly alcoholics are often in need of companionship. Thus, they may be more eager than others to substitute group therapy sessions for time spent drinking in solitude[25].

The elderly can be loosely categorized into three groups with respect to alcohol use: first, the abstainer; second, the social drinker who drinks but rarely abuses alcohol to the point of intoxication; third, the chronic alcohol abuser.

A portion of this third group started drinking late in life as a means of coping with some of the stresses of aging: isolation, loss of spouse, loss of family and friends, change of lifestyle, loss of health, or any of the myriad of other disruptions in living that comes with aging. The remainder of this group have been chronic alcohol abusers for many years and, despite the physiological toll alcohol has taken, they have survived to old age. This latter group will often exhibit remarkable constitutions. Though they may suffer the symptoms of seizures, chronic brain syndrome, cardiac disorders, gastrointestinal disorders, Wernicke's disease, and Korsakoff's psychosis, they continue to function, and many report to be satisfied with their lives. The hardiness of this group has been explained as the result of a selection process whereby many alcohol abusers die too early in life to become an elderly abuser[26].

Wernicke's disease and Korsakoff's psychosis are disorders of the central nervous system resulting from longstanding alcohol abuse along with a poor nutritional state. They are frequently found together in the elderly alcoholic. A specific lack of vitamin B_1—thiamine—is the main nutritional factor. The symptoms include delerium, unsteady gait, double vision, confused agitation, and hallucinations. Most often the sufferer is apathetic and disoriented to time and place. The condition Wernicke-Korsakoff syndrome may be complicated by other features of malnutrition including cirrhosis of liver, anemia, and skin lesions. There is a high mortality rate but most recover to some degree. Thiamine alone can reverse many of the symptoms[27].

Some alcoholic beverages, particularly beer, contribute to increased blood sugar level. For the normal individual the elevation is insignificant, but for the diabetic this blood sugar elevation will make control difficult[22]. Any elderly diabetic who repeatedly reports poor diabetic control should be questioned regarding alcohol consumption.

Alcohol Use in Extended Care Facilities

Alcohol is currently being suggested for use in nursing homes as a therapeutic agent in place of sedatives or as an antidepressant to improve sociability. Studies point to increased congeniality and co-operation following the administration of wine to test subjects[28]. Wine in amounts of four to six ounces showed no significant effect on blood glucose levels in elderly patients[29]. However, therapeutic introduction of alcohol must be handled judiciously[25].

Even modest amounts of alcohol will increase sleepiness but at the same time reduce motor skills and coordination[25]. An elderly patient, given a glass of wine for its sedative effect, may increase his risk of injury due to falling or tripping. If insomnia is the result of depression, which is quite common in the nursing home resident, alcohol, a depressant drug, is not the appropriate sedative to prescribe.

Further, alcohol is a potentially addicting drug and the elderly are more susceptible to its effects than are younger adults. Tolerance to prescribed dose levels may begin sooner and adverse behavior may be more common than might be anticipated in a younger population. As the nursing home residents begin to develop tolerance, more alcohol will be required to produce the euphoric/sedative effect. If additional alcohol is denied, the staff could face patient–management problems when the elderly seek outside channels to obtain an alcohol supply[25]. Nursing home supervisors report on many ingenious ways that the elderly manage to secure the extra alcohol they desire. When all outside sources are exhausted, they may have family and friends bring over-the-counter medications, which are essentially aqueous-alcohol solutions, to supplement therapeutically prescribed amounts of alcohol (see Table 8–3). Since many of these solutions contain 20 percent to 40 percent alcohol, their consumption cannot be ignored. (See page 184 for a further discussion of aqueous-alcohol solutions.)

Alcohol–Drug Interactions

Alcoholic beverages may react unfavorably with many drugs taken by the elderly. Routinely, the physician should question the patient on his use of alcohol when prescribing a medication or suggesting the use of over-the-counter medications[1,9]. All too often, no alcohol cautions are given and the patient is unaware of any adverse effect that could occur (see Figure 8–1).

Proprietary Name	Alcohol Content (%)	Manufacturer
Allergy Syrup (Chlortrimeton)	7%	Dow Chemicals
Breacol (mentholated)	20%	Glenbrook
Breacol (regular formula)	10%	Glenbrook
Cascara Sagrada Aromatic Fluid Extract	18%	Park Davis & Co.
Cerose Liquid	2.5%	Ives
Co-Tylenol Liquid Cough Formula	7%	McNeil
Demazine Syrup	7.5%	Schering
Digoxin Elixir	9–11.5%	generic formula
Donnagel Suspension	3.8%	Robins
Feosol Elixir	5%	Smith, Kline French
Genvitol	12%	Genovese
Geralix Liquid	12%	North American Pharmacy
Geriatric Elixir	12%	Consolidated Midland
Geri-Pen Elixir	5%	Fellows
Geroplex-FS Liquid	18%	Park Davis and Co.
Geritol	12%	J.B. Williams Co.
Gerix Elixir	20%	Abbott
Gerizyme Liquid	18%	Upjohn
Kaochlor 10% Liquid	5%	Warren - Teed
Kao-Nor Elixir	5%	North American Pharmacy
Keoparic Suspension	1%	Blue Line
Lomotil Liquid	15%	Searle
Millaril Solution	4.2%	Sands
Nembutal Elixir	18%	Abbott
Novahistine DMX	10%	Dow Pharmaceuticals
Novahistine Elixir	5%	Dow Pharmaceuticals
Pertussin 8-Hour Cough Formula	9.5%	Chesebrough-Ponds
Pertussin Plus Nighttime Cold Medicine	25%	Chesebrough-Ponds
Potassium Gluconate Elixir	5%	Philips Roxane
Quelidrine Syrup	2%	Abbott
Reserpoid	14%	Upjohn
Robitussin	3.5%	Robins
Santussin Adult Suspension	12%	Sandia
Seconal Elixir	12%	Lilly
Sedatolic	6%	Merch Sharp & Dohme
SSS Tonic	12%	SSS Company
Symptom 1,2,3 and Multi -	5%	Park Davis & Co.
Triaminic Expectorant	5%	Dorsey
Valerian	68%	Lilly
Vicks Day-Care	7.5%	Vick Chemical Co.
Vicks Formula 44	10%	Vick Chemical Co.
Vicks NyQuil	25%	Vick Chemical Co.
Vi-Gerol Elixir	12%	Columbia
Viro-med	16.63%	Whitehall Laboratories

TABLE 8-3   A chart showing alcohol content and manufacturers of various medications.

"I didn't think that a couple of drinks on top of my medication could be a problem."

·Drinking and driving don't mix. Drinking and certain medications don't mix either. Alcohol depresses your brain function. It interferes with alertness, coordination and breathing, and may cause blurring of vision. Some medications increase the effects of alcohol. So, when your doctor gives you a prescription, make sure you ask him if you can drink.

The same thing can be said if you are taking any medication that the doctor doesn't know about. Mixing medicines can cause problems if you do it yourself. Don't accept medicine from friends or relatives without checking with your doctor first. Make sure he knows all the drugs you are taking, including those you buy yourself *without* a prescription. And make sure you follow the doctor's instructions when taking your medicine. *When* you take it can be as important as *how much* you take.

Remember, mixing medicines and alcohol or other drugs on your own can be asking for trouble.

"And I'm old enough to know better."

ROCHE
ME
MEDICATION EDUCATION

Medicines that matter from people who care.

◇ROCHE◇

Roche Laboratories, Division of Hoffmann-La Roche Inc.

FIGURE 8–1   This message stressing the proper use of medication was developed as a public service by the Social Science Department of Roche Laboratories, a division of Hoffmann-La Roche Inc., Nutley, New Jersey 07110.

Even modest amounts of alcohol in combination with medications that depress the central nervous system create an intensified depressant effect. Sedatives, sleep-inducing drugs, tranquilizers, antianxiety drugs, antidepressants, and narcotics have their actions enhanced in the presence of alcohol[22]. The general result is excessive sedation and further impairment of mental performance, judgment, motor skills, and coordination. Although the drug–alcohol interaction is predictable, the intensity of the reaction varies markedly from one individual to another and from one occasion to another.

Alcohol increases the activity of liver enzymes which can affect the metabolism and duration of effect of many medications. In some instances, moderate use of alcohol can reduce drug effectiveness. When acute intoxication occurs, the alcohol may block the normal drug metabolism or detoxification resulting in a prolonged drug action. Chronic alcohol ingestion leads to a proliferation of the smooth endoplasmic reticulum[31]. The enzymes involved in the detoxification of many drugs are concentrated at this site, and enhanced metabolism of drugs can be demonstrated in chronic alcoholics.

The following discussion will serve to indicate the many and varied alcohol–drug interactions that can occur. Any drug routinely prescribed should be checked for such an interaction and the patient should be advised accordingly.

Warfarin and coumarin anticoagulants may often be taken by an elderly patient in the management of stroke or heart attack. Alcohol, used even sparingly, can either decrease or increase the effect of these drugs[32]. The individual response to the interactions of alcohol and warfarin depends on the person's sensitivity to the drug, the quantity of the drug, the type and amount of alcohol consumed, and the sequence in which drug and alcohol were taken. Heavy alcohol users, with liver damage, may be very sensitive to anticoagulants and require smaller-than-usual doses.

Meprobamate, sold under a variety of brand names such as Equanil, Kalmm, Miltown, and SK-Bamate, is classified as a mild tranquilizer or antianxiety medication. The elderly (over age sixty) are very susceptible to standard doses of this medication. With alcohol, the sedative effects of meprobamate are increased and can cause serious depression of vital brain functions[32].

Thioridazine, a strong tranquilizer, sold as Mellaril, also contraindicates the use of alcohol since the drug increases the intoxicating effect of alcohol. Alcohol can further increase the sedative action of the drug and accentuate its depressant effects on brain function[32].

Reserpine, an antihypertensive drug, may be used to reduce high blood pressure. When combined with alcohol, reserpine can increase the intoxicating effect of alcohol, thus increasing the chance of falls and injury[22]. Other antihypertensive drugs such as methyldopa (Aldomet) and the diuretic furosemide (Lasix) are often prescribed to help reduce high blood pressure in the elderly. If alcohol is ingested along with either of these medications, it can potentiate the blood pressure–lowering effect of the drug, and in some instances the alcohol–drug interaction can cause blood pressure to drop to dangerously low levels[32].

Tolbutamide, chlorpropamide, and sulfonylureas are oral antidiabetic drugs used to help correct the insulin deficiency in adult (maturity-onset) diabetes by stimulating insulin production in the pancreas. These drugs can produce a marked intolerance to alcohol and may provoke a pattern of response called the "disulfiram-like reaction"[23]. The drug interrupts the normal breakdown of alcohol by the liver, thus permitting accumulation of toxic by-products that enter the bloodstream. When sufficient levels of both alcohol and drug are present in the blood, symptoms are seen. These include flushing, severe headache, pounding heartbeat, dizziness, shortness of breath, sweating, inital rise of blood pressure, and weakness. This reaction may occur with the normal prescribed level of medication combined with cocktails before dinner. If a large amount of alcohol is taken, the reaction may progress to blurred vision, vertigo, confusion, marked drop in blood pressure, and loss of consciousness. The reaction lasts from thirty minutes to several hours. Obviously, diabetic diet instructions are incomplete without mention of the possibility of a disulfiram-like reaction following the ingestion of alcohol.

Alcohol in Pharmaceutical Products

Over 500 oral pharmaceutical preparations are aqueous-alcohol mixtures. Most of these products are vitamin tonics and antitussive-decongestant liquids ranging in alcohol concentrations from 0.5 to 68 percent[30]. Table 8–3 provides information on percentage of alcohol found in some common pharmaceutical preparations. An awareness of the alcohol content of commonly used pharmaceuticals is essential when dealing with an elderly population.

A geriatric vitamin solution may be abused by a patient because of its attractive tranquilizing effect. With a 20 percent (40 proof) alcohol content, one tablespoon of such a vitamin solution provides the same amount of alcohol as one ounce of wine[30]. It is important not only to determine if the patient is taking a vitamin solution but at what time of the day it is taken and in what amount. Often tonics are taken in the evening or right before bed and "just a little extra" is added to the suggested dose. Misuse of the vitamin solution must be considered and discussed with the patient since continued use of the vitamin solution can interfere with or react with other prescribed medications. For example, the elderly diabetic using an antidiabetic medication, such as those mentioned above, may experience a disulfiram-like reaction from ingesting a cough/cold preparation unless he is forewarned about the alcohol content of the syrup he is taking.

Aqueous-alcohol preparations also have therapeutic implications for a patient already taking sedative, antianxiety agents and mild tranquilizers. The addition of an alcohol-containing cold remedy will enhance the depressant effect on the central nervous system and can compromise the person's safety by interfering with balance, judgment, and coordination[30].

It is evident from the previous discussion that many of the aged are alcohol abusers, therefore excessive reliance on over-the-counter medication cannot be overlooked as a means for the elderly to ingest additional alcohol in a camouflaged acceptable way. These medications can further complicate alcohol intervention therapy with the elderly alcoholic[20].

CITED REFERENCES

1. Hollister, L. E. 1977. Prescribing drugs for the elderly. *Geriatrics* 32:71.
2. Leahart, D. G. 1976. The use of medications in the elderly population. *Nursing Clinics of North America* 11(1):135.
3. Lamy, P.P. 1977. What the physician should keep in mind when prescribing drugs for an elderly patient. *Geriatrics* 32:37.
4. Carson, J. S., and Gormican, A. 1976. Disease-medication relationships in altered taste sensitivity. *J. Amer. Dietetic Assoc.* 68:550.
5. Dell, R. A., ed. 1977. *Nutrition in disease-drug food interaction.* Columbus, Ohio: Ross Laboratories.
6. Roe, D. 1976. *Drug induced nutritional deficiencies.* Westport, Connecticut: Avi Publishing Co.
7. Pennington, J. 1978. *Nutritional diet therapy.* California: Bull Publishing Co.
8. Block, C. D.; Popovich, N. C.; and Black, M. C. 1977. Drug interaction in the G.I. tract. *Amer. J. of Nursing* 77(9):1426.
9. Hartshorn, E. A. 1977. Food and drug interaction. *J. Amer. Dietetic Assoc.* 70:15.
10. Lambert, M. L. 1975. Drug and diet interaction. *Amer. J. of Nursing.* 75(3):402.
11. Graham, D. M. 1978. Caffeine—its identity, dietary sources, intake and biological effects. *Nutrition Review* 36(4):97.
12. Ray, O. 1978. *Drugs, society and human behavior.* St. Louis: C.V. Mosby Co.
13. Stephenson, P. E.; Latham, M. C.; and Jones, D. V. 1977. Physiologic and psychotropic effects of caffeine on man, a review. *J. Amer. Dietetic Assoc.* 71:240.
14. Brezinova, V. 1974. Effects of caffeine on sleep: EEG study on late middle age people. *Brit. J. Clin. Pharamacology* 1:203.
15. Robertson, D., et al. 1978. Effects of caffeine on plasma renin activity, catecholamines and blood pressure. *New Eng. J. of Med.* 298(4):181.

16. Dawer, T. R.; Kannell, W. B.; and Gordon, T. 1974. Coffee and cardiovascular disease, observations from the Framingham study. *New Eng. J. of Med.* 291:871.

17. Ginsberg, R., and Weintraub, M. 1976. Caffeine in the "sundown syndrome," report of negative results. *J. of Gerontology* 31(4):419.

18. Cohen, S., and Booth, G. 1975. Gastric acid secretion and loweresophageal sphincter pressure on response to coffee and caffeine. *New Eng. J. of Med.* 293:897.

19. Statland, B. E.; Demas, T.; and Davis, M. 1976. Caffeine accumulation associated with alcoholic liver disease. *New Eng. J. of Med.* 295:110.

20. Kinney, J., and Leaton, G. 1978. *Loosening the grip, a handbook of alcohol information.* St. Louis: C.V. Mosby Co.

21. Israel, Y.; Videla, L.; and Bernstein, J. 1975. Liver hypermetabolic state after chronic ethanol consumption: Hormonal interrelations and pathogenic implications. *Fed. Proc.* 34:2052.

22. Katne, R. C., ed. 1978. *Drugs and the elderly.* The Ethel Percy Andrus Gerontology Center, California: Univ. Southern California Press.

23. Shaw, S., and Lieber, C. S. 1978. *Nutrition and alcoholic liver disease.* Nutrition and Disease, Columbus, Ohio: Ross Laboratories.

24. Fabry, T. L., and Luke, C. S. 1979. The role of zinc in alcoholism. *Nutrition and the M.D.* 5(1):3.

25. Zimberg, S. June 1974. The elderly alcoholics. *The Gerontologist* p. 221.

26. Barboriak, J. J., et al. 1978. Alcohol and nutrient intake of elderly men. *J. Amer. Dietetic Assoc.* 72:493.

27. Drefus, P. M. 1975. Nutritional disorders of the nervous system. In *Textbook of medicine,* vol. 1, eds. P. B. Beeson and W. McDermott. Philadelphia: W. B. Saunders Co.

28. Leake, C. D., and Silverman, M. 1967. The clinical use of wine in geriatrics. *Geriatrics* 22:175.

29. Murdock, H. R. 1972. The effect of table wines on blood glucose levels in the geriatric subject. *Geriatrics* 27:93.

30. Dukes, G. E.; Kuhn, J. J.; and Evan, R. P. September 1977. Alcohol in pharmaceutical products. *Amer. Family Physician* p. 97.

31. Isselbacher, K. J. 1977. Metabolic and hepatic effects of alcohol. *New Eng. J. of Med.* 296(11):612.

32. Long, J. V. 1977. *The essential guide to prescription drugs.* New York: Harper and Row.

OTHER REFERENCES

Colton, T.; Grosselin, R. E.; and Smith, R. P. 1968. The tolerance of coffee drinkers to caffeine. *Clin. Pharmacology and Therapeutics* 9(1):31.

Kosman, M. E. 1974. Pharmacokinetic drug interactions. *J. Amer. Med. Assoc.* 229(11):1485.

IIIIIIIIIIIIIIIIIIIIIIIIIIIIIIIIIIIIIIIIIIIII *9*

Dietary Supplements

The aged are often the targets of food and diet advertisements that are promoted as having cure-all qualities[1]. These foods or supplements often promise miraculous dietary cures for illness. Favorite cures often advertised are those for cancer and arthritis. If no cure is promised, such a food is often promoted as a panacea for good health and a longer life. Since the aged are at a time in life when friends and family may be chronically ill or have died, their own mortality takes on an immediate presence and the desire for a longer life becomes an urgent quest. "Health" foods do not necessarily promote good health. Some of these foods are safe and reliable and may provide benefits when added to a normal diet; others are harmful, unnecessary, and costly[2]. The elderly consumer needs education to be protected from nutrition misinformation.

The following paragraphs define and describe some commonly used dietary supplements. This information should be used as a reference when educating the elderly to the proper use of or need for special dietary supplements.

Acidophilus Milk   This milk is bacterially cultured, so that part of the milk sugar, lactose, is changed to lactic acid[3]. Acidophilus milk is effective in restoring intestinal bacteria and may be beneficial as an adjunct to antibiotic therapy which sterilizes the gut through the action of the drug. Lactose-intolerant individuals may also find this variety of milk produces less discomfort; therefore, they may be able to use it more liberally in their diet than regular cow's milk.

Alfalfa   A leguminous plant, alfalfa has been cultivated for over 2,000 years as animal forage[3]. There are claims that alfalfa roots grow deeply into the earth and probe our minerals and trace elements that shallow-rooted plants cannot reach. This claim is false. Subsoils are lower in nutrients than top soils. A 100 gm portion of alfalfa shoots provides 3,410 mcg of vitamin A, 162 mg of vitamin C, 5.4 mg of iron, and lesser amounts of other nutrients[4].

Apple Cider Vinegar   In the late 1950s, De Forest Jarvis, M.D., promoted apple cider vinegar and honey as two simple remedies for many ailments in his book *Folk Medicine: A Vermont Doctor's Guide to Good Health*[5]. Jarvis claimed apple cider vinegar was a curative due to its high potassium value. One cup of vinegar does have 240 mg of potassium but one medium orange has 300 mg, one medium banana has 550 mg, and one medium white potato has 407 mg. Jarvis advised much smaller portions than one cup in his prescriptions for treatment. He particularly recommended apple cider vinegar as a cure for arthritis. This promise is the main reason why some elderly still rely on some of Jarvis' folk medicine cures. Jarvis claimed the acid in the vinegar would remove calcium deposits in arthritic joints. He based this claim on observations of plumbers, who remove calcium deposits on pipes by the use of an acid solution. Obviously methods of treatment of household plumbing cannot be extrapolated to medical treatment for the human body.

Bioflavonoids   This group of substances is often referred to as vitamin P although the American Chemical Society, in the early 1950s, concluded that there was no such substance as vitamin P[6]. Bioflavonoid is a generic term applied to a group of flavones found mainly in the pulp and connective tissue of citrus fruits. *Rutin,* a bioflavonoid, is often sold in combination with vitamin C. There is no clinical evidence that bioflavonoids, with or without vitamin C, have a beneficial effect on rheumatoid arthritis, arteriosclerosis, hypertension, or the common cold. A recent report[7], however, did indicate that bioflavonoids along with vitamin C were beneficial in the treatment of herpes labialis (fever blisters or fever sores).

Blackstrap Molasses   This the the thick syrupy residue left behind when sugar refining is complete[8]. Regular molasses comes from the first and second extractions of sugar whereas blackstrap molasses is a product of third through fifth extractions. It is the least sweet and most impure sugar product. Blackstrap molasses began to appeal to the public in the early 1950s after Gayelord Hauser promoted it in his book *Look Younger, Live Longer*[5]. Hauser claimed the product was rich in B vitamins, calcium, and iron. All are present, but it would take between forty and seventy-five tablespoons of the molasses to meet the RDA for riboflavin, niacin, and thiamine. One tablespoon does contain 116 mg calcium and 2.3 mg iron as well as 43 Calories[9]. Claims that blackstrap molasses can prevent cancer or cure ulcers, varicose veins, and arthritis are unfounded[8]. Reliance on the excessive use of any sugar, regardless of the source or nutrient content, is unwise and should not be fostered.

Brewer's Yeast   This yeast was originally a by-product of the brewing industry. Today it is grown for human consumption and heat-treated to ensure no live organisms are present that may grow in the intestine[10]. It is a good source of protein (one tablespoon provides 3.7 gm) and B vitamins (one tablespoon provides 1484 mcg thiamine, 406 mcg riboflavin, and 3.6 mg niacin)[9]. Brewer's yeast does produce gas and may cause great discomfort to some individuals. An elderly individual should take no more than one-half teaspoon per day and gradually work up to one tablespoon if no ill effects occur. Excessive use has caused fever and problems with protein metabolism. Since the elderly are rarely protein deficient and B vitamins are available in more palatable sources, brewer's yeast is not a necessary dietary supplement.

Carob Powder   This dried and powdered seed pod of the carob tree is native to the Mediterranean area. It may be called St. John's bread, boecksur, honey locust, or locust bean[10]. Used mainly as a chocolate or cocoa substitute (although it looks like chocolate, its taste is different), it is caffeine-free, low in fat, and contains calcium and phosphorus.

Desiccated Liver   Sold in pill or powder form, it is an excellent source of vitamin B_{12}[3]. The habitual consumption of desiccated liver may conceal borderline cases of pernicious anemia and make the condition difficult to diagnose. Liver extracts such as this provide only some of the nutrients found in fresh liver. Claim that desiccated liver provides the body with all elements necessary to manufacture vitamin B_{12} are unfounded.

Garlic   According to folklore, garlic can cure intestinal disorders, gas, respiratory infections, symptoms of aging, high blood pressure, and many other chronic illnesses[8]. Garlic oil capsules are a staple of health food stores. Recent research data has suggested that large quantities of garlic and onions may lower cholesterol and serum triglyceride levels in some individuals[11]. However, if taken in large amounts, these two foods may cause the person to be socially unacceptable since the substances in garlic and onion that cause "bad breath" are absorbed into the blood stream and exhaled from the lungs. Mouthwash cannot remove the odor.

Ginseng   Sold in liquid, powder, and capsule form, ginseng is often made into a tea. The ginseng plant (the root is considered most potent) is publicized as possessing may curative powers. One teamaker used ginseng in his tea and advertised, ". . .we will guarantee joyful temper, plenty of pure red blood and relief for your irritable bladder"[5]. Others publicize its power to rejuvenate male sexuality and ease the symptoms of menopause. It is a favorite with the aged who may have bladder problems as well as sexual difficulties[12]. Fourteen persons who consumed an average of 3 gm of ginseng daily were recently studied. They suffered from insomnia, hypertension, and morning diarrhea[13]. Thus, long-term ingestion of large amounts of ginseng should be avoided.

Herbal Teas   Teas of all varieties are claimed to have curative properties. Elderberry tea is touted as being protective against witches and chamomile tea was considered by the Egyptians to be an elixir of youth. These and other folktales are harmless reasons for drinking herbal teas[12]. However, recent evidence[14] linked consumption of herbal teas with cases of abdominal cramps and profuse watery diarrhea which lasted twenty-four hours. Many herbal teas contain known cathartics such as buckthorn bark and senna which can result in the above syndrome if enough of the active ingredient is consumed.

The tannins in cinnamon tea and regular tea may help stop simple diarrhea, and peppermint tea can be a soothing and comforting way to open sinuses. However, mistletoe, nutmeg, sassafras, and horsetail teas may have dangerous side effects[15]. Burdock root and nutmeg tea have been reported to cause blurred vision and an anticholinergic syndrome (in which certain nerve impulses are blocked)[12]. Chamomile tea, made from flower heads, may cause anaphylactic shock or allergic rhinitis in individuals who have a hypersensitivity to ragweed pollen[15].

Laetrile   Often incorrectly called vitamin B_{17}, laetrile is considered to be the cure for cancer by those who believe it is a vitamin deficiency disease[16]. Although much publicity surrounds this controversial compound, no proof of its cancer-curing ability has been clearly documented. A two-year trial to end in 1980 may settle the question of laetrile usefulness once and for all. In the meantime it must be remembered that laetrile is extracted from the apricot pit and therefore the laetrile family of compounds can induce cyanide poisoning if taken in large amounts.

Lecithin   It is a phospholipid occurring in nerve and organ tissues, egg yolks, milk, soybeans, and corn. Lecithin is used as an emulsifier in foods. It is not an antidote for high serum cholesterol and cannot dissolve fatty plaques in the blood vessels that contribute to heart attacks. Lecithin is a substance formed in part from choline, a body chemical which helps transfer fat deposits from the liver to the bloodstream[10]. There is no evidence that lecithin can prevent or cure heart disease. Claims are also made that it will eliminate liver spots, relieve arthritic pain, and help dry skin and psoriasis. These claims have not been substantiated[5]. At the present time research studies are being carried out to determine the usefulness of lecithin in the diet. Recent evidence suggests that lecithin ingested in egg yolks supplies choline which helps some individuals with impaired memory function[17].

Pangamic Acid   Erroneously referred to as vitamin B_{15}, this is the newest vitamin cure. The substance does not fit the accepted definition of a vitamin (which is a substance needed in the body in small quantities, the absence of which results in deficiency symptoms). Its supporters claim it increases oxygen uptake by the blood and tissues which results in more energy, lowered blood cholesterol, and many other bodily improvements. None of these claims can be conclusively supported by research data[18]. Nonetheless, consumers are paying high prices for pangamic acid tablets. Since the name "pangamic" means "occurring everywhere" it is unlikely that anyone eating a varied, minimally processed diet would be lacking it[19].

Protein Supplements   These preparations come in pill and powder form and may be any one or a combination of more than one of the following: skim milk powder, powdered raw liver, powdered yeast, egg white, preparations from the spleen, heart, kidneys, and pancreas, soya lecithin, calcium caseinate[20]. The elderly require 0.8 gm protein per kilogram of body weight. This amount can easily be met by a normal diet, indicating no need for additional protein supplementation. On the contrary, excessive protein intakes may prove more harmful than beneficial (see chapter 4).

Wheat Germ   A rich source of vitamin E, wheat germ has been suggested as an aging preventive. It has also been claimed to cure heart disease and improve fertility and virility[3]. Wheat germ also provides B vitamins and protein and is a nutritious adjunct to a varied diet. However, by itself, it has no unusual positive health effects, and furthermore it is a concentrated source of calories.

CITED REFERENCES

1. Kilby-Kelberg, S. 1973. Aunt Libby and her cure-alls. *Amer. J. Nursing* 73(6):1056.
2. Cromwell, C. Summer 1976. Organic food—an update. *Family Economics Review* p. 8.
3. Darling, M. 1973. *Natural, organic and health foods.* Univ. of Minnesota: Agricultural Extension Service.
4. Food composition table for use in Latin America. 1961. Institute of Nutrition of Central America and Panama and Interdepartmental Committee on Nutrition for National Defense, Institutes of Health, Bethesda, Maryland.
5. Deutch, R. M. 1977. *The new nuts among the berries.* Palo Alto, California: Bull Publishing Co.
6. Goodhart, R. S. 1973. Bioflavonoids. In *Modern nutrition in health and disease,* 5th ed., eds. R. S. Goodhart and M. Shils. Philadelphia: Lea and Febiger.
7. Accelerated remission of episodes of Herpes Labialis in response to a bioflavinoid-ascorbate supplement. 1978. *Nutrition Reviews* 36(10):300.
8. Dardin, E. 1972. Sense and nonsense about health foods. *J. Am. Home Economic* 64:4.
9. Church, C. F., and Church, H. N. 1970. *Food values of portions commonly used.* Philadelphia: J. B. Lippincott Co.
10. *Glossary of health food terms.* 1974. Dairy Council of Metropolitan New York.
11. Will garlic and onions lower serum lipid levels. 1979. *Nutrition and the M.D.* IV(3).
12. Food, glorious food . . . Herbal remedies—do they work? 1979. *Environmental Nutrition Newsletter* 2(2):3.
13. Siegel, R. K. 1979. Ginseng abuse syndrome. *JAMA* 241 (15):1614.
14. News digest—not our cup of tea. 1978. *J. Amer. Dietetic Assoc.* 73:447.

15. Herbal teas . . . Often nice, sometimes noxious. 1978. *Nutrition and the M.D.* 4(14):4.
16. Jukes, T. H. 1977. Is laetrile a vitamin? *Nutrition Today* 12(5):12.
17. Schmeck, H. M., Jr. January 9, 1979. Memory loss curbed by chemicals in foods. *New York Times* Section C-Science Times, p. 1.
18. Herbert, V. 1979. Pangamic acid vitamin B15 fact or fancy. *The Professional Nutritionist* 11(1):9.
19. Nutrition update, vitamin B-15. 1978. *Environmental Nutrition Newsletter* 1(4):2.
20. Warnings outlined for protein products. 1978. *CNI Weekly Report* 7(10):5.

IIIIIIIIIIIIIIIIIIIIIIIIIIIIIIIIIIIIIIIIIII 10

Psychosocial Forces that Affect Nutrition and Food Choices

Every ninth American is a member of the group called the elderly; eleven percent of the total population is aged sixty-five and over. Every day, approximately 5,000 Americans celebrate their sixty-fifth birthday and approximately 3,600 people over sixty-five die. This result is a net increase of 1,400 aged Americans daily, or one-half million per year. Population projections suggest that by the year 2020, there will be 33 million aged.

Soon it will be necessary to divide this group into subgroups—young-old, middle-old, and very old. As more people reach age sixty-five, the proportion of middle-old and very-old grows. Over two million Americans are eighty-five years of age or older. In the past, if requested, a birthday greeting would be sent from the White House to any American celebrating his eightieth (or later) birthday. Recently, the qualifying age was raised to 100 (returned to age 80 at the time of publication), and in 1976 Social Security records listed 10,690 people aged 100 or more. This is remarkable, since the average life expectancy was forty-nine years in 1900.

Babies born in 1977 will live to an average of seventy-three; this is 68.7 years for males and 76.5 years for females[1]. The increase in life expectancy since 1900 has been achieved through a decrease in infant mortality and infectious diseases that strike the young. Less success has been realized in the battle against chronic disorders and diseases of the elderly such as cancer. Until major medical breakthroughs are made against cardiovascular disease, cancer, and other chronic conditions of the aged, the biblical lifespan of "three score and ten" will not change significantly.

As a result of the longer life expectancy of females, which has not yet been fully explained, most older Americans are women. The average for the total sixty-five-plus population is 146 women for every 100 men; in the eighty-five-plus group, there are 217 women for every 100 men. The vast majority (70 percent) of all women over seventy-five are widows who generally live alone on very meager incomes[2]. Still, when questioned as to choice of living arrangements, over one-half of all widows would rather live alone than be dependent on a relative or friend[3].

Widowers generally fare much worse living alone than do widows. Widowers are usually unprepared to take care of themselves. The remarriage rate for older widowers is higher, as many widowers find the married state to be more comfortable than single life[3].

The vast majority of the aged are satisfied with life, are happy, and lead meaningful existences[4]. This is contrary to the stereotyped view of the older person who is lonely, unhappy, and constantly complaining. Still, many elderly are economically deprived. Income is reduced at retirement and often this lowered income is not adequate to meet basic needs. One seventh (or 3.3 million) of the elderly have incomes below the official 1975 poverty threshold ($3,417 for older couples and $2,720 for older individuals), with elderly women and members of minorities overrepresented in this group[5]. Persons living on fixed incomes are hit hard by inflation. The elderly have few opportunities for improvement of personal income because of "mandatory retirement" and age-discriminatory hiring practices. In a recent survey, 37 percent of those retired said they did not stop working by choice[4].

The limited income of elderly individuals is constantly threatened by ever-increasing healthcare expenditures. In 1976, per capita health care for each older American averaged 3.5 times that spent for each person under sixty-five. The elderly 11 percent of the population incurs 29 percent of the total health care expenditures in the country[2]. Medicare covers less than half of these expenses. Older people see physicians one and one-half times as often, and have about twice as many hospital stays, as do younger people. Also, the hospital stays of the elderly tend to last twice as long as those of younger people. Yet, when questioned, 82 percent of the elderly reported no hospitalization in the previous year and 69 percent reported their health as being good to excellent[4]. Only 5 percent of the noninstitutionalized aged are housebound and only slightly over 1 percent are bedridden[2].

The myriad of psychosocial forces that affect the elderly are impossible to describe totally. The following section will deal, for the most part, with those factors that put the elderly at risk for nutritional problems. (See Figure 10–1 for a list of factors influencing nutritional status.) Those elderly who face the greatest risks are the 15 percent who are economically deprived. An additional 2.2 million elderly are "near-poor," falling into the low income population group. Collectively, the poor and near-poor number 5.5 million, or one-fourth of all persons aged sixty-five and older[5].

A. **Physical**
   1. Dental problems
   2. Excretion problems (constipation, incontinence)
   3. Physical weakness (e.g., generalized arteriosclerosis or arthritis with joint stiffness making eating painful)
   4. Lack of physical activity
   5. Loss of sensation (smell, taste)
   6. Chronic disease
   7. Lactose intolerance
   8. Drug interference (anorexia)
   9. Reduced digestive capacity

B. **Psychological**
   1. Emotional depression
   2. Anorexia
   3. Personal taste preference
   4. Lifetime eating habits
   5. Lack of socialization with meals

C. **Social**
   1. Financial constrictions
   2. Inconvenience of food preparation for one person
   3. Inability to adapt to unfamiliar surroundings (hospital or nursing home)
   4. Erroneous dietary beliefs
   5. Susceptibility to "fad nutritional" claims

FIGURE 10–1   Physical and psychosocial factors influencing the nutritional status of the elderly.

Source: Dialogues in Nutrition, Vol. 2, No. 3, "Nutritional Problems of the Elderly," Health Learning Systems Inc., Blookfield, New Jersey, 07003.

The psychosocial problems faced by these elderly—substandard housing, limited income, inadequate transportation, and social isolation—are problems that may strike any age group. These are common maladies of socioeconomically deprived minorities. It is tempting to consider the aged as a minority group. They resemble other minority groups in that they suffer from prejudice, discrimination, and deprivation. Yet, they were not born into this "minority" of deprived aged and they have little sense of group identity or political unity[6]. The elderly may form a *statistical* minority, yet they have few common identifying characteristics except advanced age, a few wrinkles, and greying hair. Herein lies the problem: the aged cannot be readily classified nor can many generalizations be easily drawn about them.

One generalization that may be drawn, however, is that many elderly are subjected to specific nutritional problems. Before intervention techniques are instituted to deal with these nutritional problems, three things must be considered[7].

1. Differences between the young and old from a therapeutic standpoint.

2. Specific age/sex/ethnic/economic differences among members of the older group.

3. Individual differences apart from ethnic/cultural/economic group association.

In short, before intervention is attempted, the elderly person's entire life experience must be considered because it may be just that experience that has created the existing problem or may be a complicating factor.

THE MEANING OF FOOD

Before any nutritional problems can be corrected, the meaning of food and the importance of food habits for that particular person must be understood.

Food is power or security, a symbol of prestige and status, an overture of hospitality and friendship, and an outlet for emotions[8]. Most people tend to define food culturally and not on the basis of the nutritional value of particular items. Food habits are learned.

They are a way for a particular culture to exert a standardizing influence on the behavior of an individual in the group so that the group comes to have common eating patterns. Food habits are established early in life and are resistant to change[9]. Familiar food and food patterns represent security to the elderly and provide a link to the past that is a source of comfort. The elderly use food to communicate and an astute health professional can translate their messages. It is important to listen carefully when an elderly person explains likes and dislikes. The elderly person has every right to expect his wishes to be respected.

For the elderly, breakfast is the most enthusiastically received and completely eaten meal of the day. Therefore, this meal, more so than lunch or dinner, should be tailored to the likes and dislikes of the person. During times of anxiety, foods that were given during infancy and childhood may provide comfort. Milk, cooked cereal, and pureed items are often requested. When a person is stressed, anxious, or confused, regression is common and may be reflected in his selection of foods. At other times, these items will be rejected because the older person does not want to be "babied"[10, 11].

Nursing home staff members can often predict an emotional episode in a patient by simply observing the foods that are or are not eaten. Increased plate waste often reflects increased emotional stress. Some patients refuse to eat anything and complain bitterly about food preparation or service during a period of unhappiness. As the emotional upset subsides, normal consumption patterns return[12].

For the institutionalized elderly as well as those who are living independently, cultural and traditional patterns of eating will affect food preferences. There have been few published studies of specific food taboos or food preferences among the aged in the United States, but health professionals who have worked with groups of ethnic elderly have made numerous observations worth noting[13].

The United States has long been divided into geographical areas that are identified with certain foods. Presentation of and encouragement to use "down home" food may foster reminiscences, which are considered psychologically important in the aged's adjustment to the final stage of the life cycle[13].

A large proportion of today's elderly were raised in a "culture of poverty" because of their rural or immigrant origins. Many may still be existing at an economic level far below the standard of living enjoyed by others. Therefore, foods associated with status—bakery items and convenience foods—may be preferred and foods identified with poverty, such as beans, may be rejected, regardless of their nutritional value.

Social scientists have also identified *age-appropriate behavior* in older persons which can affect food choices[13]. Older people, particularly older women, are often preoccupied with the health of their bodies. Whether the dysfunction or malfunction is real, imagined, or exaggerated, it will influence food selection and rejection. Digestive upsets, constipation, "poor" blood, and fatigue are often attributed to, and/or "treated" by certain foods.

Educational background is of little significance in the dietary habits of the elderly. Cultural origins and social class are better indicators. This unexpected result is related to the fact that the vast majority of the current generation over 65 had no more than eight years of formal education (and even this being of varying quality). Few received science education and none received nutrition education since nutrition science was in its youth when these people were in theirs. Their nutrition knowledge was acquired as folk myth through family and community association, with more recent information coming through the media[13]. Their lack of basic knowledge may be one reason why they are often subject to faddist notions as they may be unable to differentiate between reliable and unreliable data.

Neighborhoods in transition may interrupt eating habits of the elderly, particularly the low-income urban dweller. Nutritional crises can be precipitated when storeowners vacate, leaving aged residents in familiar but suddenly hostile neighborhoods. Where will the Jewish widow get her meat after the Kosher butcher closes his store? The Italian neighborhood that endures a wave of Puerto Rican immigration leaves little that is familiar to the aged Italians that remain[13]. When customary foods are no longer available and the person feels culturally isolated, food choices are often reduced to readily available bread, starches, and nonnutritious liquids (coffee, tea).

Frequently, the aged, caught in neighborhood decline, may be uprooted and forced to live with their acculturated American children and grandchildren. Antagonism for old-country ways on the part of children and grandchildren often results in withdrawal and exaggerated emphasis on the old ways on the part of the elderly person. Frequently, the defensive grandparent refuses to eat or participate in family meals.

It can be speculated that much of the behavior that ultimately leads to confinement of the aged in a chronic care facility is related to conflict over food and eating. Many nursing home administrators have heard a family say, "He just won't eat!" Assisting families to understand, tolerate, and support the defensive use of food by the aged may reduce the need for institutional care and in some cases may even allow the institutionalized elder to be discharged and reintegrated into the family[14].

Religious beliefs are strong in this country, particularly among the elderly who frequently firmly adhere to religious food practices[13]. An aged Catholic may still insist on "meatless" Fridays even though this practice is no longer required by his church. An elderly Jew may find a cheeseburger offensive as a lunchtime selection; although he may not actively follow the strictest observance of the dietary laws, mixing meat and milk products at the same meal may be unacceptable. Food taboos, fast periods, and holidays are important religious observances that help give structure and meaning to the lives of many people, including the elderly.

Practices of folk medicine may seem absurd to health practitioners but the aged may have great faith in home remedies. The Mexican-Americans and many Latin-Americans often subscribe to the hot-cold theory of disease[13, 15, 16]. Health is conceived as a state of balance; illness is the result of an imbalance. Foods, herbs, and medications are classified as wet or dry and hot or cold. They are used therapeutically in varying combinations to restore the body's natural balance which manifests itself as somewhat wet and warm. Cold-classified illnesses are treated with "hot" medications and foods, while hot illnesses are treated with "cool" substances. Many chronic disorders are attributed to a chill or eating excessive amounts of cold-classified foods. Arthritis is cold-classified. People who believe in the hot-cold classification and who suffer from arthritis usually will not eat orange juice, bananas, raisins, and other cold-classified foods. If an elderly arthritic patient is prescribed a diuretic and told to eat potassium-rich foods (bananas, orange juice, raisins, dried fruit) to maintain potassium balance, he generally will not follow the physician's orders. If the physician is aware of the patient's folk medicine belief, he could prescribe potassium in the form of a salt substitute or in a liquid form to be taken daily. If the physician is unaware of the patient's views, treatment may be undermined by the patient's self-manipulated diet. The hot-cold classification influences the way a patient adheres to the therapeutic regimens for hypertension, colds, ulcers, constipation, and gastrointestinal problems as well as for arthritis.

SOCIOLOGY OF NUTRITION

Old age is often a time of loss—physical, economic, and social. Food and eating are intensely social functions for the aged. Thus, sociological factors cannot be overlooked when assessing the elderly for nutritional status.

Poor nutritional status is the direct result of improper food selection, but improper food selection may be caused more by a *social* problem than a *health* problem[17]. Poor nutritional status has been correlated with economic impoverishment, poor education, and *social isolation*[10, 14]. Any combination of these three factors may be associated with malnutrition in the elderly.

Many elderly persons find themselves socially isolated. A brief discussion of the two forms of social isolation follows.

Isolates

Isolates are people who live alone by choice[3]. They may experience loneliness but they are socially adjusted. Many isolates have been "loners" most of their lives. Others have lost spouses and/or friends but choose to remain independent rather than seek a roommate or live with family.

There are more residentially isolated older women than older men. This is because women live longer than men. Those women who married usually married older men, who predeceased them. Also there are fewer chances for an older women to remarry because of the unequal sex distribution among the aged. Furthermore, women tend to be more capable than men of caring for themselves and for a home, due to their life experience[3].

Even though socially adjusted, isolates may suffer from poor nutrition simply because they are not motivated to shop, cook, and eat by themselves[18].

Desolates

Desolates are those who live alone, though not by choice[3]. These people come to live alone because of the scattering and death of relatives and friends. Each loss of a companion necessitates a re-arrangement of lifestyle. If the losses are many, or rapid in succession, there are no substitutes with whom the person can form a meaningful relationship. With no replacement for family, an elderly person may soon find no people with whom friendships may be developed. The emotional upset due to lack of association with other people may manifest itself as actual pain, somatic complaint, or constant recapitulation of the past.

The desolate aged often appear eccentric[14]. Their age precludes a future, their present has little or no meaning, so they cling to the past. Grief may be a constant companion of the desolate and takes the form of chronic depression[19]. Subgroups of the aged population most at risk for desolation are women and blacks, seventy-five years old and over[3].

Other Forms of Adjustment to Old Age

In many urban settings, the environment can have a negative effect on nutritional status. Many elderly do not have the economic, physical, or psychological resources to travel the streets. Public transportation is costly, and may be inaccessible and unadapted to those with limited mobility. Most elderly persons living in urban areas have some fear of theft and violence. Consequently, they may remain locked in their apartment or home, severely restricting shopping trips, and thus drastically altering their diets both in quantity and quality[20].

Undernutrition and malnutrition can also be related to behavior status. Extreme irritability, moodiness, anxiety, and depression can lead to an inability to make proper food choices resulting in a poor nutritional state[12].

Social and psychological differences between aged men and aged women have been reported[21]. These differences need to be understood by anyone assessing nutritional needs. In response to the changes associated with aging, many women display high levels of psychological stress. Loneliness is prevalent among older women. They tend to display higher levels of anxiety, depression, and sensitivity to criticism than younger women. Even though older women usually report their retirement as "voluntary" rather than "mandatory," sociological data shows that women enjoy retirement less than men and take a longer time to adjust to it.

Men are not as likely as women to respond to aging by becoming psychologically stressed. Among older, working class men, aging brings about an acceptable disengagement, a lessened involvement with friends and organizations. Most working class men report that they enjoy retirement. They are the "rocking chair people" who find more pleasure passively observing society than actively entering into it. They feel they have earned this time to relax and be peaceful. Yet, older men eat more meals away from home than older women, making eating one of their major social events. Older men are also willing to spend more money on weekly groceries than older women, regardless of their earnings. Conversely, women spend less on weekly groceries and this amount goes down proportionately as income increases. Thus, having adequate funds to purchase food does not automatically ensure an adequate intake[18].

It has been argued that the aforementioned sex differences are due to a tendency for women to be more willing and to find it more appropriate than men to admit that they have problems[21]. Culturally, men are assigned the capable, caretaker role, therefore older men feel it is a sign of weakness to admit to problems.

The preceding information is a compilation of conclusions drawn by varied professionals—sociologists, psychologists, gerontologists, home economists, social workers, physicians, nutritionists, and others—who have worked with the aged. The nature of this material is such that it does not easily lend itself to controlled studies. However, this observational data is believed to be of value in interpreting sociological factors affecting nutritional status of the aged.

FOOD AS A POSITIVE SOCIAL FACTOR

Eating with others is an important part of life's experiences, contributing to one's sense of belonging. Part of the goal of any nutrition program for the elderly should be to keep participants socially active and psychologically healthy as well as adequately nourished[22].

In 1969, the Senate Select Committee on Nutrition and Human Needs held hearings on "Nutrition and the Aged." Commissioner John Martin of the Administration on Aging (AoA) testified. Throughout his testimony he repeatedly emphasized that malnutrition and undernutrition of older citizens must be considered in the context of interrelated economic, social, physiologic, and psychologic elements[22]. Sensitivity to these interrelated factors must be reflected in nutrition programs for the aged.

Congregate Dining

All nutrition and feeding programs established under the Older Americans Act take into account the total living conditions of the older people who are served. The Older Americans Act supported pilot projects that developed methods and techniques that not only improved the participants' diets, but also enhanced their self-esteem and self-reliance. The success of the initial demonstration projects led to the enactment, in March 1972, of the Title VII Nutrition Program for the Elderly[22].

Title VII funds aid nutrition projects that provide the elderly at least one hot meal per day plus supportive services designed to improve the quality of their lives. The project is based in a community setting which provides congregate dining for individuals sixty years and older and their spouses of any age[23]. These centers are most effective when established near the homes of the elderly or convenient to public transportation[22]. In inner-city locations, elderly living within walking distance are most likely to use the center. Projects have been set up in schools, community centers, public housing facilities, senior citizen centers, homes for the aged, and in church basements.

Whenever possible, meals are prepared in project kitchens. When adequate kitchen facilities are unavailable, meals are purchased from commercial sources. Arrangements can be made to purchase meals from a school, home for the aged, or a commercial caterer. Purchased meals are usually delivered to the site, in bulk, and subsequently portioned into individual servings. Some sites have tested the feasibility of prepackaged meals, delivered to the site in insulated individual trays[22].

Most typically, the noon meal is the one offered to the participants, but some breakfast and a few dinner projects also exist (see Figure 10-2). The meals may be served one day a week, or as frequently as six days a week, depending on the scope and resources available to the project. However, projects funded by Title VII must provide one hot meal a day, at least five days a week, to qualify for subsidies[23].

Participants pay something for their meals. This avoids offending those elderly who would be uncomfortable accepting charity. Participants regard this as a service which they are buying, and therefore avail themselves of it without any lost pride. Cost of the meal is usually a function of one's ability to pay. No one is refused participation because of inability to pay[23]. In 1977, the most

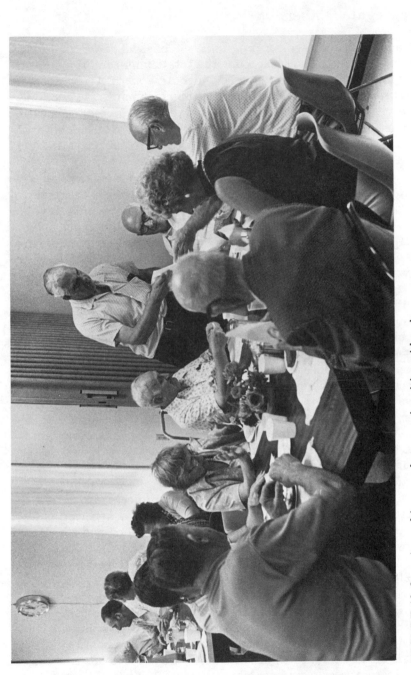

FIGURE 10-2   A meal is served at a senior citizens' lunch program.
Photo: L Miller

recent year for which statistics are available, the cost to produce a typical meal (food and nonfood) was $2.56.

Many nutrition projects use the aged participants in the meal program to help cook, set up, and serve. They may be employed full- or part-time or serve as volunteers. This increased involvement and the opportunity to earn money contributes to self-esteem and social adjustment of the participants. Most project directors enjoy the employment of senior participants since they prove to be capable and reliable employees who come with a lifetime of experience and abilities. The authors know of one case of a retired chef who was a recluse after the death of his wife until he became a cook at a senior citizen center. He went on to work, train employees, and supervise kitchen operations until his death.

Meals in all projects are planned to meet one-third of the Recommended Dietary Allowances as defined for people over age fifty-one[22]. The contribution of this one meal to the total daily intake was recently evaluated[23]. Food records showed that those eating at the meal site consumed more calories, protein, and calcium than nonparticipants and participants who did not eat at the site on the day of the record. A larger proportion of those who eat meals at nutrition sites have diets that rate good to excellent as compared to nonparticipants. Measures of "life satisfaction" and "psychological well-being" increased with the length of participation in the program.

It has been suggested that meals should be planned to provide greater than one-third of the Recommended Dietary Allowances. If a meal were planned to provide 70 percent of the individual's nutrient allowance and the person came to the program every day, one-half of the weekly nutrient needs could be obtained. Participation three times a week would ensure one-third of weekly allowances[23].

A major task of the nutrition project is to reach the socially isolated elderly in the community who most need this service. These people may need special inducements to participate[22]. Older citizens already involved in the program are most effective in recruiting other people of their age group. A sample home-delivered meal can help acquaint the uninitiated with the services and persuade them to join the group. Outreach groups, such as visiting nurses, can be helpful in acquainting the socially isolated with available services. Many centers provide transportation for those elderly who need it, and this naturally boosts participation. In 1978 there were 1,047 Nutrition Program projects serving over 383,000 meals daily. Despite the continued proliferation of programs, only a fraction of the eligible elderly have access to such a program.

Home-Delivered Meals

Delivery of meals to the homes of the handicapped and aged was one of the earliest types of feeding programs to be established. "Meals on wheels" began in England in 1939. Philadelphia became the first city in the United States to organize a "meals on wheels" program, in 1954. Currently, 15 percent of all meals served under the Title VII program are home-delivered meals to housebound elderly[24]. In addition to the federally funded Title VII "meals on wheels" programs, there are state, county, and privately operated programs as well.

Home-delivered meals provide at least one-third of the Recommended Dietary Allowances and may be adapted to suit restricted diets and, in some instances, provide Kosher meals. In addition to meeting nutritional needs, home-delivered meals help meet the social needs of the aged as well. Many meal recipients have no visitors except the volunteer deliverer who comes daily or five times a week. The volunteer provides social contact and often becomes friends with the aged recipient. In the case of temporary disability, the positive social contact resulting from the "meals on wheels" program may interest the older person in joining the congregate meals program at a local site. In the case of chronic disability, home-delivered meals may enable the individual to continue living independently and forestall institutionalization.

Many programs attempt to serve more than one meal daily. They deliver a hot lunch and leave a light supper that is cold or needs only simple heating, such as a canned main dish. Other programs deliver a hot dinner and leave sandwiches for the following day's lunch.

In order to close the significant service gaps that exist in congregate dining and home-delivered meals programs the National Aeronautics and Space Administration (NASA) was asked to use its food technology to develop a convenient, economical, shelf-stable meal system for the homebound elderly[25]. The meals were to be pleasant tasting, easily transportable, shelf-stable, and require few utensils and minimal skills to prepare. If successful, this meal system could be used when congregate or home-delivered meals are not available.

A test of the NASA program in Texas showed very favorable results, with 77 percent of the participants reporting that they "liked the program very much"[26]. The system consists of a complete meal, including main dish, fruit, vegetable, dessert, and beverage packed in one box. The meals are made up of canned, dehydrated, and freeze-dried foods, eliminating the need for refrigeration. Seven meal boxes, a week's supply, are then packed into a larger carton for delivery to the participant's home. The larger box weighed ten pounds or less when fully packed and was designed so that the mail might be used as a means of delivery in outreach areas.

The pilot project confirmed that the NASA meal system was feasible from the standpoint of user acceptability, nutritional adequacy, and cost. The meals are not yet available from retail stores but can be directly mail-ordered from a food manufacturer in Oregon. (Oregon Freeze Dry Foods, Inc., Albany, Oregon, has developed *Easy Meal* under their Mountain House label.)

Institutional Care

An elderly person with a chronic illness or degenerative disease may spend weeks, months, or the remainder of his life in a healthcare facility. Loss of independent living is a devastating event that may manifest itself in depression and anger with staff, relatives, and friends feeling the brunt of these emotions. Many individuals withdraw from personal interaction, some so completely that they may attempt suicide. For many, the regulated, routinized, impersonal environment of the health-care facility is more like a prison than their "home"[19].

There are varying types of facilities available to the aged: *medically-oriented nursing homes*, for those who require professional round-the-clock medical supervision; *health-related facilities*, for ambulatory patients who need minimal medical care but who require a caretaker for activities of daily living; and *housing facilities or proprietary homes* for those who need housekeeping and food service but are otherwise independent. No elderly person should ever be placed in a facility with *more* care provided than they need since this will often make them more dependent on others than is necessary.

It has been reported that female nursing home residents who are dissatisfied with their lives also have poor appetites[11]. They showed lower-than-normal caloric-nutrient intakes for all nutrients except ascorbic acid. If emotions are able to affect attitudes toward meals, they will thus ultimately affect general health.

Little research has been done to document the therapeutic value of a dining room in geriatric living facilities, but staff observations point toward positive effects[27]. Mealtimes become a high point in the day. Residents dress rather than spend the day in robe and slippers when a community meal is taking place. Socialization activities may evolve around meals with residents congregating in living areas for an hour or more before mealtime, waiting for the dining room to "open." Less meal-skipping and reduced plate waste have also been reported when common dining rooms are used. Complaints about food are common in all healthcare facilities but tend to occur less frequently in facilities that use dining room meal service.

Complaints regarding food service can be handled in a manner to encourage participation in group feeding. Setting up a resident's food committee to answer complaints has proven to be effective. If members of the dietary staff are present in the dining room at mealtime to answer questions and converse with residents, meals are more positively accepted. Homestyle or waitress service reduces plate waste when compared to preportioned tray service. Even disoriented residents who observed other people eating became more aware of their surroundings and in some cases began to participate in self-feeding[27]. In one reported case, the dietary supervisor established kitchen tours to prove that food was prepared on-site in a clean, well-equipped kitchen with quality food products. After most of the residents had seen the kitchen, food service complaints fell off markedly.

Geriatric Daycare

A newer concept in care for the elderly is day care, which is far less expensive than institutional care. A 1975 survey estimated that between 14 and 25 percent of all institutionalized elderly are in facilities providing more care than needed[28].

Under day care plans, participants spend the day in a program designed to serve the elderly through social and physical rehabilitation, dietary counseling, and recreational services. The participants return home at night.

All day care facilities provide a minimum of one meal a day, supplying at least one-third of the Recommended Dietary Allowances. Many programs also offer a mid-morning and mid-afternoon snack. If the day care center is located within a longterm care facility, day care participants can eat in a congregate dining room and may even be provided with individually modified diets.

Home aides may provide a type of day care in the person's home which is less structured than the aforementioned[29]. These aides help the older person perform tasks he would do for himself if he were able. Tasks include housecleaning, meal planning and preparation, grocery shopping, assisting with personal care and exercising, and reading to, and writing for the older person. Home aides are often used when an aged person has returned home after hospitalization to reduce further institutionalization during the recuperation phase of illness. Experience with this type of day care seems to indicate that it is most useful and effective for women and non-stroke patients. Men are probably less adaptive to this type of care since they have had little experience directing someone else to do homemaking tasks.

MENTAL DISORDERS

There is a wide range of disordered behavior that is frequently lumped under the category of "senility"[19]. Organic disorders as well as functional disorders occur in old age and both can affect a person's health and nutritional status.

The two main causes of chronic organic brain syndrome are senile deterioration and cerebral arteriosclerosis. Organic disorders are most frequently seen in nursing home patients. Some estimate 55 to 80 percent of all such patients have these disorders[30]. Cerebral arteriosclerosis usually starts before age sixty-five and is often referred to as the "small stroke syndrome," leaving residual damage ranging from slight to severe. Senile deterioration is an insidious process which occurs in later life and causes patchy sclerosing of brain tissue. Both conditions result in irreversible brain damage.

Depression, a functional disorder, is often viewed as a characteristic of senescence or is confused with organic disorders and consequently overlooked[19]. If a patient is ill, depression may be assumed to be part of the reaction to illness. Conversely, it may be the depression that caused the illness. It has been shown that a great number of significant life changes within a given year correlate well with a major health change the following year[31]. Loss of a spouse is the most devastating event that can occur, with widowers coping less effectively than widows. A cluster of life changes (loss of spouse, adjustment to living alone, change of residence) often immediately precedes an illness. Death, rather than coming on unpredictably in life, may follow a major life crisis[32].

Death due to depression is a real occurrence, as evidenced by the high rate of suicide among depressed, elderly, white males[33].

Depression in elderly males often reflects itself in self-aggressive, self-destructive actions. Elderly depressed women become more emotionally detached and attempt manipulative behavior. Attempted suicides by elderly women are often for manipulative rather than self-destructive purposes.

Depression in the elderly must be recognized and treated in order to stop the downward spiral of the individual's clinical state[12]. If neglected, a vicious cycle can be established and lead to apathy, isolation, poor nutrition, neglect of physical health, further depression symptomatology, and, eventually, death.

The incidence of depression in persons over age sixty-five is 8-15 percent in the general population and up to 50 percent in nursing home patient populations[12]. Most of these depressed aged also show some negative symptoms such as insomnia, anorexia, and weight loss and some behavioral disturbances such as isolation, apathy, compulsive or hostile behavior[19].

Depression frequently causes anorexia with subsequent weight loss resulting in a state of undernutrition. Undernutrition is an inadequate intake of food or an incorrect choice of food, or both. This food deprivation exaggerates the depressive behavior and may lead to a clouding of consciousness and a general state of confusion and disorientation. If allowed to proceed uninterrupted, it will lead to starvation and death[12].

Undernutrition caused by depression can be associated with many factors such as grief, social isolation, alcoholism, psychosis, poverty, and poor state of health[12].

Grief may be a constant companion to the elderly. Even people who have successfully "rolled with the punches" throughout life discover that old age can deal blows too cruel and swift to overcome. Chronic grief takes on the form of chronic depression. The elderly person often feels cheated and will often manifest these feelings in delusions about robberies or thefts. The aged begin to hold on to food and priceless objects and may insist on having them ever-present, carrying them from place to place in shopping bags. This clinging to inanimate objects is understandable in light of the ever-increasing losses the elderly person experiences. Food may be hoarded rather than eaten, and this may result in undernutrition which is clearly undesirable[14].

Depression can be causative in alcohol abuse. Elderly alcoholics are often undernourished. They will normally spend money on alcohol while neglecting food. When food is eaten, it often is of the high carbohydrate-high calorie variety resulting in minimal intakes of protein, vitamins, and minerals[12].

The psychotic elderly may refuse to eat because of delusions that the food is poisoned or crawling with insects. Hallucinations of voices may also caution against eating[19].

Overnutrition can be a direct result of depression. To cope with grief, loneliness, and feelings of helplessness, some elderly eat to reduce their anxiety and obtain comfort[12]. Some elderly eat excessively to induce sleep. Even the impoverished aged can become overweight. These people are in a paradoxical situation. They are overweight and undernourished at the same time. They often purchase "comforting" foods (candy, cake, desserts) that are high in calories but low in nutrients, leaving them deficient in protein, vitamins, and minerals. The resultant overweight condition may put the elderly at greater risk for the development of cardiovascular disease and diabetes, both of which have significant mortality rates among the aged.

PHYSICAL DISABILITIES

Since illness and physical impairment increase with age, so, predictably, does disability and limitation of activity. Of all persons sixty-five and over living outside of an institution, 85 percent reported at least one chronic disease and approximately 50 percent reported limitation in normal activity due to chronic health conditions[31].

Malnutrition and undernutrition of the elderly handicapped are major problems that must be solved[34, 35, 36, 37, 38]. Preparing, serving, and eating meals can be a major chore for the older homemaker who is handicapped. Arthritis, partial paralysis, impaired vision, and other physical conditions can make the activities of daily living unpleasant endurance events. Still, a handicap should not signal the end of independent living. When a person has a disabling physical condition, tasks must be simplified and wasted motions eliminated. One should let dishes drain dry instead of wiping them, use precut onions, peppers, and vegetables and other foods to eliminate peeling, chopping, and slicing. One should also adapt favorite recipes for convenience foods that require less physical energy to prepare and eliminate all unnecessary lifting. Instead of sliding, one should roll objects on a wheeled cart. Every task must be reduced to its essential motions[35].

Easy-open packages and flip-top cans are of no convenience to an arthritic person with limited strength or joint movement. The arthritic homemaker will tire easily and should plan activities in small sessions. One should never start a job that cannot be stopped in the middle for a rest. It makes sense to sit while doing kitchen work and use only light-weight utensils[35]. For mixing and stirring, large spoons are more easily held and reduce the stress on the hands that comes from grasping a small object. The arthritic person must learn to use the whole hand rather than just fingers to perform many tasks. Stirring can be accomplished by holding the handle of a spoon or fork between the flat palms of two hands. The heels of the hands can be used to apply pressure to package seals, such as on a milk container, to open them[35].

A stroke or surgery may result in the loss of the use of part or all of one arm. If the cause is hemiplegia—paralysis of one side of the body—this may be accompanied by loss of perception and a decreased power of quick mental recall. People with such losses must be taught to turn their heads to compensate for their visual field limitations. These people have lost sight on one side of the visual field and if they do not turn their heads to scan the entire countertop occasionally, things can be overlooked. In food preparation, an ingredient may be omitted because it cannot be seen.

To better understand this handicap, hold your hand up and out alongside your face. Now look down; on one side there will be peripheral vision but on the other side, the one that is blocked, vision is limited only to that which is immediately in front of the line of vision. Side vision is not possible without turning the head.

When a stroke results in aphasia (partial or full loss of the power of expression by speech, writing, or signs, or loss of comprehension of spoken or written language) the person must be taught to plan activities and repeat them over and over again. Easy-to-prepare foods and one-dish meals must be used. Keeping the preparation procedures the same for each meal helps to avoid confusion and frustration. Recipes such as the one presented in Figure 12–4 (see Chapter 12) make use of a repetition of skills and can be used to help reestablish the habits of meal preparation.

Hemiplegia makes relearning mealtime tasks difficult, causing the loss of the ability to stabilize food, a pot, or bowl while cooking[38]. New ways of keeping food or utensils from moving or sliding must be learned. The weak arm may be able to help if it is given some support. Holding it in a sling reduces the fatigue of holding the arm up and allows the hands and fingers to hold items. A cutting board with two stainless steel nails hammered through can secure food for cutting or peeling. A wet facecloth or spongecloth under a bowl can anchor it so it will not spin during mixing. Knees can help hold packages as they are opened or unwrapped. The knee-grasp technique works well for almost all packages other than glass screw-top jars. However, jars can be opened with one hand by putting the jar in a drawer, leaning the hip against the drawer to hold the jar securely, and twisting the top off with the free arm. Kitchen tongs work better than a fork or spoon for turning or lifting food during cooking. It is useful to place a heat-proof pad on the counter next to the range. To remove a pot from the range, it can be slid from the range to the counter to avoid lifting. It is easy to use a pitcher to fill an empty pot already on the range or have an extra-long hose attached to the sink sprayer arm, so the pot can be filled directly from the faucet. As with the arthritic patient, lightweight utensils will be the easiest and safest to use[35].

The only time an elderly person will benefit from the use of heavy utensils is when a person suffers from incoordination such as that found in Parkinson's disease[35,38]. This older patient will need to have a great deal of patience in order to complete even the simplest task. The weight of a heavy utensil will help to control excessive motion. Double-handle construction will allow one to grasp and move utensils more securely. Using many of the stabilizing techniques of a hemiplegic and resting both elbows on the counter surface during work will allow for more control.

An older person confined to a wheelchair may find the ordinary home kitchen full of architectural barriers[36]. It may be impossible to maneuver around opened cabinet doors, counters may be too high, faucets too far away to reach, burners on the range are at eye level, a clumsy and dangerous height. Architectural changes will need to be made before this person can live independently again. Today, some of the cost of training, rehabilitating, and purchasing equipment for the handicapped can be provided through local and state departments of vocational rehabilitation. Homemaking is the largest single occupation of the physically handicapped and since 1955 the disabled homemaker has qualified for state and federal funds[38].

SELF-HELP EATING DEVICES

Mealtime is more pleasant and enjoyable when a person can feed himself independently and without embarrassment. Feeding aids may be useful in assuring the independence of the older person who is having trouble handling regular utensils[34, 35].

A built-up handle on a standard eating utensil may be all that is needed to provide a secure grasp for impaired hands. Utensils of this special type can be purchased or a regular eating utensil can be adapted by slipping a foam rubber curler over the handle. The foam surface of the curler increases friction and aids in the maintenance of a steady grasp. These curlers are inexpensive and available in drug and variety stores. Handles may be angled or bent to compensate for limited motion, and a collar or band may be attached to the end of the handle which fits over the person's hand to help prevent the utensil from being dropped.

Plastic and metal plate guards and plates with rims enable the person to pick up his food by first pushing it against the raised edge. A suction cup or sponge cloth under the plate can keep the dish in place while the person is eating.

A spouted cup, extended straws, and pedestal cup can aid in drinking liquids. A two-handled drinking cup is especially useful for older persons with incoordination. Stretch terry cloth glass covers designed for use on cold drink glasses provide a secure grasp when holding a glass. These are available where picnic supplies are sold or can be hand-knit or crocheted. To hold a straw steady and in place, a pen clip can be attached to a cup, and the straw threaded through where the pen was originally held[27]. The *spork,* a combination of fork and spoon, often serrated down one edge, can replace three utensils for a person who has the use of only one hand.

The elderly blind can make use of many of these feeding aids. The lipped plate on which food is placed in a prescribed clockwise fashion is often used to train the blind to feed themselves.

Figures 10–3(a), (b), (c), and (d) show a variety of these eating aids. It is important to remember that the ability to feed oneself is a most important factor in feeling independent. It is uncomfortable, humiliating, and embarrassing for an older person to be fed, and every effort should be made to encourage self-feeding. When necessary, eating devices should be provided and the person taught to use them effectively[27, 35].

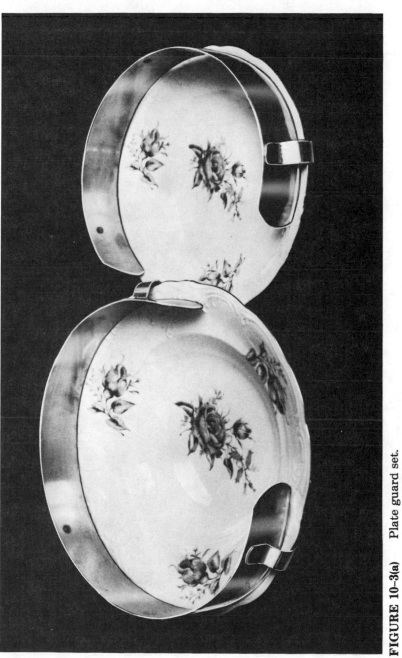

FIGURE 10-3(a)   Plate guard set.

Source: Reprinted by permission of © J. A. Preston Corp., 1978.

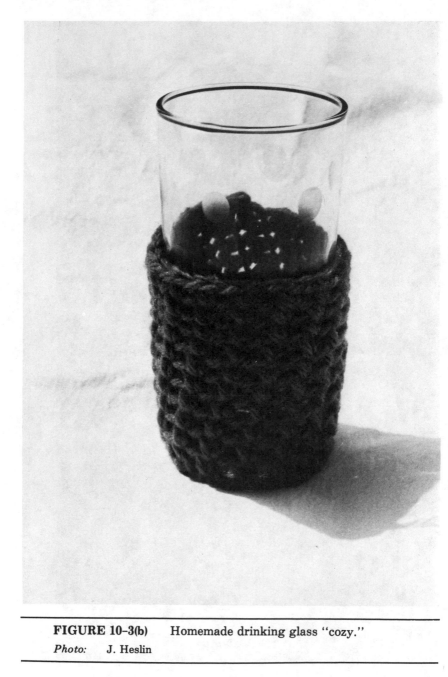

FIGURE 10–3(b)   Homemade drinking glass "cozy."
Photo: J. Heslin

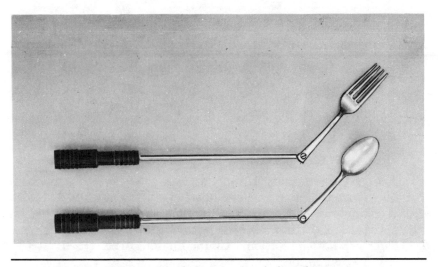

FIGURE 10–3(c)   Angled extension fork and teaspoon.

Source: Reprinted by permission of © J.A. Preston Corp., 1978.

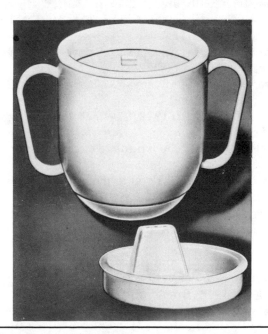

FIGURE 10–3(d)   Twin-handled spouted drinking cup.

Source: Reprinted by permission of © J.A. Preston Corp., 1978.

CITED REFERENCES

1. The graying of every 10th American or every 9th American, taken from *Part I Development in aging: 1977.* 1978. Washington: US Government Printing Office.
2. Harris, C. S. 1978. *Fact book on aging: A profile of America's older population.* National Council. Aging, Inc. 1828L Street, N.W., Washington, D.C.
3. Troll, L. E. 1971. Eating and aging. *J. Am. Diet Assoc.* 59:456.
4. Harris L. Pres. Louis Harris and Associates. 1974. Who the senior citizens really are. Speech presented at Annual Meeting of National Council on the Aging, Oct. 2, 1974, Detroit, Michigan.
5. Fowles, D. G. 1977. Income and poverty among the elderly. *CNI Weekly Newsletter* 8(24):4.
6. Palmore, E. 1978. Are the aged a minority group? *J. Amer. Geriatrics Soc.* 26(6):214.
7. Brotman, H. B. March 1972. The fastest growing minority: The aging. *Family Economics Review* p. 10.
8. Chappelle, M. 1972. The language of food. *Amer. J. of Nursing* 72(7): 1294.
9. Todhunter, E. N. 1972. Food is more than nutrients. *Food and Nutrition News* 43(6–7):1.
10. Sherwood, S. October 1973. Sociology of food and eating: Implications for action for the elderly. *Am. J. Clin. Nutri.* 26:108
11. Harrill, I.; Erbes, C.; and Schwartz, C. 1976. Observations on food acceptance by elderly women. *Gerontologist* 16(4):349.
12. Garetz, F. K. 1976. Breaking the dangerous cycle of depression and faulty nutrition. *Geriatrics* 33:73.
13. Howell, S. C., and Loeb, M. B. 1969. Nutrition and aging, chapter III, culture, myths and food, preferences among aged. *Gerontologist* 9(3):66.

14. Weinberg, J. April 1972. Psychologic implications of the nutritional needs of the elderly. *J. Am. Diet Assoc.* 60:293.
15. Currier, R. L. 1966. The hot-cold syndrome and symbolic balance in Mexican and Spanish-American folk medicine. *Ethnol.* 5:251.
16. Harwood, A. 1971. The hot-cold theory of disease implications for treatment of Puerto Rican patients. *J. Amer. Med. Assoc.* 216(7):1153.
17. Hanson, G. 1978. Considering "social nutrition" in assessing geriatric nutrition. *Geriatrics* 33:49.
18. Brown, E. L. 1976. Factors influencing food choices and intake. *Geriatrics* 31:89.
19. Epstein, L. J. 1976. Symposium on age differentiation in depressive illness, depression in the elderly. *Journal of Gerontology.* 31(3):278.
20. Bengtson, V. L., and Haber, D. 1976. Social forces and aging individuals: An overview. In *Nursing and the aged,* ed. I. M. Burnside. New York: McGraw-Hill Book Co.
21. Atchley, R. C. 1976. Selected social and psychological differences between men and women in later life. *J. of Gerontology* 31(2):204.
22. Pelcovits, J. 1971. Nutrition for older americans. *J. Amer. Dietetic Assoc.* 58(1):17.
23. Kohrs, M. B.; O'Hanlon, P.; and Eklund, D. 1978. Title VII–nutrition program for the elderly. *J. Amer. Dietetic Assoc.* 72:487.
24. Lawmakers plan new funding for the elderly. 1978. *Institutions* 82(4).
25. Delicious hot meals without cooking. 1978. *Food Engineering* 50:ef–22.
26. Rhodes, L. 1977. NASA food technology, a method for meeting the nutritional needs of the elderly. *The Gerontologist* 17(4):333.
27. Rankin, G. 1975. The therapeutic value of a dining room program in a geriatric setting. *J. Gerontological Nursing* 1(3):5.
28. O'Brien, C. L. 1977. Exploring geriatric day care: An alternative to institutionalization. *J. of Gerontological Nursing* 3(5):26.
29. Neilson, M., et al. 1972. Older persons after hospitalization: A controlled study of home aide service. *Amer. J. of Public Health* 62(8):1094.
30. Schwab, M. 1973. Caring for the aged. *Amer. J. Nursing* 73(12):2049.

31. Shanas, E., and Maddox, G. L. 1977. Aging, health and the organization of health resources. In *Handbook of the psychology of the aging,* eds. J. E. Birren and J. E. Schaie. New York: Van Nostrand Reinhold Co.

32. Rahe, R. H.; McKean, J. D.; and Arthur, R. J. 1967. A longitudinal study of life change and illness patterns. *J. Psychosomatic Research* 10:355.

33. Latorre, R. A., and McLeoad, E. 1978. Machiavellianism and clinical depression in a geriatric sample. *J. Clin. Psychology* 34(3):659.

34. Klinger, J. L.; Frieden, F. H.; and Sullivan, R. A. 1970. *Mealtime manual for the aged and handicapped,* New York: Essandes Special Editions, Simon and Shuster, Inc.

35. Klinger, J. L. 1978. Mealtime manual for people with disabilities and the aging. Camden, New Jersey: Campbell Soup Corp.

36. Agan, T., et al. 1977. Adjusting the environment for the elderly and the handicapped. *J. Home Economics* 69(5):18.

37. Green, K. B. 1978. Coping daily with the handicapped and the elderly. *J. Home Economics* 70(40):15.

38. Rusk, H. A. 1970. Nutrition in the fourth phase of medical care. *Nutrition Today* 5:24.

OTHER REFERENCES

Kuhn, M. 1978. Insight on aging. *J. Home Economics* 70(40):18.

Lee, R. J. 1976. Self images of the elderly. *Nursing Clinics of North America* 11(1):119.

Lewis, C. 1978. *Nutrition: Nutritional consideration for the elderly.* Philadelphia: F.A. Davis Company.

Montgomery, J. E. 1978. Quality of life for the aging, home economics role. *J. Home Economics* 70(40):12.

‖‖ 11

Nutrition Education in Later Years

Nutrition education has been defined as a means of accomplishing "the control of health insofar as it is affected by the food we eat." It is hoped that with nutrition education, people will make rational decisions about food so that all will enjoy a wide variety of food, eaten healthfully and moderately[1]. With this goal, nutrition education is more than an isolated learning experience, it is an ongoing, lifelong process. Hopefully, the process is initiated in the cradle and is continued throughout life.

Most educators feel that children's habits are the most easily modified. Although one is never too old to learn, a person with a history of sixty, seventy, or eighty years of established eating habits will often be more resistant to change and the change may take longer to accomplish than in a younger person. However, modification of food habits *is possible* at any stage in the life cycle[2].

Nutrition education programs specifically designed for the elderly are new in concept. The Older Americans Act (Public Law 92–258), amended in 1972, clearly established nutrition education for the elderly as a primary goal[3]. Unfortunately this well-intentioned law has not had the impact that was originally hoped simply because the elderly have not been responsive to established modalities for the presentation of nutrition information.

Many things must be considered when planning a nutrition education program for the older person. First and foremost, established, lifelong food preferences must be respected[4]. Food habits are a link with one's culture, youth, family, and religion. A well-planned program of education will never attempt to reeducate the elderly to a new style of eating but rather will attempt to modify existing habits and present new combinations that will meet nutritional needs and satisfy established food preferences.

The paramount concern of most older people is the maintenance of good health. They value their independence and fear any illness that may cause them to be handicapped, homebound, or institutionalized. An astute nutrition educator can use this concern to advantage by promoting the axiom that proper nutrition is essential to good health[4]. The elderly will be far more receptive to new ideas if they feel that such acceptance will help keep them well and living independently.

An important, but often overlooked, fact is that the elderly do not constitute a homogeneous group[4]. Quite the contrary, as the only thing many members of an elderly group have in common is their age. Therefore, the successful nutrition educator must know the group he is working with: who they are, how they live, what their past eating habits constitute, and their educational level. The more the educator knows about the needs of a particular group, the more useful and meaningful the educational program will be.

The realities of living conditions must be considered before a suitable and useful educational program can be planned. For each individual, it must be determined if food preparation is possible, if there is adequate money to purchase food, and if the individual lives alone[4]. Teaching a group of older people about the advantages of cooking food in batches and freezing the food in single portions for future use is ludicrous if most of the audience does not have a freezer. Often the nutrition educator is disheartened because a well-planned and well-presented topic was poorly received by an elderly group largely because the presentation concerned practices that were too expensive or otherwise unrealistic for the group members.

It has been stated that the elderly frequently have a negative attitude toward attempts at nutrition education[4]. This perception of a negative attitude and lack of motivation to learn is most often a misinterpretation of what is actually a reaction to the manner in which the material is presented. Some of the nutrition education material used for the aged seems to have been prepared for young children with only the titles changed. It is true that older adults have slower reaction times, may speak and move less quickly, and may take longer to perceive a thought than younger adults, but elderly people are definitely not children. They are demeaned when subjected to simplistic audiovisuals and when they are spoken to as if they were children.

In 1977, 47 percent of the aged in America had not completed one year of high school. Nine percent, or 2.2 million, were "functionally illiterate" (having less than five years of schooling)[3]. Nutrition education programs have often been presented in an oversimplified manner so as to ensure that even the most poorly educated, psychologically "slow" individuals would be reached. What the educator has often failed to recognize is that what the aged lack in physical capabilities and education they partially make up for in "life experience." Anyone who has survived for six, seven, or eight decades has accumulated a body of practical knowledge to use in solving problems. The nutrition educator should use this knowledge and experience as the basis for new learning and should encourage the elderly to rely heavily on what they already know to help them find workable solutions to existing problems[5].

Poor attendance at nutrition information sessions is a problem. The aged have a number of reasons why they cannot attend. "They tell me I can't eat things I like." "I can't hear what they say." "They lecture during lunch when I want to talk to my friends." Listening carefully to these excuses will provide clues to some of the problems that need to be solved by the effective educator[4,5,7].

The following sections will deal in depth with changes that occur with aging that influence learning. It is important to recognize that the onset of age as well as the rate of decline of functions differs markedly among the elderly[5], and the suggestions that are presented should serve as guidelines rather than absolute rules.

CHANGES THAT AFFECT LEARNING

Vision

With advanced age, a yellowing of the lens of the eye occurs that may prevent older people from discriminating between colors that are similar in hues. The discrimination between blue, blue-green, and violet may be particularly difficult. When visuals are employed, they should be colored in different and distinct colors, especially if a colored bar graph is shown. One should try to avoid the use of shadings of color[5]. For example, color shadings are often used in certain tests, such as the urine test for the presence of sugar. The older person with a visual problem could easily misinterpret the results of such a test.

Visual acuity also declines with age, making the perception of detail increasingly difficult. Visuals should be planned that are uncluttered so that the details of the picture or graph do not blur into each other. The important figures in the visual should be large and distinctively outlined. Projected images from films, filmstrips, and opaque projections may prove to be more frustrating than instructive to older people[5].

Prior to an audiovisual presentation, the educator can also gently remind those in the group who wear glasses to put them on to be sure that they will not miss anything. An older person who just started to wear glasses may often forget when to wear them.

Audition

As with vision, there is a loss of auditory sensitivity that occurs with age. The older person suffers high tone hearing loss accompanied by poor discrimination of consonants, particularly s, z, t, f, and g. The inability to clearly hear phonetically similar words may cause difficulty in following normal conversation[5]. Noisy settings make it even harder to perceive sounds clearly and rapid speech reduces intelligibility[4,5].

Therefore, when teaching older adults, auditory implications must be considered. It is important never to exceed a normal word rate (140 words/minute). Background noise such as the clattering of dishes should also be avoided. It is also important to position the speaker in front of the group and minimize the movement of the speaker[5]. A lecturer who paces back and forth before the group will find his aged audience having difficulty grasping his material because the sound of his voice is constantly moving.

The speaker must be alert to nonverbal clues that the audience is having difficulty. A person may lean forward, cup his ear, or turn his "good ear" to the speaker. Other older persons will look directly at the speaker's mouth and not divert their eyes while he is talking. They are lipreading, using their visual sense to compensate for their impaired-auditory sense[5]. A speaker should always ask the group whether he is speaking too softly, too fast, or too indistinctly. Checking with the audience two or three times during the presentation is wise to be sure the rate and level of sound remain constant.

Intelligence

Verbal abilities and the ability to store and recall information show little change, if any, in the elderly. Psychomotor skills do depreciate with age. An older person's intelligence is often underestimated because his loss of audition makes him appear "slow"[5].

Aged adults do have longer reaction times and appear to need more time to process information than do younger adults. Some research indicates further that older people also have increased error proneness[5]. However, most elderly function quite efficiently in real situations. It has been suggested that this actual efficiency is due to the role of experience in compensating for biological changes in mental capacity.

When teaching older adults, particular attention should be paid to the age composition of the group. The pace of discussion that is satisfactory for individuals in their sixties might be too rapid for an eighty-year-old. The slow rate needed by the eighty-year-old may prove annoying and boring to the sixty-year-old[6]. The best retention of information occurs when the learning can be self-paced. Visual aids and tapes that can be operated at varying paces by the aged person have a marked advantage over presentations paced to accomodate an entire group[5].

Memory

Memory is a multifaceted function. Research suggests that the memory function begins to decline in the late thirties and forties and continues until senility. Short-term memory is the least effective as a person grows older. Short-term memory appears to be the least effective when distractions are present at the time material is presented[5].

The most effective teaching–learning situation is one that is arranged in a setting with a minimum of simultaneous activity and background noise[5]. The extraneous noise in the lunchroom of a senior citizen center makes this setting inappropriate for learning[2,4]. Although group learning has many advantages for the older adult, in some cases the activity of a group of people may produce too many competing inputs to permit effective learning. The type of learning most appropriate for an audience must be carefully evaluated[8]. With an extremely old population, small groups of four to six people may prove less distracting, and result in greater retention of material.

Other Factors Related to Learning

Many individual and situational variables may influence the elderly's ability to learn: motivation, life experience, education, ethnic background, religion, socioeconomic status, and condition of health[5,9]. The importance of some or all of these cannot be ignored. They must be considered as variables in an effective teaching–learning situation.

THE LEARNING
ENVIRONMENT

Nutrition education should be initiated as part of the regular routine of a group meals program[2] or incorporated into any group activity that routinely has aged participants: YMCA-YWCA, church or temple groups, auxilliaries, community education programs, neighborhood associations.

Sessions should be held at least once a week, preferably at the same hour and day each week. Experience has shown that just before or after lunch is the best time. Mid-afternoon sessions inevitably have poor attendance as many older people enjoy an afternoon nap. Sessions should never be held during lunchtime itself, since the noise and activity will make the learning ineffectual and prevent vital socialization with others during the meal[2].

Older people tire easily. Sessions of thirty minutes to an hour are sufficiently long, and it is important to avoid letting sessions run overtime. The elderly find this stressful and will become anxious and frustrated, reducing the effectiveness of the teaching. To avoid this stress, it is important to adjourn the session on time and invite any who wish further information or have questions to remain afterwards.

The most effective nutrition education programs actively involve the elderly in the planning, directing, and carrying out[2]. Often, a nutrition committee is formed to coordinate the nutrition education program (see Figure 11–1). The nutrition educator serves primarily as a source of guidance and expertise.

The elderly should be able to formulate the list of topics to be pursued[4,6]. The nutrition educator then directs and coordinates the activities. For example, rather than lecture on the merits and drawbacks of the use of convenience foods, the educator can set up a tasting session. The group might be given assignments to buy convenience foods that can be used by a diabetic or a person on a low sodium diet or to show how a TV dinner can be complemented to provide complete nutrition. The items are then prepared for tasting. The vast array of new and convenience foods can be bewildering. Guidance in the selection and appropriate use of suitable convenience foods can lead to a good discussion[2].

One of the main purposes of nutrition education for the elderly is to help them make wiser food selections[6]. An unstructured, informal discussion session often allows the educator to impart a great deal of information that would be difficult to organize into a lecture format[4]. The elderly, by asking questions, find the information more meaningful because by taking part in a dialogue, they are more likely to feel they are learning what they want to know. In a lecture situation, the audience is passive[6]. The discussion format allows for greater and more active involvement and usually results in better retention of material.

The educator should never lose sight of the fact that the older person is a voluntary participant in the nutrition education program[6]. He has decades of living and eating experience behind him. He is not a young, impressionable student and will find little or no interest or value in learning about vague concepts or generalizations regarding nutrition. He will be most interested in nutrition information that has immediate usefulness and application[2].

A recent survey determined those topics which would be of most value and interest to an elderly population[6]. Of the thirty-one topics identified, the following ten topics were the ones in which the elderly had the greatest interest.

1. Cooking for one

2. Shopping for one

3. Thrifty use of leftovers

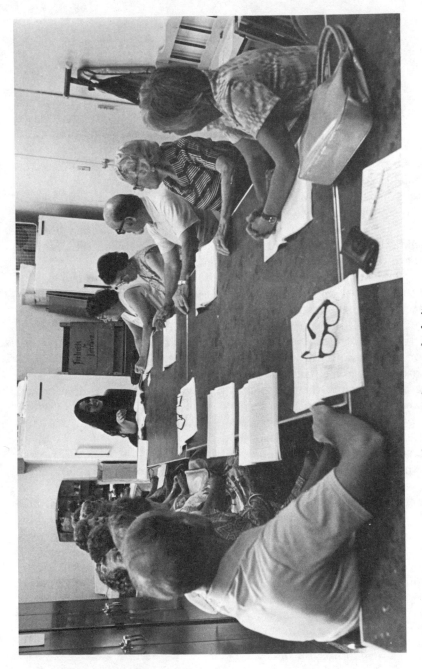

FIGURE 11-1 A nutrition committee meeting at a feed site.

4. Using color and flavor garnishes in meals

5. Nutritious between-meal snacks

6. Knowledge about brand names

7. Preparing a cookbook for senior citizens

8. What supermarket shopping means to the senior citizen

9. Quick tricks with soup, chowders, and stews

10. Ways to economize on the use of meat, poultry, and fish

Once the needs of the group have been established, the first nutrition education session will be the most important. The topic of discussion should be specific, and the material to be presented should be carefully planned and the session thoroughly publicized[4].

	Can a Coupon Clipper Really Save Money?
Nutrition Education Class	Nutrition Education Class
11:30 A.M.—Tuesday	11:30 A.M.—Tuesday
West Patio	West Patio
Everyone Welcome	Everyone Welcome
POOR PUBLICITY	GOOD PUBLICITY

The first session may be poorly attended. However, even if only three or four people attend, the program should be conducted with as much enthusiasm as if the room were filled. If the participants enjoy the session, the attendance will gradually increase. Whenever possible, at least one appropriate handout should be provided for each session. It may summarize in a few sentences key points of the session and can be reproduced in an inexpensive form such as by a ditto machine. If the material is typed, all capital letters should be used as well as double or triple spacing wherever possible. The elderly will place more value on what is learned if they have something to take home with them from the session. These handouts can be a link between sessions, providing a quick review of what was learned last session at the beginning of each new session. This review and recall of the past material helps to reinforce the learning. The group might even decide to compile a nutrition information handbook containing all the handouts provided, adding their own hints, experience, and recipes.

NUTRITION EDUCATION MATERIALS

As was mentioned above, nutrition education for the elderly has only recently been given attention; consequently, teaching aids are limited[6,10]. Appendix 2 provides a list of printed materials that may prove useful. Although most of these booklets were developed for an aged audience, few are in large type. Appendix 3 lists some audiovisuals produced for the aged themselves and others designed to be used to educate those who work with the aged.

The paucity of visual materials should stimulate more educators to produce their own audiovisual aids[6]. This can become a group project, and the use of local people and local scenes adds a dimension that commercially produced audiovisuals lack. Attendance at nutrition education sessions may increase as the curious come to see if they are featured in a given day's showing. Very little investment is needed to produce a good slide presentation[6]. The following equipment is necessary:

1. 35 mm camera (an inexpensive instamatic camera can be used)

2. flash attachment

3. four or five rolls of 35 mm slide film

4. slide projector

5. screen (a white or light-colored wall, or sheet tacked to the wall, can be used)

One of the participating senior citizens may be an amateur photographer. A committee of elderly can take the pictures, write the script, and even present the slide program. By involving the elderly in the preparation of the visuals, the concepts to be learned will be continuously reinforced during the process of producing the visual aid.

Figure 11-2 (pp. 235-238) shows a sample slide production, "Rules to Shop By," developed at the New England Gerontology Center[6]. The left hand column is a suggested script. The right hand column suggests the type of pictures to take.

Visual aids not specifically produced for an aged population can still be used with an older group. However, before any visual is

Rules to Shop By: A Sample Slide Presentation

Suggested Script	*Title and/or Scene*
1. A food dollar is *precious*. Used *wisely*, it will bring food to your table that is not only attractive and tasty but can help you become the energetic and *healthy* individual you want to be.	PICTURE OF MONEY
2. To get "more for less" calls for penny-pinching with know-how. A little knowledge about how to shop with careful *planning* can do much to insure that you get the best value for your dollar when you shop for food.	FOOD IN ARMS OF OLDER PERSON
3. "Shopping is an art" says Bess Myerson, New York City's Director of Consumer Affairs. "You have to do your homework. You cannot go totally unprepared. The more you know, the more you can save.	"THE MORE YOU KNOW, THE MORE YOU CAN SAVE"
4. The first rule for shopping is to purchase food from a prepared list.	"SHOP FROM A LIST"
5. Plan your meals (in writing) for 2 or 3 days or a week. This will help you avoid impulse buying when you get to the store.	PICTURE OF SHOPPING
6. Keep a memo pad handy in the kitchen; when you run low on a food item, jot it down.	HAND WITH PENCIL IN KITCHEN
7. The second rule to shop by is to check newspaper ads.	"CHECK NEWSPAPER ADS"
8. The good buys are in big type. The great ones are heralded as if they were the second coming.	NEWSPAPER AD #1 NEWSPAPER AD #2
9. Compare prices of similar items and add these sale items to your shopping list.	PAD IN HAND, NEWSPAPER IN BACKGROUND
10. Take advantage of "cents off" coupons, but don't buy a product if you don't need it.	PICTURE OF COUPONS

(continued)

Rules to Shop By: Continued

Suggested Script	*Title and/or Scene*
11. If there is more than one supermarket in your community, learn from experience, friends, and by comparing ads in the various stores. . .	PICTURE OF SUPERMARKET #1
12. . . .of which ones consistently have the lowest prices. If you have the energy, shop in several stores for the best prices.	PICTURE OF SUPERMARKET #2
13. As a general rule, small neighborhood grocery stores have higher prices, but may offer services which the larger supermarkets cannot. For example:	PICTURE OF NEIGHBORHOOD STORES
Deliveries......................	BOY CARRYING BAGS
Ethnic foods...................	IMPORTED FOODS
Convenience...................	WOMAN WALKING TO URBAN STORE
14. When you go to the market, start early. Stores are generally less crowded in the mornings. Be prepared with your shopping list. Check to be sure you have your glasses.	WOMAN WALKING INTO A STORE
15. Select a cart that rolls and steers easily.	WOMAN PUSHING CART
16. Buy foods in season. In-season sales are better for the budget than out-of-season temptations.	"BUY FOOD IN SEASON" PICTURE OF PRODUCE SALE
17. Besides being reasonably priced, in-season foods are at their peak of quality—but don't forget, buy only the quantities you need.	PICTURE IN PRODUCE AISLE
18. Shop for variety	"SHOP FOR VARIETY"
19. Instead of having mashed potatoes day after day, have them baked, boiled, oven-browned, or scalloped. Don't forget sweet potatoes.	WOMAN SELECTING SWEET POTATOES
20. If you are in the rut of only eating the "good old standby's" of peas and carrots, treat yourself to broccoli, whole beets, lima beans, asparagus, squash, brussel sprouts.	WOMAN SELECTING FRESH BROCCOLI

(continued)

Rules to Shop By: Continued

Suggested Script	Title and/or Scene
21. Variety makes meals interesting and increases the chances that you will meet your body's need for the various nutrients.	PICTURE OF SHOPPING CART FILLING UP
22. Another rule is to eat whole grain breads.	"SELECT WHOLE GRAIN BREADS."
23. Rye, pumpernickel and whole wheat specialty breads have a taste edge over the white breads besides having those extra vitamins.	SPECIALTY BREADS
24. While smaller loaves may cost more than large loaves, they may be a better buy if you cannot eat a larger loaf before it goes stale.	WOMAN SELECTING BREAD
25. Don't overlook biscuits and muffins for variety.	PICTURE OF VARIETY AT THE BREAD COUNTER
26. The next rule is "Don't be bashful, Demand Service."	"DEMAND SERVICE"
27. Ask the supermarket staff any questions that occur to you. . .	WOMAN ASKING FOR HELP HOLDING A PKG. OF 4 PORK CHOPS
28. . . .if you need one pork chop, a 1/2 lb. of ground beef or only a few potatoes, ask to have the product repackaged. . .	BUTCHER HANDING PKG. OF ONE PORK CHOP TO WOMAN
29. Many stores already provide this service for their customers.	SHOW MEAT PKG. FOR ONE IN CASE.
30. The next rule is to compare prices.	"COMPARE PRICES"
31. Bargain-hunt like mad. If you have unit pricing in your area (it is spreading fast), be sure to use it as a guide.	SHOW UNIT PRICING STICKER
32. The next rule is to shop for store brands.	"SHOP FOR STORE BRANDS"
33. Most chain stores have their own brands, which are cheaper than nationally advertised ones. . .	SHOW NATIONAL AND STORE BRANDS SIDE BY SIDE

(continued)

Rules to Shop By: Continued

Suggested Script	Title and/or Scene
34. . . .compare prices. Don't be totally loyal to one brand. If you can get another brand of similar quality at a lower price, buy it.	TOP VIEW WITH DIFFERENT PRICES
35. Another rule is to buy only the quantities you need.	"BUY ONLY THE QUANTITIES YOU NEED"
36. Avoid impulse buying. Resist the unplanned "extras" that can run up your bill and may add little food value to meals.	"AVOID IMPULSE BUYING." PICTURE IN POTATO CHIP AISLE
37. Avoid those foods that are high in sugar, fat, or salt content. Go easy on soft drinks, cake, and pastry items. . .	SOFT DRINK AISLE
38. . . .these products are expensive when you consider their low nutritional value.	CANDY AISLE
39. In place of those high sugar-fat-salt snacks, select fruit juices, dairy products and fresh fruit and vegetables. . .	V-8 JUICE IN SMALL CANS
40. . . .when chilled, they make a wonderful mid-afternoon or evening pick-me-up.	PLATE OF FRESH FRUIT GLASS OF MILK AND COOKIES
41. Buy only enough food which you can carry home safely.	WOMAN CARRYING A SMALL BAG
42. Watch the cash register as the cashier rings up your purchases. His mistakes cost *you* money!	WOMAN AT CHECK OUT COUNTER
43. To make mealtime more enjoyable, invite a friend over to dinner.	"INVITE A FRIEND TO DINNER." MAN AND WOMAN HAVING DINNER

FIGURE 11-2   Sample slide production, describing a suggested script and accompanying slides, appropriate as a visual aid in nutrition education for the elderly.

Source: Reprinted with permission from Joseph Carlin, *Serving the Elderly, The Technique Part IV: Nutrition Education for the Older American,* pp. 12–14, Chapter IV, Published by the New England Gerontology Center.

used it should be previewed and evaluated for usefulness[8] with the following criteria in mind:

Is the content accurate?

Is the material presented appropriate for the educational and economic level of the group?

Is the background music disruptive to the narration?

Is the narrative clear and moderately paced?

Are the visuals clear, distinct, and in sharp contrasting colors?

Is the concept to be learned clear and reinforced throughout the visual?

Is visually depicted printed material large, clear, and distinctively outlined from the background?

Is the viewing length short to moderate?

USING TELEVISION FOR NUTRITION EDUCATION

In one study, the elderly were asked to identify sources of nutrition information which had been most helpful to them in the past. In descending order, those most frequently mentioned were: television, physicians, magazine articles, and cookbooks[9]. The potential effectiveness of television as a tool for disseminating nutrition information should be considered, particularly for the homebound who are unable to participate in group nutrition education programs[11,12].

Watching television is a popular leisure activity of the elderly, with news and information shows leading the list of preferred programs[11]. This fact is borne out with the popularity of "Over Easy," a half-hour television show funded through the Older Americans Act. Begun in late 1977, the show currently has two million viewers each day and is aired on 254 public broadcasting stations. No other program, public or commercial, is aired on that many networks[3]. The sheer number of people that can be reached through television must be considered and nutrition educators should not hesitate to contact local television stations to explore the possible use of this medium to present nutrition information[13].

The Federal Communications Commission, which issues licenses to radio and television stations, requires that the media give noncommercial interests access to a designated amount of free air time. This means that nonprofit, tax-exempt groups (social, educational, religious, civic, and charitable) are eligible to use free air time to publicize activities[13].

The days and times allowed for public service announcements (PSAs) vary from station to station but can be determined by a telephone call to local stations in an area. Most PSAs are brief, varying in length between 10–60 seconds. A basic PSA includes *who, what, where, when,* and *why* plus important names and, when necessary, a telephone number. This information is submitted, typed, to the public service director at each station. Advanced planning is necessary so the station may reserve an appropriate time slot for the PSA[13].

One study that explored the use of PSAs and the elderly found that these announcements were most useful in providing publicity for a nutrition program, offering further sources of nutrition information, or providing money-saving tips. However, the PSAs had no measurable impact on the eating behavior of the elderly subjects studied[11]. Perhaps the short time span of the PSAs is an inappropriate tool to use for conveying general nutrition messages. However, the usefulness of television as a nutrition education tool has not been fully explored, so further research is needed.

NUTRITION EDUCATION PROGRAMS

Nutrition education programs for the elderly can be established by a legislative mandate, as was the case with the Older Americans Act, Title VII, Nutrition Program for the Elderly in 1972[3,4,6]. Alternatively, nutrition education programs can be loosely organized informal programs, established at the local level[7,11]. The main purpose of nutrition education for the elderly is to influence them to make better decisions regarding their food selections and meal patterns. Almost any method that achieves this end should be considered valid. The following is a brief discussion of some model approaches to nutrition education for the older person.

A vegetable garden project can be started to communicate nutrition knowledge and consumer economics. The elderly provide the know-how—many were raised in rural settings or grew Victory Gardens during World War II. The local Cooperative Extension Service can provide information for inexperienced gardeners, and local service groups or commercial companies are sources for available land plots. It should be noted that *eligible food* under the Food Stamp Act includes seeds and plants for use in gardens to produce food for personal consumption[6].

Food cooperatives have been established primarily to fight inflation but can also serve as a vehicle for nutrition education. The elderly retired, with substantial amounts of free time, can organize and operate a cooperative that can service any interested families or individuals in a given area. Along with lower prices and the availability of fresher produce, a nutrition educator can use the co-op site for informal classes, cooking demonstrations, and sample taste-tests of unusual foods[6]. Often, an organization of interested members can evolve these informal classes into regular sessions on food economics and nutrition education. The weekly market order sheet can carry buying tips, recipes, and nutrition facts. Using the elderly members to organize and run the cooperative gives them a sense of usefulness and purpose and provides a setting in which they can rejoin the mainstream of community activity.

Printed materials on food and nutrition are available for distribution to the public[14]. This readily available information can be easily adapted to the needs of the elderly and incorporated into newsletters and newspapers published just for this group[15].

Sunkist Growers, Inc. has begun a newspaper called *Happiness Is* to provide nutrition, health, and food information to the senior citizen. Many state, county, and local groups serving the elderly put out periodicals and would welcome articles of interest to their readers. Often daily and weekly newspapers have a regular column or section devoted to activities and interests of the elderly members of the community who make up part of their readership. The nutrition educator should contact such newspapers to see if nutrition articles could be featured in this section.

Finally, nutrition education for the elderly can be achieved indirectly. Instead of teaching the elderly themselves, programs can be set up to educate those who deal with the elderly. An excellent example of how this can be accomplished is in educating local restaurant owners to adapt their menu selections to fit the restrictions of modified diets[16,17]. With slight, easily-managed variations, many menus can be adapted to meet the needs of cardiac patients, diabetics, hypertensives, weight-watchers, and others. The special menus might include a section like the following:

On a special diet? Tell your waiter and don't hesitate to request:

skim milk

low-salt soup

low-salt salad dressing

margarine made with liquid vegetable oil

decaffeinated coffee

low-cholesterol salad dressing

water-packed fruits

See our special diabetic luncheon plate and the low-fat sandwich selection featured today.

Additional patrons mean greater profits so the restaurant owner will be motivated to adapt the menu if the variations are simple and not costly. The elderly, many of whom must eat their meals in restaurants because of lack of cooking facilities, will be more likely to follow their diet restrictions if an eating establishment encourages them to do so. The menu also serves as a reminder of their necessary diet modifications and encourages the elderly to continue to make rational decisions about food, which is the ultimate goal of nutrition education.

CITED REFERENCES

1. Hill, M. M. 1976. Nutrition education. *Nutrition Program News*, U.S. Dept. of Agriculture.
2. Hill, M. M. 1972. Modification of food habits. *Food and Nutrition News* 44(1–2):1.
3. *A report of the Special Committee on Aging, United States Senate, Part I. Developments in aging: 1977.* 1978. Washington: U.S. Government Printing Office.
4. Pelcovits, J. 1973. Nutrition education in group meals for the aged. *J. Nutrition Education* 5(2):118.
5. Hallburg, J. C. 1976. The teaching of aged adults. *J. of Gerontological Nursing* 2(3):13.
6. Carlin, J. M. *Nutrition education for the older american, serving the elderly, the technique Part 4.* Durham, New Hampshire: New England Gerontology Center.
7. Pao, E. M., and Hill, M. M. 1974. Diets of the elderly, nutrition labeling and nutrition education. *J. Nutrition Educ.* 6(3):96.
8. Hicks, B. M. 1977. Selecting educational materials—Part I. *Food and Nutrition News* 49(1):3.
9. Grotkowski, M. I., and Sims, L. S. 1978. Nutritional knowledge, attitudes and dietary practices of the elderly. *J. Amer. Dietetic Assoc.* 72:499.
10. *Nutrition Education Materials.* 1977. Washington, D.C.: The Nutrition Foundation, Inc.
11. Fitzgibbons, J. J., and Garcia, P. A. 1977. TV. PSAs, nutrition and the elderly. *J. Nutrition Educ.* 9(3):114.
12. Welczuk, P. 1973. The Senior Chef. *J. Nutrition Educ.* 5:142.
13. Nutrition in the news: A communications manual. The Potato Board, 1385 South Colorado Blvd., Suite 512, Denver, Colorado 80222.
14. Virginia Council on Health and Medical Care. 1978. *Nutrition education for the elderly,* Richmond, Virginia.
15. Leonard, B. B. 1978. Small newspaper builds older americans network. *Community Nutrition Institute Weekly Report* 8(11)4.

16. Holmberg, R. 1978. Nutrition in neon, Part II: Cash in on diet menus. *Institutions* 82:118.
17. Scott, L. W., et. al. 1979. A low cholesterol menu in a steak restaurant. *J. Amer. Dietetic Assoc.* 74(1):54.

||||||||||||||||||||||||||||||||||||||||||| 12

Appropriate Food Selection

During older adulthood, one's food selection may change drastically. A couple in their forties is often actively raising a family at a time when they have reached the peak of their earnings. Their meals are large, and they spend liberally on food each week. Enormous quantities of food are bought each week and stored in the house, especially if growing adolescents are at home. These adolescent children, however, grow to young adulthood and depart for college, career, or marriage, leaving behind a household composed of two mature adults who require far less food per meal and each week than does an active family. Retirement years are approaching for the members of the two-person household, and a retirement income, regardless how liberal, usually means reduced spending power.

In the elderly, chronic health problems may appear, heart disease, diabetes, arthritis, and obesity often imposing diet modifications on the family's food selection. The loss of a spouse leaves the survivor a single person household. The widower may never have shopped, stored, or prepared food. His spending power may remain constant after his wife's death but his practical knowledge of food and nutrition may be sketchy or nonexistent.

A widow may be a more competent homemaker. Her income, however, may be cut drastically; monthly social security payments may prove to be her only source of income, if she does not receive benefits from her husband's pension. Her weekly food budget will reflect her lowered income. She will have to learn to make lower cost food selections and many of her favored items may disappear from her weekly shopping list.

It is obvious that during older adulthood both food selection and food budgets will undergo many changes as family size and spending power decrease. It is wise, therefore, for both husband and wife to be knowledgeable about budgeting, shopping, and preparing food.

BUDGETING

With continued inflation and the escalating food prices of the 1970s, few consumers purchase food without forethought. Food budgets, even flexible ones, are a fact of life.

The United States Department of Agriculture (USDA) has developed Family Food Plans to serve as guides for estimating food needs and food costs for individuals and families[1]. Food plans have been in existence for more than 40 years and are revised periodically, the last revision having been done in 1974. Originally there were three food plans—"low cost," "moderate cost," and "liberal." An "economy" food plan was instituted at the inception of the Food Stamp Program. In January 1976, this economy food plan was replaced by a "thrifty" food plan[2]. The thrifty plan offers an assortment of food which very closely approximates average food consumption of families who spend limited amounts on food.

The food plans list amounts of foods of different types that a family should use to provide nutritious diets for the family members at the four different levels of cost. Tables 12-1, 12-2, 12-3, and 12-4 present the USDA Family Food Plans based on estimated cost per week for food at the four levels. It must be noted that the food plans were developed for individuals in a model four-person family. To use these plans for budgeting with the aged, who generally have smaller households, the following adjustments are necessary: one person—add 20 percent; two persons—add 10 percent; three persons—add 5 percent.

The nutritional basis for the food plans is the 1974 Recommended Dietary Allowances (RDA). If followed carefully, the plans will provide adequate amounts of energy, protein, calcium, iron, vitamin A, thiamine, riboflavin, niacin, and ascorbic acid for all age/sex groups. Fat will comprise no more than forty percent of the food energy.

Low-cost food plan: Amounts of food for a week[1]

Family member	Milk, cheese, ice cream[2]	Meat, poultry, fish[3]	Eggs	Dry beans and peas, nuts[4]	Dark-green, deep-yellow vegetables	Citrus fruit, tomatoes	Potatoes	Other vegetables, fruit	Cereal	Flour	Bread	Other bakery products	Fats, oils	Sugar, sweets	Accessories[5]
	Qt	Lb	No.	Lb	Lb	Lb	Lb	Lb	Lb	Lb	Lb	Lb	Lb	Lb	Lb
Child:															
7 months to 1 year	5.70	0.56	2.1	0.15	0.35	0.42	0.06	3.43	0.71*	0.02	0.06	0.05	0.05	0.18	0.06
1–2 years	3.57	1.26	3.6	.16	.23	1.01	.60	2.88	.99*	.27	.76	.33	.12	.36	.68
3–5 years	3.91	1.52	2.7	.25	.25	1.20	.85	2.95	.90	.30	.91	.57	.38	.71	1.02
6–8 years	4.74	2.03	2.9	.39	.31	1.58	1.10	3.67	1.11	.45	1.27	.84	.52	.90	1.43
9–11 years	5.46	2.57	3.9	.44	.38	2.13	1.41	4.81	1.24	.62	1.65	1.20	.61	1.15	1.89
Male:															
12–14 years	5.74	2.98	4.0	.56	.40	1.99	1.50	3.90	1.15	.67	1.88	1.25	.77	1.15	2.61
15–19 years	5.49	3.74	4.0	.34	.39	2.20	1.87	4.50	.90	.75	2.10	1.55	1.05	1.04	3.09
20–54 years	2.74	4.56	4.0	.33	.48	2.32	1.87	4.81	.93	.71	2.10	1.47	.91	.81	2.11
55 years and over	2.61	3.63	4.0	.21	.61	2.38	1.72	4.92	1.02	.62	1.73	1.23	.77	.90	1.16
Female:															
12–19 years	5.63	2.55	4.0	.24	.46	2.17	1.17	4.57	.75	.63	1.44	1.05	.53	.88	2.44
20–54 years	3.02	3.21	4.0	.19	.55	2.34	1.40	4.17	.71	.55	1.31	.94	.59	.72	2.13
55 years and over	3.01	2.45	4.0	.15	.62	2.54	1.22	4.57	.97	.58	1.24	.86	.38	.64	1.11
Pregnant	5.25	3.68	4.0	.29	.67	2.80	1.65	4.99	.95	.66	1.52	1.06	.55	.78	2.56
Nursing	5.25	4.16	4.0	.26	.66	2.99	1.67	5.33	.78	.61	1.55	1.16	.76	.91	2.70

[1] Amounts are for food as purchased or brought into the kitchen from garden or farm. Amounts allow for a discard of about one-tenth of the *edible* food as plate waste, spoilage, etc. Amounts of foods are shown to two decimal places to allow for greater accuracy, especially in estimating rations for large groups of people and for long periods of time. For general use, amounts of food groups for a family may be rounded to the nearest tenth or quarter of a pound.

[2] Fluid milk and beverage made from dry or evaporated milk. Cheese and ice cream may replace some milk. Count as equivalent to a quart of fluid milk: Natural or processed Cheddar-type cheese, 6 oz.; cottage cheese, 2 1/2 lbs.; ice cream, 1 1/2 quarts.

[3] Bacon and salt pork should not exceed 1/3 pound for each 5 pounds of this group.

[4] Weight in terms of dry beans and peas, shelled nuts, and peanut butter. Count 1 pound of canned dry beans—pork and beans, kidney beans, etc.—as .33 pound.

[5] Includes coffee, tea, cocoa, punches, ades, soft drinks, leavenings, and seasonings. The use of iodized salt is recommended.

*Cereal fortified with iron is recommended.

TABLE 12-1 The USDA Low-cost Family Food Plan.

Source: Peterkin, B. "USDA Family Food Plan, 1974," *Family Economics Review,* Agricultural Research Services, USDA, Winter 1975.

Moderate-cost food plan: Amounts of food for a week[1]

Family member	Milk, cheese, ice cream[2] Qt	Meat, poultry, fish[3] Lb	Eggs No.	Dry beans and peas, nuts[4] Lb	Dark-green, deep-yellow vegetables Lb	Citrus fruit, tomatoes Lb	Potatoes Lb	Other vegetables, fruit Lb	Cereal Lb	Flour Lb	Bread Lb	Other bakery products Lb	Fats, oils Lb	Sugar, sweets Lb	Accessories[5] Lb
Child:															
7 months to 1 year	6.46	0.80	2.2	0.13	0.41	0.49	0.06	3.98	0.64[6]	0.02	0.06	0.05	0.05	0.19	0.08
1–2 years	4.04	1.69	4.0	.15	.29	1.24	.59	3.44	1.03[6]	.26	.81	.33	.12	.28	.79
3–5 years	4.74	1.88	3.0	.22	.30	1.46	.85	3.51	.74	.27	.82	.73	.41	.81	1.42
6–8 years	5.79	2.60	3.3	.34	.37	1.94	1.17	4.39	.84	.39	1.14	1.11	.56	1.03	1.97
9–11 years	6.68	3.31	4.0	.38	.45	2.61	1.40	5.76	1.03	.51	1.47	1.51	.66	1.31	2.63
Male:															
12–14 years	7.02	3.77	4.0	.48	.48	2.44	1.52	4.66	.94	.56	1.69	1.54	.85	1.34	3.65
15–19 years	6.65	4.65	4.0	.29	.47	2.73	2.00	5.45	.80	.67	1.98	1.82	1.05	1.15	4.41
20–54 years	3.38	5.73	4.0	.29	.59	2.92	1.94	5.93	.76	.65	1.97	1.65	.95	.96	2.95
55 years and over	2.97	4.64	4.0	.19	.70	2.91	1.69	5.88	.89	.53	1.58	1.45	.87	1.05	1.50
Female:															
12–19 years	6.22	3.32	4.0	.24	.53	2.62	1.21	5.38	.68	.56	1.34	1.22	.56	.97	3.36
20–54 years	3.35	4.12	4.0	.19	.62	2.84	1.35	4.94	.54	.49	1.28	1.08	.65	.81	2.89
55 years and over	3.35	3.21	4.0	.14	.72	3.09	1.17	5.50	.81	.52	1.20	.98	45	.73	1.39
Pregnant	5.44	4.57	4.0	.25	.91	3.52	1.60	6.13	.73	.83	1.77	1.28	.46	.85	3.50
Nursing	5.31	5.01	4.0	.26	.91	3.76	1.73	6.52	.74	.81	1.84	1.42	.69	1.00	3.79

[1]Amounts are for food as purchased or brought into the kitchen from garden or farm. Amounts allow for a discard of about one-sixth of the *edible* food as plate waste, spoilage, etc. Amounts of foods are shown to two decimal places to allow for greater accuracy, especially in estimating rations for large groups of people and for long periods of time. For general use, amounts of food groups for a family may be rounded to the nearest tenth or quarter of a pound.

[2]Fluid milk and beverage made from dry or evaporated milk. Cheese and ice cream may replace some milk. Count as equivalent to a quart of fluid milk: Natural or processed Cheddar-type cheese, 6 oz.; cottage cheese, 2 1/2 lbs.; ice cream, 1 1/2 quarts.

[3]Bacon and salt pork should not exceed 1/3 pound for each 5 pounds of this group.

[4]Weight in terms of dry beans and peas, shelled nuts, and peanut butter. Count 1 pound of canned dry beans—pork and beans, kidney beans, etc.—as .33 pound.

[5]Includes coffee, tea, cocoa, punches, ades, soft drinks, leavenings, and seasonings. The use of iodized salt is recommended.

[6]Cereal fortified with iron is recommended.

TABLE 12-2   The USDA Moderate-cost Family Food Plan.

Source: Peterkin, B. "USDA Family Food Plan, 1974," *Family Economics Review*, Agricultural Research Services, USDA, Winter 1975.

Liberal food plan: Amounts of food for a week[1]

Family member	Milk, cheese, ice cream[2]	Meat, poultry, fish[3]	Eggs	Dry beans and peas, nuts[4]	Dark-green, deep-yellow vegetables	Citrus fruit, tomatoes	Potatoes	Other vegetables, fruit	Cereal	Flour	Bread	Other bakery products	Fats, oils	Sugar, sweets	Accessories[5]
	Qt	Lb	No.	Lb	Lb	Lb	Lb	Lb	Lb	Lb	Lb	Lb	Lb	Lb	Lb
Child:															
7 months to 1 year	6.94	0.97	2.3	0.14	0.43	0.60	0.06	4.71	0.64*	0.02	0.05	0.06	0.05	0.20	0.09
1–2 years	4.26	2.07	4.0	.17	.31	1.50	.59	4.10	1.07*	.28	.82	.35	.13	.27	.95
3–5 years	5.08	2.35	3.1	.23	.32	1.77	.85	4.18	.76	.27	.79	.78	.45	.85	1.74
6–8 years	6.25	3.18	3.4	.36	.40	2.35	1.18	5.21	.85	.39	1.08	1.23	.60	1.08	2.41
9–11 years	7.21	4.04	4.0	.39	.48	3.15	1.41	6.83	1.04	.51	1.39	1.67	.71	1.38	3.21
Male:															
12–14 years	7.57	4.57	4.0	.50	.51	2.94	1.52	5.52	.95	.56	1.60	1.71	.92	1.40	4.47
15–19 years	7.18	5.59	4.0	.31	.50	3.29	2.01	6.45	.84	.69	1.92	2.05	1.07	1.20	5.36
20–54 years	3.64	6.83	4.0	.32	.62	3.51	1.95	6.99	.79	.66	1.91	1.86	.95	1.00	3.54
55 years and over	3.24	5.54	4.0	.19	.76	3.52	1.68	6.97	.89	.54	1.49	1.57	.94	1.09	1.82
Female:															
12–19 years	6.72	3.97	4.0	.25	.56	3.15	1.21	6.34	.71	.59	1.31	1.35	.54	.98	4.09
20–54 years	3.62	4.86	4.0	.20	.66	3.41	1.35	5.81	.56	.51	1.24	1.22	.66	.84	3.47
55 years and over	3.65	3.79	4.0	.15	.76	3.71	1.14	6.42	.74	.54	1.17	1.12	.48	.77	1.66
Pregnant	5.91	5.43	4.0	.26	.96	4.22	1.57	7.17	.70	.87	1.70	1.45	.46	.87	4.20
Nursing	5.76	5.97	4.0	.28	.97	4.51	1.72	7.66	.75	.84	1.76	1.58	.68	1.02	4.52

[1]Amounts are for food as purchased or brought into the kitchen from garden or farm. Amounts allow for a discard of about one-fourth of the *edible* food as plate waste, spoilage, etc. Amounts of foods are shown to two decimal places to allow for greater accuracy, especially in estimating rations for large groups of people and for long periods of time. For general use, amounts of food groups for a family may be rounded to the nearest tenth or quarter of a pound.

[2]Fluid milk and beverage made from dry or evaporated milk. Cheese and ice cream may replace some milk. Count as equivalent to a quart of fluid milk: Natural or processed Cheddar-type cheese, 6 oz.; cottage cheese, 2 1/2 lbs.; ice cream, 1 1/2 quarts.

[3]Bacon and salt pork should not exceed 1/3 pound for each 5 pounds of this group.

[4]Weight in terms of dry beans and peas, shelled nuts, and peanut butter. Count 1 pound of canned dry beans—pork and beans, kidney beans, etc.—as .33 pound.

[5]Includes coffee, tea, cocoa, punches, ades, soft drinks, leavenings, and seasonings. The use of iodized salt is recommended.

*Cereal fortified with iron is recommended.

TABLE 12-3   The USDA Liberal Family Food Plan.

Source: Peterkin, B. "USDA Family Food Plan, 1974," *Family Economics Review,* Agricultural Research Services, USDA, Winter 1975.

Thrifty food plan: Amounts of food for a week[1]

Family member	Milk, cheese, ice cream[2] Qt	Meat, poultry, fish[3] Lb	Eggs No.	Dry beans and peas, nuts[4] Lb	Dark-green, deep-yellow vegetables Lb	Citrus fruit, tomatoes Lb	Potatoes Lb	Other vegetables, fruit Lb	Cereal Lb	Flour Lb	Bread Lb	Other bakery products Lb	Fats, oils Lb	Sugar, sweets Lb	Accessories[5] Lb
Child:															
7 months to 1 year	4.95	0.39	1.2	0.15	0.41	0.55	0.09	2.49	1.02[a]	0.02	0.08	0.04	0.04	0.19	0.05
1–2 years	3.30	.83	3.3	.17	.22	.89	.65	2.26	1.02[a]	.31	.78	.24	.11	.30	.37
3–5 years	3.54	.95	2.5	.28	.20	.92	.88	2.28	1.03	.37	.94	.53	.38	.74	.59
6–8 years	4.22	1.27	2.4	.49	.22	1.10	1.23	2.50	1.12	.62	1.42	.79	.51	.94	.84
9–11 years	4.92	1.61	3.4	.53	.28	1.52	1.48	3.38	1.34	.81	1.82	1.10	.60	1.20	1.10
Male:															
12–14 years	5.18	1.79	3.6	.67	.33	1.45	1.59	3.30	1.22	.81	2.07	1.13	.77	1.21	1.45
15–19 years	5.08	2.35	4.0	.43	.32	1.70	2.10	3.43	.98	.99	2.36	1.46	1.00	1.05	1.73
20–54 years	2.57	3.03	4.0	.44	.39	1.80	2.02	3.69	.89	.92	2.29	1.33	.95	.86	1.24
55 years and over	2.37	2.45	4.0	.25	.51	1.85	1.75	3.77	1.09	.80	1.90	1.12	.79	.94	.73
Female:															
12–19 years	5.35	1.80	3.8	.28	.42	1.74	1.22	3.61	.72	.76	1.49	.84	.51	.74	1.36
20–54 years	2.81	2.41	4.0	.27	.52	1.86	1.51	3.39	.90	.67	1.41	.67	.57	.57	1.18
55 years and over	2.85	1.84	4.0	.19	.60	2.02	1.26	3.73	1.12	.68	1.30	.58	.37	.45	.66
Pregnant	5.25[7]	2.69	4.0	.42	.56	2.17	1.89	4.03	1.13	.58	1.41	.66	.59	.58	1.48
Nursing	5.25[7]	3.00	4.0	.38	.57	2.36	1.92	4.27	.98	.63	1.56	.82	.80	.75	1.54

[1]Amounts are for food as purchased or brought into the kitchen from garden or farm to prepare all meals and snacks for the week. Amounts allow for a discard of about 5 percent of the edible food as plate waste, spoilage, etc.

[2]Fluid milk and beverage made from dry or evaporated milk. Cheese and ice cream may replace some milk. Count as equivalent to a quart of fluid milk: Natural or processed Cheddar-type cheese, 6 oz.; cottage cheese, 2 1/2 lbs.; ice cream or ice milk, 1 1/2 quarts; unflavored yoghurt, 4 cups.

[3]Bacon and salt pork should not exceed 1/3 pound for each 5 pounds of this group.

[4]Weight in terms of dry beans and peas, shelled nuts, and peanut butter. Count 1 pound of canned dry beans—pork and beans, kidney beans, etc. Count 1 pound of dry beans and peas, shelled nuts, etc.—as .33 pound.

[5]Includes coffee, tea, cocoa, soft drinks, punches, ades, leavenings, and seasonings.

[a]Cereal fortified with iron is recommended.

[7]For pregnant and nursing teenagers, 7 quarts is recommended.

TABLE 12-4   The USDA Thrifty Family Food Plan.

Source: The Thrifty Food Plan, Consumer and Food Economics Institute, Agricultural Research Services, USDA, Sept. 1975.

During the second half of life, a couple might make use of any one of the four cost levels appropriate to their family's income. The liberal plan provides for a greater variety of food, more expensive choices within the groups, and a larger use of animal products, fruits, and vegetables. A greater allowance for food waste is also assumed for the liberal plan. The moderate-cost plan allows for meals of more variety, more meat, vegetables, and fruit, and less home preparation than does the low-cost plan. It also provides for more frequent purchases of higher-priced cuts of meat and out-of-season foods. The low-cost plan calls for the use of smaller amounts of foods, especially milk, cheese, ice cream, meat, poultry, fish, fruit, vegetables (other than potatoes), and bakery products. In the low-cost plan it is assumed the consumer will select the lower cost foods within a food group—ground meat rather than steak, bread rather than pastry. This plan stresses the use of larger amounts of cereal, flour, bread, and dried beans. These foods are filling, inexpensive sources of calories, and important as sources of iron and B vitamins[1].

The lowest-cost food plan is the thrifty food plan. Prior to 1974, the estimated cost of this plan was 80 percent of the low-cost plan. Its cost basis is no longer dependent on the low cost food plan. Compared to the low-cost plan, the thrifty plan includes less milk, cheese and ice cream, meat, dried peas and beans, fruits and vegetables (except potatoes), and bakery products. The amount of eggs allowed in one week is the same as the low-cost plan, while quantities of cereal, flour, bread, fats, and oils are increased[3].

In addition to the USDA's Family Food Plans, the United States Department of Labor provides information on budgeting for retired couples[4]. The Department of Labor defines a retired couple as a husband over sixty-five years of age and his wife, both of whom are self-supporting, in reasonably good health, and living in an urban area. Table 12–5 gives figures provided by the U.S. Department of Labor for a suggested budget of a retired urban couple at three different levels of living. These levels of living can coincide with the use of the food cost plans proposed by the USDA at the low cost, moderate, and liberal levels.

The greatest portion of money available to a retired couple is spent on food and housing. The percentage spent on these increases as income decreases. It must be noted that in 1977, the U.S. poverty threshold was $3,417 per couple per year, and $2,720 per person per year. One-seventh or 3.3 million elderly in the U.S. have incomes below these official poverty thresholds. With such meager incomes,

	Lower Budget	*Moderate Budget*	*Higher Budget*
*Total Budget**	$5,031	$7,198	$10,711
Food	30.5%	28.2%	23.8%
Housing	34.7%	35.0%	36.7%
Transportation	6.7%	9.1%	11.3%
Clothing	4.3%	5.0%	5.1%
Personal care	2.9%	3.0%	2.9%
Medical care**	12.5%	8.8%	5.9%
Other family consumption	4.2%	4.8%	6.4%
Other items	4.3%	6.0%	7.6%

*Because of rounding, sums of individual items may not equal 100%.

**The autumn 1977 cost estimates for medical care contain preliminary estimates for "out-of-pocket" costs for Medicare.

TABLE 12-5   Annual budgets for retired urban couples at three income levels, 1977.

Source: Adapted from "Summary of annual budgets for a retired couple at three levels of living, urban, U.S.," Autumn 1977, U.S. Department of Labor.

they cannot meet the expenditures of the lowest budget suggested by the Bureau of Labor Statistics.

Many older people fail to realize that they can stretch their limited budget by the use of USDA Food Stamps. The purchasing power of Food Stamps is greater than the price paid for them. Eligibility for Food Stamps is based on monthly net income and is revised periodically[5]. In 1978, a household with one adult was eligible for assistance if the monthly income did not exceed $277. In a household of two people, the maximum allowable monthly income was $363.

Complete information on the USDA Food Stamp Plan is available at local welfare offices. However, a person who is eligible for the benefits of the Food Stamp Plan need not be on welfare. Older Americans often do not avail themselves of participation in the Food Stamp Program because it reminds them of the dole of the Depression years. Senior citizens' groups frequently conduct drives to inform the elderly about Food Stamps and recruit their participation in the program.

MARKETING

Consumer studies have shown that half the food items bought on a weekly shopping trip are bought on impulse and 65 percent of all grocery shopping is done after 4:30 P.M. (i.e., when the consumer is either hungry or tired). These and many other poor shopping practices can be wasteful of food dollars[5,6]. A typical large chain supermarket may stock over 10,000 items, a staggering amount to select from. Temptation awaits the consumer at every turn. In addition, staples such as meat and dairy products are often placed at the rear of the store so the shopper must pass by many other food items before he selects that item which he originally intended to buy.

The first decision an elderly shopper must make is where to shop. The type of store in which a person shops will often influence the size of the grocery bill. Supermarkets and large chain stores usually offer more food items at lower prices than small independent stores[5]. If such a large store is convenient to use, its patronage should be encouraged. A recent study showed that many elderly like to shop and, that rather than being a chore, it provides recreation, exercise, and sensory benefits[7]. However, it is important to recognize that some aged people find the modern, spacious, noisy supermarket atmosphere overwhelming and confusing. They become intimidated by the seemingly limitless variety and impersonal behavior of the employees. Their confusion may lead to disorientation, and shopping in such a situation can be difficult.

The aged consumer may need to consider many factors when selecting a food market. Does he drive? Can he walk the many and long aisles of a supermarket? How will he carry the bundles home? Does the store accept Food Stamps? Will the store cash Social Security or pension checks?

For a disabled shopper, the convenience of telephoning in an order and having it home-delivered may be worth the few pennies more per item he might pay to a small local grocer. This service might be a critical factor in determining whether or not this person can continue to function in an independent, self-sufficient household. Credit may also be extended by a neighborhood grocer. The luxury of paying for groceries on a monthly basis may help the budgeting of a retired person who does not have a weekly pay check to depend on.

Some communities have organized volunteer groups to help the elderly do their marketing. They may provide transportation to and from the market, or may shop for and deliver groceries to the homebound person. Whenever possible, the elderly should be encouraged to do their own marketing, even if they need to be accompanied while doing so. Every opportunity to participate in activity outside the home should be fostered.

The use of a preplanned grocery list will cut down on impulse buying[5,8,9]. A grocery list should not be made up the day before a shopping trip but should be the result of a continuing inventory check on household food supplies. Keeping a pad and pencil handy in the kitchen and encouraging the homemaker to jot down items as they are used up or as the quantity begins to run low will help to keep a continuing check on household supplies, especially staples. Then with this replacement list as the basis of the weekly grocery list, the homemaker can plan menus for the week. These weekly menus should take into consideration items on hand, leftovers in the refrigerator or freezer, and weekly special sales.

Supermarket specials can save money but they must be evaluated carefully. Turkey may be the special of the week and one of the least expensive meat protein sources the consumer can buy that week. However, one person may not have use for a 14-lb turkey. In this case, the weekly special is not a bargain, and neither is the purchase of 10 pounds of potatoes or the large economy size of cereal. No matter how inexpensive their price, the size of these items could necessitate waste, thus offsetting the monetary saving. Alternatively, to avoid waste of these large purchases, it would be necessary to use the food repetitively, causing one's diet to be monotonous.

Store-hopping for weekly specials may appear pennywise, but unless the stores are close together it can be costly in time, limited energy, gasoline, or bus fare.

"Cents off" coupons may be used, when available, to purchase needed food. They are usually offered on brand name food items. One should always compare the price of the store brand with the brand name product after the brand name item has been discounted by the coupon value. Often it will be found that the store brand was the better value all along. Money-back offers are also tempting but the postage and the number of packages that must be bought before a consumer is eligible for a refund must be considered when evaluating the potential savings.

Some supermarket chains are beginning to offer lower-cost generic food[10]. Generic foods are lines of fruits, vegetables, and other foods sold in plain wrappers at prices 33 percent lower than national brands and between 10 and 20 percent lower than the store's private brand. For example, if a 15½-oz can of brand name green beans sells for 39¢ per can, the store's private label would be 29¢ and the generic product would be 23¢ (for a 15½-oz can). The generic foods usually carry a lower government grade than do name brands. National and private brands are from "fancy" or "choice" government grades of food. Generic products consist of "extra standard" and "standard" grade items. As government grading is based on aesthetic quality rather than nutritional quality, generic brands are a nutritious and economical consumer choice. Consumers have demonstrated a preference for the lower cost generic items in supermarkets where they are offered. Therefore, the slightly inferior asthetic qualities are not a major deterrent to many consumers.

In spite of a budget, a shopping list, and premium offers, the aged consumer may still find it difficult to buy food economically for one or two people. Often they cannot take advantage of sales because of package size or because a particular food, no matter how economical, is prohibited on their modified diet. In every category of food, however, there are some choices that will provide more value for each food dollar spent[11]. The following tips should be stressed when offering marketing suggestions.

Milk

Nonfat dry milk is less expensive than fluid milk. It can be reconstituted in small amounts and, in the powdered form, will remain fresh for months on the cupboard shelf when stored in an airtight container. Even if mixed half-and-half with fluid whole milk it is still less expensive than the fluid milk.

Milk Products

Natural cheese costs more than processed cheese. Grated cheese costs more than a solid piece of the same cheese. Cottage cheese with fruit or vegetables is more expensive than regular cottage cheese. Yogurt, ice cream, and pudding can substitute for milk but at an added cost. For example, ¾ cup of ice cream may cost three times as much as the ½ cup of whole milk it replaces.

Fruits and Vegetables

Fresh produce is least expensive when it is in season. These perishable foods should be bought in limited amounts even at bargain prices. One should look for a store that sells loose rather than prepackaged produce. There is nothing wrong with buying two potatoes, one banana, and two apples if that is all one needs. If a larger amount must be purchased, such as a bag of onions, one might consider splitting the amount and cost with a neighbor. Medium-sized cans of fruits and vegetables are the best buy because they are more economical than a small-sized can and yet are not so large that the food cannot be used in a reasonable period of time. Leftover vegetables can be used to make soup more hearty or as a cold salad. Pureed leftover fruit can be served as a warm sauce over plain cake or pudding. Frozen vegetables in a bag are a better buy than those in a box. The bag can be opened, one serving poured out, then the bag can be resealed and returned to the freezer. Such a resealable freezer container is convenient and offers a lower price per serving than a smaller package.

Meat

Weekly specials should be taken advantage of when possible. One should try to select cuts of meat, fish, and poultry that give the most servings of cooked lean meat per pound. Bony, fatty cuts should be avoided; excessive waste increases the cost per edible portion. Variety meats like chicken liver can be used. Leftover meat, fish, and poultry can be used in sandwiches, salads, soups, and casseroles; even two tablespoons of leftover meat will add variety to plain vegetables or rice.

Breads and Cereals

The use of whole grain or enriched products should be encouraged. Cereals that must be cooked are less expensive than ready-to-serve cereals in individual boxes or multipacks. Highly fortified cereals are also usually more expensive, and the added nutrients in the fortified cereals are not needed as part of a well-balanced diet. Prepackaged rice and macaroni mixes are more expensive than regular rice or macaroni seasoned at home. Day-old bread is less costly than fresh bread. Naturally, homebaked goods are less expensive than storebought goods of the same type.

Convenience Foods

Labels should be read carefully; ingredients are listed in order of amount contained. *Beef stew: water, potatoes, beef, carrots, tomato sauce, etc.* is not as good a buy as one which lists beef as the first ingredient. One needs to watch for ingredients such as salt or fat that must be eliminated or limited in the diet. If milk and eggs need to be added, during preparation, then the cost of a convenience mix increases. However, when prices are compared, some convenience foods are less expensive than buying small amounts of many ingredients. Wise selection of convenience foods can save money, time, and energy.

Comparison shopping is an important key to staying within the prescribed limits of a set food budget. However, a controversial new computerized checkout system may make comparison shopping harder to do[12]. The new system will rely on identification of the Universal Product Code (UPC) symbol on the food package by a scanner at the checkout counter. The UPC symbol consists of a series of bars of varying widths, unique to that product and readable by the computers (see Figure 12-1). The electronic system "reads" the symbol, identifies the product, "rings up" the price, and prints the price and description of the items on the customer's cash register receipt. The price will not appear on each item but will be shown on the shelf where the items are selected. Many consumer groups fear that item price removal will make it more difficult to keep track of changing costs and reduce the consumer's ability to comparison shop. They also fear that the excessive costs of installing this system will make already escalating food prices go even higher. In the spring of 1977, there were approximately fifty scanning sites in the United States, with more being planned.

The UPC system might be very unpleasant to an elderly shopper. The faster checkout and the impersonal computer "ring-up" might prove too technologically overwhelming for the older consumer, especially if he is uncomfortable with high speed data processing. Careful explanation of the use of this type of pricing system will be absolutely essential for the elderly shopper if he is to make use of and feel comfortable with this new checkout system.

CUSTOMER CASH REGISTER RECEIPT

```
    ....  STORE  NAME  ....

          GRAPEFRUIT     .48
          SWEET PEAS     .39
          MILK 1/2 GAL   .89
          FR COCKTAIL    .47
          BACKEYE PEAS   .29
          STEW TOMATO    .32
          V-8 JUICE      .49
        3 RITZ CRACKER  1.41
  3.59# APPLES .21/#    .75
          LISTERINE     1.19
          T BONE STEAK  3.87
          TV LG EGGS     .87
   .30D COCA-COLA        .91
          TAX DUE        .11

          TOTAL        12.44

          LISTERINE     1.19-
          TAX DUE        .05

          TOTAL        11.19

          FS BAL DUE     9.76

          FS TEND        9.00

          BAL DUE        2.19

          CK TEND        5.00

          FS CHG          .00

          CHG DUE        2.81

            STAMPS        89

   1/30/74 10:05  64/6 1
   THANKS--PLEASE COME BACK
```

The Universal Product Code consists of a 10-digit number. The first 5 numbers identify the manufacturer.
The second 5 numbers identify the contents and package size. There are 2 additional coded characters in the symbol. The one at the extreme left is called the number system character and it signifies the product category type. "0" indicates regular grocery items.

On the extreme right is the only character that does not have a human readable equivalent. This is a check character providing a fail-safe method of checking the accuracy of the code and will signal in-store symbol tampering.

When the scanner reads the symbol, it signals the equipment to look up the price of that particular item. (This price has previously been programmed into the computer by the retailer.) The electronic equipment will then instantly "write out" the name of the item and its price on the cash register tape. At the same time, the equipment can note if the shelves need to be restocked on this particular item and can indicate the need to reorder the item.

FIGURE 12-1   Illustration and description of the use of the Universal Product Code.

Source: Loding, J. B. "UPC (Universal Product Code) Issue," white paper, New York City Home Economists in Business, Spring 1977.

STORAGE

Many older people have already lived through hard times. Some may have been children or struggling young adults during the Depression. They vividly remember bare cupboards and half-empty stomachs after dinner was eaten, and they are determined never to face this situation again. Other older homemakers may have spent most of their lives feeding a large family, needing and using very large quantities of food weekly. For whatever the reason, many older people find comfort in possessing overflowing cupboards filled with food. At times, items may have to be discarded because they become stale or spoiled. Having sufficient supplies and keeping a few frozen dinners on hand for nights when no one feels like cooking makes sense, but hoarding food is expensive and impractical. A good hint is: *store but don't be a squirrel.*

Generally, it would be practical to keep one or two pounds of staples—flour, sugar, coffee. Most other foods should be bought in the smaller sizes that can be eaten by one or two people in a short period of time. After shopping, older items are best moved to the front of the cupboard to be used sooner than the more recent purchases.

It is often a good idea to repackage items in smaller quantities. For example, if 8 oz of Swiss cheese is bought in a chunk, it can be cut into two pieces. One piece can be put in the refrigerator for immediate use and the second piece wrapped in wax paper, put in a sealed plastic bag, and frozen for future use. It is also a good idea to divide and freeze meat in recipe-size pieces. Ground beef can be shaped into patties and placed, unwrapped, on a tray in the freezer. Once the patties are frozen they can be wrapped individually and put into a plastic bag. Then, the bag can be closed, dated, and returned to the freezer. The individual portions can then be used as needed and will defrost more quickly than the original portion because of their smaller size.

Eggs are often used up very slowly by older people. To keep a carton of eggs fresher longer, eggs should be left in the carton and stored on the coldest refrigerator shelf. Eggs should not be stored uncovered on the refrigerator door. The vibration of opening and closing the door plus the temperature changes will adversely affect quality. For long storage, the carton of eggs should be kept in a sealed plastic bag. This double packaging slows down the loss of moisture through the porous eggshell. With this extra packaging, whole eggs will remain in good condition for three weeks on the refrigerator shelf.

Even a small loaf of bread may become stale or moldy before it is eaten. If it is stored in the refrigerator it will not mold, but it will become hard and dry. A practical solution is to freeze an entire loaf, removing one or a few slices as needed. The slices will defrost quickly at room temperature and be equal in freshness to a recently purchased loaf of bread. The frozen bread will retain good quality for up to three months.

Both the refrigerator and freezer can be helpful in extending the storage life of food products[13]. See Figure 12-2 for ideas on maximizing the use of these two pieces of kitchen equipment.

The elderly person should be encouraged to keep screw-top jars such as wide-mouth mayonnaise jars. They make excellent storage receptacles for rice and dried beans, and they will safely store leftovers in the refrigerator.

It cannot be presumed that every elderly homemaker will have a freezer. In some cases, even a refrigerator may not be available. If there is no refrigeration, canned and dried foods will need to be relied upon heavily. Nonfat dried milk can be made as needed. Single-serving sizes of canned items should be bought to avoid leftovers. There are even single-serving rehydratable casseroles on the market. These foods, however, are generally high in carbohydrate and sodium and low in protein. Although they can be used occasionally, they should be avoided totally by people who need to restrict their sodium intake. Protein foods (meat, milk, eggs, cheese, poultry, and fish) cannot be held safely without refrigeration for longer than two hours. After this time, the chance of bacterial contamination becomes too great for safety. The elderly are particularly susceptible to food-borne illness, so every precaution should be taken to handle food carefully.

The Center of Disease Control (CDC) in Atlanta, Georgia, is the national agency which records the incidence of food-borne disease[14,15]. The CDC estimates that in this country over two million people each year suffer from food-borne or food-transmitted illness. Often mild indisposition is mistakenly labeled as a case of "24-hour virus." Staphylococcal food intoxication and food-borne illnesses caused by clostridium perfringens and salmonella are the most common food-borne diseases afflicting people in the United States[16].

In the United States, staphylococcus aureus is the bacteria that causes more cases of food-borne disease than any other microorganism. Staphylococcal food intoxication is a food poisoning. It is sometimes inappropriately called *ptomaine poisoning*, a term first

Items that will keep longer in the refrigerator than in the cupboard
Bread crumbs
Catsup
Coffee, regular and instant
Crackers
Dried fruit
Fresh fruit
Jam
Jelly
Nuts
Onions
Peanut butter
Potatoes
Raisins
Salad oil
Shortening
Whole wheat flours

Items that will keep longer in the freezer than in the refrigerator
Baked goods
Butter
Cheese
  Cheddar
  Cream cheese
  Farmer cheese
  Mozzerella
  Muenster
  Swiss
  Other firm cheese
Coffee, instant or regular
Leftovers
Margarine
Pastry

FIGURE 12-2   Food item storage information.

applied to food poisoning in 1887[14]. The bacteria enters the food from human or animal contamination. (It is found on the skin and in body openings such as the nasal cavity.) The poison produced by the bacteria is an enterotoxin. It causes inflammation and irritation of the lining of the stomach and intestine. The symptoms occur quickly—two to four hours after the food is consumed—and the person suffers from severe diarrhea, vomiting, and abdominal cramps which last about twenty-four hours until the poison is eliminated from the system. Staphylococcal food poisonings generally arise from improper handling of cooked foods. Puddings, sandwiches, poultry, fish, and egg salads are frequently involved. These foods should be kept refrigerated whenever possible and never allowed to stand at room temperature for any length of time.

Salmonellosis is a food-borne infection. The microorganisms salmonellae are found in the intestines of humans, animals, and insects. Meat, poultry, and eggs are often contaminated, thus these foods should never be eaten raw. Cooking will destroy the bacteria but improperly handled cooked food can become recontaminated. Therefore, leftovers should be kept refrigerated and heated thoroughly, brought to boiling, and held at 212°F (100°C) for at least one minute, to be sure the bacteria are destroyed. The symptoms of salmonellosis occur eight to seventy-two hours after the food is eaten and include diarrhea, nausea, abdominal pain, chills, fever, and vomiting. The intensity of the symptoms can range from mild discomfort to very severe pain and fever requiring hospitalization. Salmonellosis has a mortality rate of 1 percent, most often striking infants, older people, and those suffering from other disease.

Clostridium perfringens is a microorganism widely distributed throughout the environment. Meat, poultry, gravies, and soups are its most favored targets. The organisms will grow very rapidly if any of these foods are prepared ahead of time and held warm before serving, cooled at room temperature, or merely warmed up rather than reheated thoroughly when the foods are used as leftovers. The symptoms of clostridium perfringens food-borne illness are very mild and often not recognized as being due to contaminated food. The symptoms include intestinal gas, diarrhea, cramps, and occasional nausea. These symptoms occur eight to twelve hours after eating and continue for six to twelve hours.

The elderly are more susceptible to food-borne illness than younger adults and they should be given a careful explanation of what symptoms to expect and be instructed to always report these symptoms to their doctor. The effects of vomiting and diarrhea are serious health hazards to the elderly; in some cases hospitalization may be necessary. Proper handling of food—keeping hot things hot, cold things cold, and avoiding eating foods raw (eggs or ground beef)—will greatly reduce the risk of illness from contaminated food.

Another way to become ill from eating contaminated food is to eat food with mold on it[17]. Certain species of mold can cause serious eye, ear, sinus, and respiratory tract infections, which have lead, in some cases, to blindness and death. Mold also causes allergic reactions such as hay fever and rashes.

No one likes to throw food in the garbage, so it seems logical to cut away the mold and eat the remaining food. The fluffy, cottony substance, which can be any color, is actually the "bloom" of the mold; the roots may have spread throughout the food. Therefore, even portions without obvious mold may be contaminated. Whenever mold is found, the entire piece of food should be discarded (except, of course when the mold appears on a piece of cheese or other such foods which may contain mold purposely introduced during processing). Cooking will destroy the mold itself but not the toxin the mold produced, so cooking a food that shows signs of mold will not necessarily reduce the health hazard. Musty odors are a signal that mold is present, but a healthy sniff to check for this odor may send mold spores directly into the respiratory tract, which is an even greater hazard than eating the mold.

In a household of one or two people, food may not be used up quickly, and thus ample time for the growth of mold is allowed. The elderly should be cautioned *never* to try to be frugal and make use of food that has the appearance of mold. They could be inviting a health hazard with fatal consequences.

FOOD PREPARATION

The various losses associated with increasing age often make simple tasks difficult and time consuming. Older persons must readjust to new ways of doing things so that they can continue to live independently. This is especially true of food preparation.

Eating is one of the true pleasures of life, and one that should continue throughout life. Food preparation can also be an enjoyable, or at least a beneficial, activity in which an older person may engage. The simple exercise of preparing and serving a meal can help keep arthritic joints limber or help to fill lonely hours with purposeful activity.

Before meal preparation can be made a constructive, enjoyable activity many things have to be considered. Does the individual know basic food preparation skills? Are there facilities for cooking, such as a hot plate, oven, or complete kitchen? What kinds of utensils are available? Have heavy and large utensils been replaced with equipment suited to the smaller amounts of food now being pre-pared? Are utensils arranged within easy reach to avoid uncomfort-able stretching or climbing? Is there a pleasant place to eat? Does the person have someone else to eat with at least occasionally? Are there any dietary limitations that must be considered?

Appropriate Equipment

It is easy to prepare attractive, tasty meals in a complete and well-equipped kitchen. However, many older people have moved from big homes to smaller apartments, mobile homes, or furnished rooms where cooking equipment may be limited. Still, attractive and tasty meals can be made with a small amount of equipment and a little in-genuity.

For one person, a one-burner hot plate, a toaster oven, and 1.5 cu ft refrigerator can serve as a complete kitchen. Add a small table to work on and a bathroom sink for cleanup and anyone can prepare tasty meals that are well-balanced.

A double boiler is a useful piece of equipment for someone with a one-burner hotplate. One food can be cooked on the top of the double boiler and a second food can be made in the lower portion at the same time. For example, a piece of frozen fish could be poaching in the top section while a vegetable cooks in the lower portion. A pot with a steamer tray/basket can also be put to dual use. One can sim-mer a salisbury steak patty in the pot while steaming one or two vegetables on the tray.

An electric skillet or crockpot can be adapted to many types of cooking. Even a frozen TV dinner can be heated in a covered electric skillet, and some manufacturers provide recipes for baking in this appliance as well.

Convenience foods can save on equipment by reducing pre-paration steps and avoiding the need for a variety of utensils. These convenience items can also help add variety to a meal. Many come in single or double portion servings, which are particularly useful if cooking for one or two people.

As a person grows older, safety in the kitchen becomes particu-larly important. The elderly are constantly at risk of an injury, which may be minor but could cause a major crisis. A person who has impaired vision or is unsteady on his feet must take extra pre-cautions to avoid falls or accidents. A rubber mat in front of the sink avoids slipping. A wheeled cart eliminates carrying and can provide some support for balance control. A stool to sit on relieves pressure on the legs and hips. Utility stools are a good choice since they have a step on which to rest the feet for added comfort and a small section to support the back. A light sponge mop, long handled dustpan, and broom eliminate stooping and bending for cleanup.

Clothing should also be appropriate. Sturdy shoes reduce fatigue and provide more secure balance. Slippers are a poor choice for an older person while working in the kitchen. Shoes provide better support and may prevent slips and falls. Flammable fabrics, as often found in nightgowns and bathrobes, can be a hazard when lighting the oven or reaching for a pan on a back burner.

Burns are a special danger for the elderly. If the hot water thermostat is set too high, the temperature of the water flowing from the tap may scald the elderly person. Similarly, grasping a hot pot may burn the skin. Perception of touch and heat are impaired by normal aging changes in sensory organs[18]. This can lead to reduced sensitivity and the inability to localize pain. A very thick or well-insulated pot holder should be kept in a convenient place and always used when holding hot objects.

Reduction in olfactory sensation may make gas ranges dangerous for the elderly. Over 50 percent of those sixty-five years and older are unable to smell domestic gas if it is escaping from an open but unlit gas jet. Studies show that over three-quarters of the deaths due to domestic gas poisoning are of persons over sixty years of age[18]. An aged person using a gas range should be cautioned to check the range controls several times throughout the day.

DAILY FOOD GUIDE

The nutritional needs of the elderly are generally the same as those of young adults, with a reduction in caloric need (see Chapter 4). Because of the lowered caloric need, the meal plan of the geriatric person has less room for empty-calorie and high-calorie food. Therefore, in old age more than ever, the daily food guide emphasizing the four food groups will serve as a pattern for the recommended daily food intake. Selecting the recommended adult servings from each of the four food groups provides a daily meal plan of approximately 1,200 calories with sufficient protein, vitamins, and minerals. Additional foods and fats can be added to the basic plan depending upon the individual's caloric need.

DAILY FOOD GUIDE

Food Group	*Recommended Daily Intake*
Milk Group	two cups
Vegetable-Fruit Group	four servings
Meat Group	two (2-oz) servings
Bread-Cereals Group	four servings

Milk and Dairy Products

The need for milk and milk products does not decrease with age, yet milk is a food often missing in the daily meal pattern of the elderly. Foods from this group supply protein, calcium, riboflavin, and phosphorus. Two 8-oz cups per day is the adult requirement. The older person should try very hard to include this full 16 oz of milk per day, but when not possible, the minimum intake should be 1 cup of milk or its equivalent. Milk may be ingested in the form of cheese, cottage cheese, yogurt, pudding, custard, cream soup, or ice cream. The following is a list of some common milk equivalents:

1 cup yogurt equals 1 cup milk

½ cup evaporated milk plus ½ cup water equals 1 cup milk

1 ounce natural cheese equals ¾ cup milk

½ cup cottage cheese equals ⅓ cup milk

½ cup ice cream equals ¼ cup milk

For the person with lactose intolerance (see Chapter 4), smaller portions than those listed might be better tolerated. In this case, one should use 4-oz (½ cup) portions of milk as a serving rather than 8 oz (1 cup). Fermented milks, yogurt, and acidophilous milk are often better tolerated. During fermentation, part of the milk sugar, lactose, has been converted to lactic acid, leaving less lactose and therefore making the milk product easier for the lactose-intolerant person to digest. Cheese may also be better tolerated than milk by the lactose-intolerant individual. During cheesemaking, milk is divided into curds and whey. The cheese itself is made mostly from the curd; the liquid whey is removed and with it, the dissolved milk sugar, lactose. The harder the cheese variety, the more whey has been removed during processing. Swiss, cheddar, parmesan, and other hard varieties of cheese contain little or no carbohydrate—and therefore little or no lactose—and thus these cheeses are tolerated better by the lactose-intolerant individual.

Vegetable and Fruit Group

Fruits and vegetables are valuable in the diet because of the variety of vitamins and minerals they contain. Four servings should be included daily from this group in the form of juice or fresh, canned or frozen fruits, and/or vegetables. One serving is ½ cup of juice or ½ cup of cooked vegetable or canned fruit. One serving may also be a portion as commonly served such as one medium apple, peach, orange or potato, half of a medium grapefruit, or a wedge of canta-loupe, honeydew, or other melon. Within the four servings daily, one serving should be from a fruit or vegetable rich in vitamin C. In ad-dition to oranges or orange juice, there are many good sources of vitamin C to choose from: cantaloupe, grapefruit or grapefruit juice, honeydew melon, mango, papaya, fresh strawberries, tangerine and tangerine juice, broccoli, green and sweet red peppers, potato and sweet potato cooked in their skins, raw cabbage, and tomato and tomato juice. One vitamin A-containing fruit or vegetable should be included at least every other day, or a minimum of three times a week. Vitamin A is found in fresh produce that is deep yellow and dark green in color, such as: apricots, broccoli, cantaloupe, carrots, spinach and other dark green leafy vegetables, pumpkin, sweet potato, and winter squash.

Bread and Cereal Group

This food group provides a small but worthwhile source of protein and iron, plus B vitamins and food energy in the form of calories. All types of enriched or whole grain breads and cereals—both ready-to-eat and cooked—fall into this group, as do cornmeal, crackers, grits, macaroni, spaghetti, noodles, rice, cracked wheat, and quick breads. Making use of any combination of the above choices, at least four servings should be included in each day's meal plan. One serving would be: one slice of bread, 1 oz of ready-to-eat cereal (approxi-mately ¾ to 1 cup), or ½ cup cooked cereal, cornmeal, macaroni, noodles, rice, or spaghetti. The best foundation for a limited budget is a diet that makes good use of milk and enriched or whole grain bread and cereal. A glass of milk and a slice of toast or a bowl of cereal are good food choices at any time of the day.

Meat and Meat Alternatives Group

The foods in this group are valued for their protein, B vitamins, iron, zinc, and phosphorus contents. For many reasons, the elderly often eat diets low in protein. An adult should eat at least two 2-oz servings from this food group daily. The serving could be made up of 2-oz of lean meat, fish, poultry, or shellfish. These are all excellent sources of protein but, as they are expensive sources, the elderly may use them less than they should. Consequently, the use of meat alternatives as sources of protein should be encouraged. Two oz of cooked lean meat is the protein equivalent of: two eggs, 2 oz of cheese, ½ cup cottage cheese, 1 cup cooked dried peas or beans, 4 tablespoons peanut butter or ¼ cup peanuts, ⅓ cup of nuts (cashews, walnuts, pecans, etc.), ⅓ cup of seeds (pumpkin, sesame, sunflower, etc.), ¾ cup soybean curd, and 3 oz of prepared meat analog or textured vegetable protein (TVP)[19].

Some of the meat alternatives suggested above may be unusual or unknown sources of protein to the older consumer. A careful explanation of their use and their value as protein sources should be stressed to maximize their use in the diet.

Eggs and cheese are obvious meat alternatives. Most older people who use four eggs per week have four ounces of excellent quality protein. Cheese, too, is a high quality protein and 1 oz goes a long way, providing 7.5 gm of protein.

Nuts contain an average of approximately 15 percent protein in the edible portion[20]. Due to dental problems, nuts may not be easily eaten by older people. However, nuts can easily be ground to a powder in the blender and the powder offers no difficulty in chewing. A tablespoon of nut powder sprinkled on a bowl of hot or cold cereal adds flavor as well as protein. It is easy to incorporate ¼ cup nut powder into pudding mixes, pancakes, rice pilaf, and other combination dishes. As with cheese, a little goes a long way.

Peanut butter offers a good source of protein, providing 4 gm per tablespoon[21]. Because of its sticky consistency, many older people do not find it pleasant to eat, especially if they have dentures. Therefore, suggesting the use of peanut butter sandwiches, though they are nutritious, is often not practical. The health professional needs to seek out ingenious ways to get peanut butter into the meal pattern. It is best to try recipes in which peanut butter can be melted down and incorporated into the product. For example, a powdered pudding mix can accommodate ¼ cup of peanut butter along with the regular amount of milk called for on the package directions. The new flavor created by the addition of peanut butter is interesting and the sticky character of the peanut butter is masked by the smoothness of the pudding. With the added peanut butter, each ½-cup serving of pudding supplies approximately 8 gm of protein—4 gm of protein from the additional 1 tablespoon of peanut butter per serving, and 4 gm of protein from the ½ cup of milk in each serving. The stickiness of peanut butter can also be reduced by mixing it with other ingredients to make a sandwich spread. The following are some sandwich spread suggestions using peanut butter.

Peanut Butter Sandwich Spreads   With all the following combinations, simply mix ingredients together, in the amounts indicated, until the mixture is thoroughly combined. Store in the refrigerator in a covered container.

> 1 can (2¼ ounces) deviled ham + ½ cup peanut butter
>
> ½ cup ground ham, bologna, or luncheon meat + ½ cup peanut butter
>
> 1 ripe mashed banana + ⅓ cup peanut butter
>
> ¼ cup applesauce + ½ cup peanut butter
>
> ¼ cup stewed fruit + ¼ cup peanut butter
>
> ¼ cup applesauce + ¼ cup cottage cheese + ½ cup peanut butter
>
> ¼ cup stewed fruit + ¼ cup cottage cheese + ½ cup peanut butter
>
> ⅓ cup cottage cheese + ½ cup peanut butter

Peanut butter can also be used in main dish recipes. The following is an example of one such recipe.

PEANUT–RICE LOAF

1 cup peanut butter
1 cup cooked rice
1 cup soft bread crumbs
2 cups milk

1 egg, well beaten
1 teaspoon salt
1/8 teaspoon pepper

Preheat oven to 350°F

Grease a 9″ × 5″ × 3″ loafpan.

Mix all ingredients until thoroughly blended. Pack into loaf pan.

Bake 45–50 minutes. Turn out on a platter and cut into slices to serve. Makes four servings.

Serve with cream soup base sauce such as celery or mushroom, if you wish.

Soybean curd is often called soy cheese or tofu[21]. It is the precipitated curd of mashed soybeans, white in color, soft in texture and with a delicate flavor. It is sold in slices fresh, or canned. One slice (2½″ × 2¾″ × 1″) contains 86 calories, 9.4 gm of protein, and 150 mg of calcium with lesser amounts of other nutrients. The fresh and canned varieties can be found in oriental specialty food shops, health food stores, and occasionally in supermarkets with a large selection of "ethnic" foods. Soybean curd is a low-cost protein, with a soft easy-to-chew texture similar to that of cream cheese or farmers' cheese. It can be added to almost any cooked combination dish to increase protein value. Soybean curd can also be used for a sandwich spread.

TOFU–PEANUT BUTTER SPREAD

¼ lb. soybean curd, drained
   & mashed
½ cup peanut butter

2 T. honey or applesauce
¼ cup raisins (optional)

Combine all ingredients and blend well. This makes a light, fluffy spread which should be refrigerated.

Many older people avoid the use of dried beans as alternatives to meat because of flatulence. The elderly should be encouraged to try using beans since many varieties are not gas-producing. Soybeans in particular are lower in carbohydrate than other bean varieties and less likely to cause flatulence. Split peas, lima beans, and lentils are also easy to digest[20]. Beans are a very versatile food. They can be used to make soups, salads, casseroles, sandwich spreads, or dips for crackers. Because they require long cooking times, the trick is to cook them only once or twice per week and draw on a refrigerated supply as needed. The cooked quantity can also be frozen in small batches to be used as needed. The electric slow cooker can provide a very simple way to cook beans. Beans can be easily eaten for breakfast with whole-grain toast or a corn muffin. This is the perfect time in the day for a hearty meal and the preparation can be done overnight in the electric slow cooker. Beans of many varieties are available at the supermarket, precooked, in cans, or in frozen 10-oz and 2-lb packages. The canned beans are purchased ready-to-eat and the frozen variety takes only minutes to prepare, making beans readily available for meals.

Beans can also be eaten as bean sprouts[20]. Mung beans, garbanzos, whole dried peas, lentils, alfalfa seeds, and soybeans are among the thirty varieties of dried beans or grains that can be sprouted. An elderly gardener might enjoy growing a crop of bean sprouts. For a few minutes' time and a few cents' investment, he will reap a versatile and nutritious food. Sprouts are not gas producers, have a natural, sweet flavor, and are rich in vitamin C.

One quarter of a cup of dried beans will yield about two cups of sprouts. To sprout beans, soak them overnight. In the morning, rinse the soaked beans and drain them thoroughly. Place moist paper towels or a dampened washcloth over the beans and cover the container. Twice a day for the next three to five days—depending on what type of beans are being sprouted—uncover the beans, rinse and drain them thoroughly, and replace the dampened towel and container cover. The crop can be harvested in three days when sprouting mung beans, lentils, and soybeans, and in four to five days when sprouting alfalfa seeds.

All sprouts have a delicate flavor and texture; they are a natural salad choice for anyone who finds crunchy greens difficult to chew. Mixed with cottage cheese, they make an instant garden salad, adding only about 25 calories for a ½ cup of sprouts[20]. They also make an excellent quick-to-prepare vegetable. All sprouts can be stir-fried in a small amount of oil or margarine plus a favorite herb and onion, or steamed for approximately five minutes until they are limp.

Meat analogs or textured vegetable protein (TVP) may be used in place of, or to extend, meat for a meal. TVP is usually used as a meat extender. The vegetable protein is from the soybean which is processed and texturized to resemble meat, poultry, or chicken. The TVP is sold dry and needs to be reconstituted with water during preparation. Lipton and other large food manufacturers have promoted these products in the supermarkets principally as extenders of ground beef. However, TVP lends itself to use in spaghetti sauce, chili, baked beans, and many other casserole-type dishes.

Meat analogs can also be found in the supermarket, canned or frozen. They are nonmeat, meat-like foods derived from vegetable protein (usually soy, gluten, or nut protein). Egg white is often added to the vegetable protein to increase the protein value. The Seventh Day Adventists were the first to experiment with soybean foods in the early 1930s and today the consumer can choose from over fifty such products available as chicken, ham, frankfurters, beef, pork, sausage, and bacon[22]. A 3-oz serving of a meat analog is usually equivalent to a 2-oz serving of meat, fish, or poultry. However, products vary and labels should be read carefully. In most cases, meat analogs do not offer a great saving over the price of a comparable amount of meat. Also, since analogs are *manufactured* foods, they contain many food additives, sodium, and added fat. Salt and sodium-containing food additives are used extensively in all analog products, making them an unacceptable choice for anyone on a sodium-restricted diet.

It should be kept in mind that it is not necessary to increase the protein content of meals for most elderly people. Protein intake should approximate 12-14 percent of the total daily caloric need. (See Figure 12-3 for examples of meals planned to provide adequate protein and other nutrients.) Additional protein, added to food as suggested above, is neither necessary or desirable in many cases. These suggestions are useful for situations in which protein intake is limited because of unusual dietary practices or budgetary restrictions, or when protein intake must be increased temporarily.

Understanding and using the Daily Food Guide including the milk group, meat group, vegetable and fruit group, and bread and cereal group will ensure that the older person or older couple eat nutritious meals consisting of a variety of foods. Figure 12-3 (pp. 273-275) gives an example of three days' choices and how those meals meet the recommendations of the daily food guide.

Sample Menus

Day 1

Breakfast:
  Cooked Prunes
  Puffed Wheat and Milk
  Whole Wheat Toast and Jelly
  Coffee or Tea

Lunch:
  Hard Cooked Eggs with Cheese Sauce on Toast
  Sliced Tomato
  Steamed Carrot Sticks
  Pound Cake
  Milk

Dinner:
  Lamb Stew
  Bean Sprout Salad
  Biscuit
  Jello and Fruit
  Tea

Daily Assessment

Milk
  with cereal, ½ cup
  cheese sauce, ½ cup   Total 2 cups
  as beverage, 1 cup   (2 cups minimum)

Vegetable-Fruit
  Prunes
  Tomato
  Carrots
  Stew Vegetables
  Sprout Salad   Total 6 servings
  Fruit in Jello   (4 servings minimum)

Meat or Alternative
  Eggs   Total 2 servings
  Lamb   (2 servings minimum)

Bread-Cereal
  Puffed Rice
  Whole Wheat Toast
  Toast at Lunch   Total 4 servings
  Biscuit   (4 servings minimum)

(continued)

Day 2

Breakfast:
  Orange
  Breakfast Beans
  Corn Muffin
  Hot Chocolate

Lunch:
  Tuna Salad Sandwich
  Cold Vegetable Salad
  Banana
  Milk

Dinner:
  Creamed Fish Chowder
  Carrot-Raisin Salad
  Bread and Butter
  Baked Apple
  Tea

Daily Assessment

Milk
  Hot Chocolate, 3/4 cup
  Creamed Soup, ½ cup   Total 2¼ cups
  as beverage, 1 cup   (2 cups minimum)

Vegetable–Fruit
  Orange
  Vegetable Salad
  Banana
  Carrot-Raisin Salad   Total 5 servings
  Baked Apple   (4 servings minimum)

Meat or Alternative
  Breakfast Beans   Total 2½ servings
  Tuna Fish   (2 servings minimum)
  Fish Chowder

Bread–Cereal
  Corn Muffin
  Sandwich Bread   Total 4 servings
  Bread at dinner   (4 servings minimum)

(continued)

Day 3

Breakfast:
  Grapefruit Sections
  Oatmeal
  Raisin Bread Toast
  Coffee

Lunch:
  Creamed Dried Beef on Toast
  Waldorf Salad
  Vanilla Pudding and Cookies
  Tea

Dinner:
  Filet of Flounder, broiled
  Rice
  Broccoli
  Dinner Roll
  Canned Apricots
  Milk

Daily Assessment

Milk
  Creamed Beef, ½ cup
  Pudding, ½ cup   Total 2 cups
  as beverage, 1 cup   (2 cups minimum)

Vegetable-Fruit
  Grapefruit Sections
  Waldorf Salad
  Broccoli   Total 4 servings
  Apricots   (4 servings minimum)

Meat of Alternative
  Dried Beef   Total 2 servings
  Flounder   (2 servings minimum)

Bread-Cereal
  Raisin Toast
  Toast at Lunch
  Rice   Total 4 servings
  Dinner Roll   (4 servings minimum)

FIGURE 12-3   Three days' sample menus developed to satisfy the
recommendations of the daily food guide.

COOKING FOR ONE
OR TWO

If a person eats alone a great deal of the time he is apt to forget how pleasant eating can be. A person who lives alone should be encouraged to take the time to set the table, use a nice placemat, or put a flower in a vase. If the kitchen atmosphere is lonely, he should take a tray to an armchair near a window and watch the neighborhood. Eating with the TV or radio on can offer some company. Instituting a once or twice a week "share-a-meal" dinner can bring back imagination to meal preparation. It would not be a bad idea to have two or three elderly singles or couples prepare a pot luck supper. One would make the vegetable, one the salad, and one the main dish casserole. Each one will fuss more on their single item than they would if they had to prepare the whole meal. This idea can introduce everyone to new dishes while also fostering socialization. Turns can be taken each week making different items and even setting goals for the meal—no-meat, low cost, or low-fat.

During retirement the homemaker makes many adjustments, but one of her most surprising ones may be that she now has to *share* her kitchen with her husband. At first, the husband may just linger after meals to prolong the time together and the conversation, but slowly he may start doing kitchen jobs such as drying dishes, setting or clearing the table, peeling onions. Some women resent this intrusion into their territory. However, a husband's active participation in meal preparation should be encouraged for many reasons. First, since both husband and wife may have somewhat limited energy and mobility, the shared activity of meal preparation and cleanup can relieve the homemaker of the total burden. The husband may not mind clearing the table and washing the dishes while the wife enjoys a second cup of coffee. During meal preparation, the husband will quickly see how much food is used and what it costs, making it easier for him to budget their limited funds. Last, and possibly most important, is that this experience will serve the husband if the wife ever becomes disabled or dies and he must take over complete responsibility for meal preparation. Often, men find themselves totally confused when left to their own resources in a kitchen. An apprenticeship in meal preparation served under the tutelage of an experienced wife will undoubtedly prove valuable.

Anyone who cooks relies on favorite dishes which he prepares time and time again. Favorites are fine but monotony in meals will cause a person to lose interest in eating. Due to limited funds, the need for small quantities, and possibly due to the lack of companionship, many older people need to have their imaginations rekindled to add variety to their meals. The importance of structured meals at regular times should be emphasized to be sure that a variety of food is eaten and that the person does not rely on readily available snacks[6].

The health professional should try to provide elderly homemakers with a few recipes that can be varied in flavor without changing the basic preparation skills and techniques. Soups, stews, and casseroles are dishes that easily lend themselves to adaptations. It is best to provide one basic recipe showing options for other ingredients. Figure 12–4 is an example of a recipe for a top-of-the-stove casserole that uses the same directions to produce countless meals that vary in color, texture, and flavor. This method of teaching food preparations encourages the person to actively use his imagination in selecting the ingredients while cooking. It is especially useful for the single, elderly man who may feel ill at ease in the kitchen and frustrated because there are so many different methods of preparing food. After he has made the recipe once, he will be comfortable with the procedure. Then each subsequent time the dish is prepared, the procedure will remain the same but the ingredients can be changed depending on what is available or preferred. The recipe procedure will become easy and simple to use and can be relied on time and time again. Top-of-the-stove casserole dishes are particularly useful since they need less energy for preparation than casseroles cooked in an oven, which many elderly homemakers do not have.

Lack of exercise, aging taste buds, difficulty in chewing, or intestinal discomfort from certain foods causes many people to lose their appetite as they grow older. Not all of these problems can be corrected but interest in eating must be maintained[6].

The following suggestions can be used to increase interest in meals:

Use foods that vary in texture when the taste sensation is dull.

Drink a small glass of wine before dinner to stimulate the appetite.

Eat regular meals at regular times.

Have the big meal of the day at breakfast or lunch; keep dinner small.

Endless Variety Skillet Casserole

CARBOHYDRATE
- 2/3 C rice, uncooked
- 1 C fine or medium noodles, uncooked
- 1 C elbow macaroni, uncooked
- 2 C diced raw potatoes*

PROTEIN
- ½ C cooked, cut-up chicken, or turkey, or beef, or veal or pork
- ½ C cut-up ham
- ½ C flaked tuna
- 1 C cooked, cut-up breakfast sausage
- ½ C cut-up luncheon meat
- ¼ lb. raw chopped meat
- ⅔ C cooked or canned chickpeas
- ¾ C soy bean curd, diced

VEGETABLES
- ½ C fresh or frozen carrots, or peas, or corn, or green beans, or chopped broccoli, or mixed vegetables
- ½ C canned vegetables (same variety as above)

LIQUID
- 2¼ C beef or chicken broth
- 2½ C tomato sauce or puree
- 2¼ C canned gravy
- 1 can (11–12 oz) condensed cream of mushroom, or cream of celery, or cream of chicken, or cream of tomato soup (mix all of above with 1 soup can water)
- 1 can (11–12 oz.) condensed barley-mushroom soup (mix with 1 soup can water)

SEASONING
- 1 T dehydrated onion, or parsley, or chives or celery
- ¼ C frozen diced green pepper or onion
- 2 T diced pimento

TOPPING
- ¼ C seasoned bread crumbs
- ¼ C crushed cornflakes or other dry cereal
- ¼ C crushed potato chips or corn chips
- ¼ C grated parmesan, or cheddar, or American cheese
- 1 hard cooked egg, finely chopped
- 2 T wheat germ
- ¼ C cracker crumbs

1. In a 10-inch skillet combine 1 carbohydrate, 1 protein, 1 vegetable, 1 choice of liquid, and 2 choices of seasoning; stir to combine thoroughly.
2. Bring mixture to a boil, reduce heat to simmer, cover and continue cooking 25–30 minutes, stirring occasionally.
3. When casserole is done, transfer to a serving dish and sprinkle with selected topping and serve. Yield: 3 cups or two 1½ cup servings

*When selecting potatoes as the casserole carbohydrate do not use beef or chicken broth as the liquid.

FIGURE 12–4   An easy-to-prepare casserole recipe that can produce countless meals using the same basic directions.

Serve some hot and some cold foods at each meal; this will enhance the food's appeal.

Avoid repetition of the same food in many meals.

Avoid repetition of the same flavor in one meal.

Chop, grind, or mechanically blend foods that are hard to chew.

Mash cooked vegetables; shred raw vegetables.

Use baby foods; strained meat and melted cheese on bread make an easily eaten sandwich.

Share meals with a friend; make this a regular habit.

Take a daily walk to increase your activity and appetite.

Plan five or six small meals per day.

Drink at least six glasses of fluid a day to prevent constipation and dehydration; eat ample whole grain cereals, fruits, and vegetables.

Eat slowly and chew thoroughly.

Avoid food that is high in fat or overly spiced.

Eat out occasionally; have a meal at a senior center or a restaurant which features senior citizen discount days.

Serve food attractively; food tastes better if it looks good to eat.

CITED REFERENCES

1. Peterkin, B. Winter 1975. USDA family food plans, 1974. *Family Economics Review* p. 3.
2. Peterkin, B.; Chassy, J; and Kerr, R. 1975. The thrifty food plan. Consumer and Food Economics Institute, Agricultural Research Service, U.S. Dept. of Agriculture.
3. Agricultural Research Service. 1976. *Food for thrifty families.* U.S. Department of Agriculture.
4. Three budgets for a retired couple, Autumn, 1973. August 27, 1974. U.S. Dept. of Labor, Bureau of Labor Statistics.
5. Food Stamp Program: Maximum Monthly Allowable Income Standards and Basis of Coupon Issuance: 48 States and District of Columbia, Part 271-Participation of State Agencies and Eligible Households, Federal Register 43(95)-May 16, 1978.
6. Young, C. N. May 1974. Nutritional counseling for better health. *Geriatric* 83.
7. Mason, B., and Bearden, W. 1978. Profiling the shopping behavior of elderly consumers. *Gerontologist* 18:454.
8. Tennessee Commission on Aging. 1973. *Grand food for grandparents.* Nashville, Tennessee.
9. *For older people eating right for less.* 1977. Mt. Vernon, New York: Consumers Union.
10. Barmash, I. June 4, 1978. Inflation puts the squeeze on supermarkets, too. *New York Times* Section 3, Page 1, Column 1.
11. United States Dept. of Agriculture. 1972. *Food guide for older folks.* Home and Garden Bulletin No. 17, Washington, D.C.: U.S. Government Printing Office.
12. Loding, J. B. 1977. *The UPC (Universal Product Code) issue.* Home Economists in Business, New York City Group.
13. Washborn, M. 1968. *Cooking for one.* Cornell Miscellaneous Bulletin 93, Cooperative Extension, Cornell University, Ithaca, New York.
14. Zottola, E. A. September 1977. "Food-borne disease I." *Contemporary Nutrition* 2.

15. Zottola, E. A. January 1978. "Food-borne disease II." *Contemporary Nutrition* 3.
16. *Food facts from Rutgers.* 1967. New Brunswick, New Jersey: Rutgers College of Agriculture and Environmental Science.
17. Please don't eat the mold. April 1978. *Cooperative Extension, Home Economics Newsletter* Cornell Univ., p. 3.
18. Busse, E. W. 1978. How mind, body and environment influence nutrition in the elderly. *Postgraduate Medicine* 63(3):118.
19. Smith, E. B. 1975. A guide to good eating the vegetarian way. *J. of Nutrition Educ.* 9:109.
20. Robertson, L.; Flinder, C.; and Godfrey, B. 1976. *Laurel's kitchen.* California: Niligiri Press.
21. Aykroyd, W. R., and Doughty, J. 1964. *Legumes in human nutrition.* Rome: Food and Agriculture Organization.
22. Peterson, T. October 1974. The bean that's making meat obsolete. *Popular Mechanics* p. 82.

Afterword

Old age is a positive period in life if accompanied by the continuing respect of younger people and a minimum of physical decline and loss of status. The founding fathers of this country recognized and respected the wisdom that comes with age by writing into the Constitution the stipulation that a President must be at least thirty-five years of age. In practice, most presidents have been in their fifties or sixties when they served. William Henry Harrison was sixty-eight when he took office.

Elderly persons have a need to remain respected, active, independent members of the community. They have a need for companionship and for self-respect. However, some elderly persons today are living without any of these needs being met. Much of this is due to *ageism*, or prejudice against the elderly because of their age. People of all ages are guilty of this prejudice, even the elderly themselves. The idea that elderly persons are cantankerous, stubborn, infirm, demented, and unproductive leads many of the elderly to be outcast from their communities and to look negatively upon themselves.

Many elderly enjoy vibrant health and social, busy days. Moreover, 63 percent of the elderly feel that they are open-minded and adaptable. Only 23 percent report that they are infirm[1].

[1] Harris, L., 1974. Speech: Who The Senior Citizens Really Are, Annual Meeting of National Council on the Aging, Detroit, Michigan.

As the current surge of interest in bettering the life of the elderly continues, it is hoped that increasing numbers of people in this country will eschew ageism in favor of a more realistic, positive view of the final stage of the life cycle. This may amount to a revolution in current popular thinking. We hope to have contributed in some small way to this change.

ABN
JH
AJN

||||||||||||||||||||||||||||||||||||||||||||||||||| APPENDIX 1

Organizations, Advocacy Groups, and Referral Agencies

Action for Independent
  Maturity
1909 K St. NW
Washington, D.C.   20006

Advisory Committee on Aging
Administration on Aging
Social and Rehabilitation
  Service
Washington, D.C.   20201

American Aging Association
University of Nebraska Medical Center
42nd and Dewey Ave.
Omaha, Nebraska   68105

American Association of
  Homes for the Aging
1050 17th St. NW
Suite 770
Washington, D.C.   20045

American Association of Re-
  tired Persons (AARP)
National Retired Teachers
  Association (NRTA)
1225 Connecticut Ave. NW
Washington, D.C.   20036

American Dietetic Association
Gerontological Nutrition Prac-
  tice Group
Janette C. Martin, R.D.,
  M.P.H.
Office on Aging, Room 1004
State Office Building
301 W. Preston Street
Baltimore, Maryland   21201

American Geriatrics Society
10 Columbus Circle
New York, New York   10019

American Nurses Association,
   Inc.
Division on Geriatric Nursing
   Practice
Kansas City, Missouri   64108

American Nursing Home
   Association
1101 17th St. NW
Washington, D.C.   20045

Department of Health,
   Education and Welfare
Administration on Aging
330 Independence Ave. SW
Washington, D.C.   20201

Food and Nutrition Service
U.S. Department of Agricul-
   ture
Washington, D.C.   20250

Gerontological Society
1 Dupont Circle, Suite 520
Washington, D.C.   20036

Grey Panthers
3700 Chestnut St.
Philadelphia,
   Pennsylvania   19104

Homecall, Inc.
30 E. Patrick St.
Frederick, Maryland   21701

International Federation on
   Aging
1909 K St. NW
Washington, D.C.   20049

International Senior Citizens
   Association
11753 Wilshire Blvd.
Los Angeles, California   90025

National Association of Retired
   Federal Employees
1909 Q St. NW
Washington, D.C.   20009

National Caucus for the Black
   Aged
4400 W. Girard Ave.
Philadelphia,
   Pennsylvania   19104

National Center for Voluntary
   Action
RSVP (Retired Senior Volun-
   teer Program)
21735 I St. NW
Washington, D.C.   20006

National Clearinghouse on
   Aging
U.S. Dept. of Health, Educa-
   tion and Welfare
Human Development Services
Administration on Aging
Washington, D.C.   20201

National Congress of American
   Indians
Suite 312
1346 Connecticut Ave. NW
Washington, D.C.   20036

National Council of Senior Citizens
1511 K St. NW
Washington, D.C.   20005

National Council on Aging
1828 L St. NW, Suite 501
Washington, D.C.   20036

National Institution of
  Aging—National Institute of
  Health
Building 31, Room 5C02
9000 Rockville Pike
Bethesda, Maryland   20014

National Senior Citizen's Law
  Center
1709 West 8th St.
Los Angeles, California   90017

Retired Professional Action
  Group
2000 P St. NW
Suite 711
Washington, D.C.   20036

Senate Special Committee on
  Aging
Dirkson Senate Office Building
Room 223
Washington, D.C.   20510

Senior Advocates
  International, Inc.
1825 K St. NW
Washington, D.C.   20006

Western Gerontological Society
785 Market St.
Suite 1114
San Francisco,
  California   94103

‖‖‖‖‖‖‖‖‖‖‖‖‖‖‖‖‖‖‖‖‖‖‖‖‖‖‖‖‖‖ APPENDIX 2

Resources: Part A

FOR THE PROFESSIONAL

Active and Alert: Learning Experiences for Older Adults

Rotrock, L. and L.D. Miller
New England Gerontology Center
15 Garrison Ave.
Durham, New Hampshire   03824
058

1974
This booklet introduces the reader to the concept and principles of learning for the older adult.

Aging (periodical)

Superintendent of Documents
Government Printing Office
Washington, D.C.   20402

Offical periodical of the National Clearinghouse on Aging. Published bimonthly, reports on programs for, by, and with the elderly in state and local areas and in foreign countries.

Aging and Human Development

Greenwood Press, Inc.
Periodicals Division
51 Riverside Avenue
Westport, Connecticut   06880

Concerned with psychological and social studies of aging, with special emphasis on research.

A Guide to Nutrition and Food Service for Nursing Homes and Homes for the Aged

U.S. Dept. Health, Education and Welfare
Public Health Service
Health Resources Administration
Bureau of Health Services Research
Rockville, Maryland   20852
DHEW Publication No. (HRA) 74-3124

1971
Booklet provides guidance on the operation of a food service in addition to explaining principles of nutrition.

A Home Delivered Meals Program for the Elderly

U.S. Dept. of Health, Education and Welfare
Administration on Aging
Washington, D.C.   20201
DHEW No. (SRS) 73-20234

1971
A report on a demonstration project in St. Petersburg, Florida set up to deliver meals to the homebound aged. This project could be used as a model for setting up similar programs, since guidelines are complete and detailed.

Developing Insights into Aging

Minnesota Home Economic Association
Garrett Russell
452 Upton Ave S.
Minneapolis, Minnesota   55405

1978
A resource book listing booklets, books, articles, speakers, and audiovisuals useful in working with or to better understand the aged. Covers all areas of concern for the aged: health, clothing, psychological well-being, shelter, and so on.

Diets for Use in Homes for the Aged—Public Homes and Private Proprietary Homes for Adults

New York State Board of Social Welfare
Bureau of Adult Institutions
1450 Western Ave.
Albany, New York   12203

Information on the most common dietary modifications, i.e., low-sodium, diabetic, low-fat, etc.

Enhancing Title VII Nutrition Programs with USDA Food Commodities

Missouri Office of Aging
Department of Social Services
Jefferson City, Missouri   65101

Booklet of recipes utilizing 16 USDA food commodities. Recipes written to serve fifty portions. Large print for easy use by senior volunteers.

Geriatric Focus

Knoll Pharmaceutical Co.
386 Park Avenue South
New York, New York   10016

A monthly publication devoted to problems of aging and the aged.

Gerontologist

Gerontological Society
1 Dupont Circle
Washington, D.C.   20036

Source for the most recent studies and research conducted in the field of aging.

Gerontopics

Publications Desk
New England Gerontology Center
New England Center for Continuing Education
15 Garrison Ave.
Durham, New Hampshire   03824

A practitioner's news journal covering management, funding, education, and service delivery for the aging.

Good Eating, Meeting Nutritional Needs for Aged Persons in Residental Care Homes

Documents and Publications
Ordering Dept.
P.O. Box 20191
Sacramento, California   95820

1971
Information on budgeting, food management, food preparation, menu planning, and basic nutrition.

Group Meals for Senior Citizens in a Community Setting, a Procedural Manual

CAFE Co-op
119 9th Ave.
New York, New York   10011

1972
Information on home-delivered meals, program planning and evaluation.

Guide for Developing Nutrition Services in Community Health Programs

U.S. Dept. Health, Education and Welfare
Public Health Service
Health Services Administration
Bureau of Community Health Service
Rockville, Maryland   20857
DHEW No. (HSA) 78-5103

1978
A guide for information about developing and implementing nutrition services: planning the program, providing services; policy statements; personnel; and financing. Not specifically geared to the aged but providing useful information appropriate to many age/cultural groups.

Guidelines for Meals on Wheels and Congregate Meals for the Elderly

Pennsylvania Dietetic Association
P.O. Box 608
Camp Hill, Pennsylvania   17011

1973
Guidelines for menu planning; using volunteers and cook helpers; catering.

Let's End Isolation

AoA
330 C. St., SW
Washington, D.C.   20402

1971
Information on senior centers, food programs, home-delivered meals, and program planning and evaluation.

Mealtime Manual for People with Disabilities and the Aging

J.L. Klinger
Campbell Soup Corporation
Camden, New Jersey

1978
Thorough manual on ways to help disabled to live, prepare food, and eat independently. Illustrated and referenced.

Menu-Maker for Homes for the Aged

Federation of Protestants Welfare Agencies, Inc.
Division on Aging
281 Park Ave. South
New York, New York   10010

1968
A listing of approximately 100 dinner and supper menus, appropriate for an aged population. Consideration is taken to insure flexibility and variety while maintaining a tight budget. Useful time saver in small- or mid-sized homes where dietitian may not be on-site.

NCOA Publications List

National Council on the Aging, Inc.
1828 L. Street NW
Washington, D.C.   20036

A periodically issued listing of books, brochures, pamphlets, periodicals, tapes, and films useful to those who deal with the aged.

Nutrition and Aging: A Selected Bibliography

Ruth B. Weg
Ethel Percy Andrus Gerontological Center
University of Southern California
University Park
Los Angeles, California   90007
#051

1977
A bibliography with references covering the years 1969–1977. Listing is divided into subheadings: nutritional adequacy, theories of
aging, etc.

Nutrition and the Aged

Nutritional Perspectives No. 6
Mead Johnson & Company
Evansville, Indiana   47721

1975
Booklet focuses on nutrient needs for people 65 and older.

Nutrition Education for the Elderly

Virginia Council on Health and Medical Care
P.O. Box 12363, Central Station
Richmond, Virginia 23241

1978
Handbook providing lessons on nutrition, shopping, food information, diet, and cooking geared to elderly. Appendix gives information on techniques for teaching older adults.

Nutrition Education for the Older American

New England Gerontology Center
15 Garrison Ave.
Durham, New Hampshire   03824

A guide on nutrition education for the elderly. Developed for professionals working with the National Nutrition Program for the Elderly (Title VII).

Nutrition in Old Age

United Fresh Fruit & Vegetable Association
1019 Nineteenth Street NW
Washington, D.C.   20036

1968
Abstracts of literature on the aged through 1968.

Nutrition—Nutritional Considerations for the Elderly

Clara Lewis
F.A. Davis Company
1915 Arch St.
Philadelphia, Pennsylvania   19103

1978
A programmed-learning text describing physiologic and psychosocial parameters which may have an influence on the nutritional status of the elderly. Material is not presented in depth, but text would be useful for a basic overview of geriatric nutritional needs.

Nutritional Problems of the Elderly

Mead Johnson & Company
Evansville, Indiana   47721

September 1977
Audiotape and printed newsletter in which a panel of experts discuss nutrition problems of institutionalized elderly patients.

Senate Special Committee on Aging Memorandum

G-233 Senate Office Building
Washington, DC   20510

Serves as a supplement to activities (hearings, studies) of the committee; has excellent legislative coverage, gives status of bills, and describes new programs.

The Journal of Gerontology

Gerontological Society
1 Dupont Circle, Suite 520
Washington, DC   20036

Journal has a scientific research orientation.

The Senior Citizens News

National Council of Senior Citizens
1511 K St. NW
Washington, DC   20005

A monthly publication that has very good legislative coverage.

Training Volunteer Leaders

New England Gerontology Center
15 Garrison Ave.
Durham, New Hampshire   03824

1974
Concepts of leadership and principles of training are outlined, discussed, and applied to situations in which volunteers are recruited, organized, and monitored.

Your Money's Worth in Foods

U.S. Department of Agriculture
Superintendent of Documents
U.S. Government Printing Office
Washington, D.C.   20402
Stock No. 001-000-03580-1

1976
Information on meal planning and food shopping to help families of different sizes (1-6 members) with varying incomes get the most out of their food money.

Resources: Part B

FOR THE AGED

A Guide for Food and Nutrition in Later Years

Society for Nutrition Education
2140 Shattuck Ave.
Suite 1110
Berkeley, California   94704

1976
Comprehensive booklet providing information on nutrients and their food sources, marketing hints, dietary problems, supplements, and a bibliography of resource programs and publications.

A Guide to Budgeting for the Retired Couple

Home and Garden Bulletin No. 194
Superintendent of Documents
U.S. Government Printing Office
Washington, D.C.   20402
Stock No. 001-000-02963-1
Catalog No. Al.77:194/3

1973
General information on estimating retirement income and expenses.

Cooking for One

Cornell Miscellaneous Bulletin 93
New York State College of Human Ecology
Cornell University
Cooperative Extension
Ithaca, New York   14850

1968
Information on foods needed daily and how to include them in your
meals if cooking facilities and money are limited.

Cooking for One or Two in Leisure Years

Clemson University
Cooperative Extension Service
Clemson, South Carolina   29631

1978
General information on how to make food preparation and meal
acceptance more pleasant for the elderly single person.

Cooking for Two

Superintendent of Documents
U.S. Government Printing Office
Washington, D.C.   20402
Stock Number 0100–03327

1974
Large print booklet provides recipes, hints on planning and serving
meals, and general information on nutrition.

Delicious Low-Sodium Diets

Standard Brands, Inc.
625 Madison Ave.
New York, New York   10022

1976
General information on following a low-sodium diet plan; table of sodium content of foods; sample menus; recipes.

Food Guide for Older Folks

Home & Garden Bulletin No. 17
Superintendent of Documents
U.S. Government Printing Office
Washington, D.C.   20402
Stock No. 0100–1515

1972
Explanation and application of four food groups, shopping and cooking information, recipes.

Food Is More Than Just Something to Eat

U.S. Department of Agriculture
Home & Garden Bulletin No. 216
Superintendent of Documents
U.S. Government Printing Office
Washington, D.C. 20402
Stock No. 001–000–03564

Large print. Discusses major nutrients, calories, nutrition and life cycles, labeling, and daily food guide. Simplistic yet comprehensive.

Food to Keep Fit as Years Go By

Con Edison
Consumer Affairs
4 Irving Place
New York, New York

Leaflet on daily food needs and common food problems of the aged.

For Older People Eating Right for Less

Consumers Union
Mount Vernon, New York   10550

1977
Large print. Information on general nutrition and common health problems of aged. Extensive purchasing information on all types of food.

Grand Food for Grandparents

Tennessee Commission on Aging
Capitol Tower Apartment
510 Gay Street
Nashville, Tennessee   37219

1973
General nutrition information with emphasis on basic food groups.
Suggested low-cost Tennessee menus for one person.

Happiness Is!

Consumer Services
Sunkist Growers, Inc.
76–16 Box 7888
Van Nuys, California   91409

A newspaper for senior citizens with information on food, health,
nutrition, and recipes.

Meal Planning for the Golden Years

General Mills
Nutrition Service
Minneapolis, Minnesota   55440

1977
General nutrition information; how to add and subtract calories
from food plans, plus marketing and meal planning suggestions.

News

New York State Office of the Aging
Agency Bldg. 2
Empire State Plaza
Albany, New York   12223

A newsletter devoted to information on aging, legislation, programs, and general information.

Nutrition for Older Adults

Project IN-STEP
Division of Aging
Department of Health & Rehabilitative Services
1323 Winewood Boulevard
Tallahassee, Florida   32301

A series of 7 pamphlets dealing with nutrition information. Titles of individual pamphlets include: Preparing Food Safely; Plan Ahead and Save; Eating-out Tips.

Nutrition for Seniors

University of Minnesota
Institute of Agriculture
Agriculture Extension Service
St. Paul, Minnesota   55108

1977
A set of four leaflets dealing with the aging process, daily food selection, dental health, and the importance of daily activity. All leaflets feature the maintenance and repair of an antique automobile.

Protection for the Elderly

FTC Buyer's Guide No. 9
Federal Trade Commission
6th St. & Pennsylvania Ave., NW
Washington, D.C.   20580

Discussion of areas where elderly are vulnerable to deception. Shows how to avoid being deceived and losing money.

Recipes for Fat-Controlled, Low Cholesterol Meals

American Heart Association
44 East 23rd Street
New York, New York   10010

1973
Recipes to be used for a fat-controlled, low cholesterol diet.

Retirement Living

99 Garden Street
Marion, Ohio   43302

News and views on topics of interest to senior adults. Monthly features include nutrition, health, activity, travel, philosophy, retirement planning, and social network articles.

The Golden Spoon—Recipes for One or Two

Retired Senior Volunteer Program (RSVP)
1505 Park Ave.
Minneapolis, Minnesota   55404

1975
Large-type cookbook. Extensive selection of main dish recipes including low-sodium, no-sugar, and low-cost foods.

The Cookbook That Tells How, the Retirement Food and Nutrition Manual

H.E. Zaccarelli
CBI Publishing Company, Inc.
51 Sleeper Street
Boston, Massachusetts   02210

1972
A hardbound book containing purchasing, preparation, menu planning, and recipes for modified diets.

To Your Health . . . In Your Second Fifty Years

Dairy Council of Metropolitan New York
60 East 42nd Street
New York, New York   10017

1977
Leaflet offering many suggestions to the aged on general nutrition and meal planning, preparation, and storage.

Your Retirement Food Guide

American Association of Retired Persons
National Retired Teachers Association
215 Long Beach Blvd.
Long Beach, California   90801

1976
Basic nutrition information; tips on supplements, faddism, shopping, and menu planning. Aimed at 55–75 age group.

||||||||||||||||||||||||||||||||||||||||||| APPENDIX 3

Audiovisual Aids

1. AGING
   16mm   1973
   CRM Films
   McGraw Hill
   Hightstown, New Jersey
   Refutes common stereotypes.

2. BIOLOGIC CHANGES: FUNCTION AND CAPACITY
   filmstrip + cassette   20 minutes   1976
   Trainex Corporation
   P.O. Box 116
   Garden Grove, California   92642
   Defines the normal physiological changes that occur during the aging process.

3. BIOLOGIC CHANGES: PHYSICAL APPEARANCE AND SPECIAL SENSES
   filmstrip + cassette   23 minutes   1976
   Trainex Corporation
   (see address #2)
   Shows physiological changes of appearance and stature and defines those changes that normally occur in the senses during aging.

4. CRISIS IN AGING

slides + cassette   14½ minutes

Trainex Corporation
(see address #2)

Shows the impact of institutionalization on an elderly diabetic and on his son, both of whom have just endured the loss of wife/mother. No nutrition information is given but valuable for understanding the emotional impact of this situation.

5. DON'T STOP THE MUSIC

16mm   17½ minutes

Department of Health, Education and Welfare
Modern Talking Pictures
2323 New Hyde Park Road
New Hyde Park, New York   11040

Challenges myths and stereotypes of older persons, shows ways the community can respond to their needs.

6. FOOD FOR OLDER FOLKS

filmstrip   1972

Double Sixteen Co.
P.O. Box 1616
Wheaton, Illinois   60187

For use with general public; discusses basic food selection.

7. GERI AND JERRY GERONTOLOGY PRESENT: THE OLDER AMERICANS ACT

slides + 2 cassettes   29 minutes

Scripps Foundation Gerontology Center
Timothy H. Brubaker
218 Harrison Hall
Miami University
Miami, Ohio   45056

Explains programs covered by Titles I, II, III, IV, V, VII, and IX.

8. GROW OLDER—FEEL YOUNGER

16mm   color   10 minutes

New York State Office for the Aging
Empire State Plaza
State Agency Building #2
Albany, New York

Film hosted by Victor Borge to motivate older persons to improve and maintain their physical and mental well-being.

9. HELP YOURSELF TO BETTER HEALTH

16mm   16 minutes   1976

Nutrition Education Clearing House
Society for Nutrition Education
2140 Shattuck Ave. Suite 1110
Berkeley, California   94704

Shows how good nutrition is possible despite limited budgets, varying food habits, and limited cooking facilities. Leader's guide and large type booklet accompany film.

10. MORE THAN BREAD ALONE

16 mm   27 minutes

New York State Office for the Aging
(see address #8)

Film describes the Title VII Nutrition Program for the Elderly; may be used for professional and lay adult groups.

11. NUTRITION AND AGING—WHERE OLD AGE BEGINS

11 slides + script   1967

No. TA-2

Nutrition Today, Inc.
Director Educational Services
703 Giddings Ave.
Annapolis, Maryland   21404

Explores theories of aging from a nutritional viewpoint. For use with professionals.

12. NUTRITION FOR SENIORS

slide set #118

Visual Film Library
University of Minnesota
442 Coffey Hall
University of Minnesota
St. Paul, Minnesota   55108

An antique automobile lectures on daily needs, maintenance, physical activity and social needs.

13. OLD, BLACK AND ALIVE!

16mm   28 minutes

National Center on Black Aged
1725 Desales St.
Suite 402
Washington, D.C.   20036

The film provides insights into social stratification among elderly blacks. It depicts problems of this group and ways to resolve them.

14. OUR ELDERS: A GENERATION NEGLECTED

2 color/sound filmstrips   1972

Prentice-Hall Media Inc.
Marketing Assistant
150 White Plains Rd.
Tarrytown, New York   10591

Directed at a teenage audience.
Teacher's guide included

15. PERSPECTIVES ON AGING—IMPLICATIONS FOR TEACHING

filmstrip + cassette   26 minutes   1973

Concept Media
1500 Adams Ave.
Costa Mesa, California   92626

Surveys the physiological, sociological, and psychological factors affecting the learning ability of the elderly, presenting specific teaching techniques to overcome these factors.

16. PERSPECTIVES ON AGING—MYTHS AND REALITIES

filmstrip + cassette   24 minutes   1973

Concept Media
(see address #15)

Presents several common misconceptions about the aged.

17. PERSPECTIVES ON AGING—PHYSICAL CHANGES AND THEIR IMPLICATIONS

filmstrip + cassette   32 minutes   1973

Concept Media
(see address #15)

Shows how body systems and functions are affected by the physical changes that accompany aging.

18. POSITIVE LIVING IN THE SENIOR YEARS

74 slides + script   1976

Media Services
Office of Visual Communications
412 Roberts Hall
Cornell University
Ithaca, New York   14853

For use with the general public. Slide set is divided into 4 sections: Aging and Today's Senior Citizen; The Body and Aging; Food Needs of the Elderly; Feelings and Food.

19. RIGHTS OF AGE, THE

16mm   28 minutes

International Film Bureau, Inc.
332 South Michigan Ave.
Chicago, Illinois   60604

A story of an elderly widow, cut off from society, living on a meager diet; discusses protective services available to her.

20. SEASONS

16mm   16 minutes   color   1973

Consolidated Film Industries
959 Seward St.
Hollywood, California   90028

Film deals with health and rehabilitation of older people, including nursing home conditions.

21. STEP ASIDE, STEP DOWN

16mm   20 minutes

Consolidated Film Industries
(see address #20)

Film depicts problems of the aged—income, housing, nutrition—and programs designed to solve them.

22. TO HELL WITH GRANDMA

4 filmstrips + cassettes

Audio Visual Narrative Arts., Inc.
St. Paul Book and Stationery Co.
1233 W. County Road E.
St. Paul, Minnesota   55112

Explores the effects that forced retirement, segregation from society, poverty, and loneliness have on over 20 million individuals in our society. Teacher's guide included.

23. TRIGGER FILMS ON AGING

16mm

University of Michigan Television Center
Instructional Media Center
Towsley Center for Continuing Education
University of Michigan
Ann Arbor, Michigan   48104

A series of 5 brief films dramatizing situations common to older people, designed to trigger discussion. (Titles: To Market, To Market; Mrs. P.; The Center; Dinner Time; Tagged.)

APPENDIX 4

Nutritional Analyses of Fast Foods

Source: Young, E. A., Brennan, E. H. and Irving, G. L., Perspectives on Fast Foods, *Dietetic Currents,* 5:23, 1978, Ross Laboratories, Columbus, Ohio.

	Wt (g)	kcal	PRO (g)	CHO (g)	FAT (g)	Chol (mg)	Vit A (IU)	Vit B1 (mg)	Vit B2 (mg)	Nia (mg)	Vit B6 (mg)	Vit B12 (µg)	Vit C (mg)	Vit D (IU)	Ca (mg)	Cu (mg)	Fe (mg)	K (mg)	Mg (mg)	P (mg)	Na (mg)	Zn (mg)	Mois-ture (mg)	Crude Fiber (mg)
BURGER CHEF																								
Big Shef	186	542	23	35	34	-	282	0.34	0.35	5.4	-	-	2	-	189	-	3.4	384	-	278	622	-	-	0.3
Cheeseburger	104	304	14	24	17	-	266	0.22	0.23	3.2	-	-	1	-	156	-	2.0	220	-	198	535	-	-	0.2
Double Cheeseburger	145	434	24	24	26	-	430	0.25	0.34	4.8	-	-	1	-	246	-	3.1	361	-	351	691	-	-	0.2
French Fries	68	187	3	25	9	-	tr	0.09	0.05	2.1	-	-	14	-	10	-	0.9	581	-	76	4	-	-	0.7
Hamburger, Regular	91	258	11	24	13	-	114	0.22	0.18	3.2	-	-	1	-	69	-	1.9	210	-	102	393	-	-	0.2
Mariner Platter	373	680	32	85	24	-	448	0.37	0.40	7.3	-	-	24	-	137	-	4.7	1278	-	396	882	-	-	1.5
Rancher Platter	316	640	30	44	38	-	367	0.30	0.37	8.7	-	-	24	-	57	-	5.1	1370	-	326	444	-	-	1.3
Shake	305	326	11	47	11	-	10	0.11	0.57	0.3	-	-	2	-	411	-	0.2	548	-	319	167	-	-	-
Skipper's Treat	179	604	21	47	37	-	303	0.29	0.30	3.7	-	-	1	-	201	-	2.5	284	-	288	783	-	-	0.3
Super Shef	252	600	29	39	37	-	763	0.37	0.43	6.7	-	-	9	-	240	-	4.2	590	-	371	918	-	-	0.5

Source: Burger Chef Systems, Inc. Indianapolis, Ind. 1978 (analyses obtained from USDA Handbook No. 8).

	Wt (g)	kcal	PRO (g)	CHO (g)	FAT (g)	Chol (mg)	Vit A (IU)	Vit B1 (mg)	Vit B2 (mg)	Nia (mg)	Vit B6 (mg)	Vit B12 (µg)	Vit C (mg)	Vit D (IU)	Ca (mg)	Cu (mg)	Fe (mg)	K (mg)	Mg (mg)	P (mg)	Na (mg)	Zn (mg)	Mois-ture (mg)	Crude Fiber (mg)
BURGER KING																								
Cheeseburger	-	305	17	29	13	-	195	0.01	0.02	2.20	-	-	0.5	-	141	-	2.0	219	-	229	562	-	-	-
Hamburger	-	252	14	29	9	-	21	0.01	0.01	2.20	-	-	0.5	-	45	-	2.0	208	-	119	401	-	-	-
Whopper	-	606	29	51	32	-	641	0.02	0.03	5.20	-	-	13.0	-	37	-	6.0	653	-	205	909	-	-	-
French Fries	-	214	3	28	10	-	0	0.01	0.01	2.42	-	-	16.0	-	12	-	1.0	666	-	87	5	-	-	-
Vanilla Shake	-	332	11	50	11	-	9	0.01	0.05	0.27	-	-	tr	-	390	-	0.2	520	-	303	159	-	-	-
Whaler	-	486	18	64	46	-	141	0.01	0.01	1.04	-	-	1.3	-	70	-	1.0	130	-	91	735	-	-	-
Hot Dog	-	291	11	23	17	-	0	0.04	0.02	2.00	-	-	0	-	40	-	2.0	170	-	117	841	-	-	-

Source: Chart House, Inc. Oak Brook, Ill. 1978.

	Wt (g)	kcal	PRO (g)	CHO (g)	FAT (g)	Chol (mg)	Vit A (IU)	Vit B1 (mg)	Vit B2 (mg)	Nia (mg)	Vit B6 (mg)	Vit B12 (µg)	Vit C (mg)	Vit D (IU)	Ca (mg)	Cu (mg)	Fe (mg)	K (mg)	Mg (mg)	P (mg)	Na (mg)	Zn (mg)	Mois-ture (mg)	Crude Fiber (mg)
DAIRY QUEEN																								
Big Brazier Deluxe	213	470	28	36	24	-	-	0.34	0.37	9.6	0.38	2.55	<2.5	30	111	0.21	5.2	-	45	262	920	5.5	-	-
Big Brazier Regular	184	457	27	37	23	-	-	0.37	0.39	9.6	0.34	2.29	<2.0	31	113	0.18	5.2	-	42	223	910	5.4	-	-
Big Brazier W/Cheese	213	553	32	38	30	-	495	0.34	0.53	9.5	0.35	2.89	<2.3	36	268	0.19	5.2	-	47	359	1435	5.9	-	-
Brazier W/Cheese	121	318	18	30	14	-	-	0.29	0.29	5.7	0.11	1.20	<1.2	13	163	0.10	3.5	-	26	192	865	2.8	-	-
Brazier Cheese Dog	113	330	15	24	19	-	-	-	0.18	3.3	0.07	1.22	tr	23	168	0.08	1.6	-	24	182	-	1.9	-	-
Brazier Chili Dog	128	330	13	25	20	-	-	0.15	0.23	3.9	0.17	1.29	11.0	20	86	0.13	2.0	-	38	139	939	1.8	-	-
Brazier Dog	99	273	23	23	15	-	-	0.12	0.15	2.6	0.08	1.05	11.0	16	75	0.79	1.5	-	21	104	868	1.4	-	-
Brazier French Fries, 2.5 oz	71	200	2	25	10	-	tr	0.06	tr	0.8	0.16	-	3.6	24	tr	0.04	0.4	-	16	100	-	tr	-	-
Brazier French Fries, 4.0 oz	113	320	3	40	16	-	tr	0.09	0.03	1.2	0.30	-	4.8	-	tr	0.08	0.4	-	24	150	-	0.3	-	-

Item																					
Brazier Onion Rings	85	300	6	33	17	-	tr	0.09	tr	0.4	0.08	-	2.4	8	20	0.08	0.4	-	16	60	-	0.3
Brazier Regular	106	260	13	28	9	-	-	0.28	0.26	5.0	0.13	1.03	<1.0	13	70	0.11	3.5	-	23	114	576	2.3
Fish Sandwich	170	400	20	41	17	-	tr	0.15	0.26	3.0	0.16	1.20	tr	40	60	0.08	1.1	-	24	200	-	0.3
Fish Sandwich W/Cheese	177	440	24	39	21	-	100	0.15	0.26	3.0	0.16	1.50	tr	40	150	0.08	0.4	-	24	250	-	0.3
Super Brazier	298	783	53	35	48	-	tr	0.39	0.69	15.6	0.69	4.97	<3.2	65	282	0.27	7.3	-	61	518	1619	10.5
Super Brazier Dog	182	518	20	41	30	-	tr	0.42	0.44	7.0	0.17	2.09	14.0	44	158	0.18	4.3	-	37	195	1552	2.8
Super Brazier Dog W/Cheese	203	593	26	43	36	-	-	0.43	0.48	8.1	0.18	2.34	14.0	44	297	0.18	4.4	-	42	312	1986	3.5
Super Brazier Chili Dog	210	555	23	42	33	-	-	0.42	0.48	8.8	0.27	2.67	18.0	32	158	0.21	4.0	-	48	231	1640	2.8
Banana Split	383	540	10	91	15	-	750	0.60	0.60	0.8	0.50	0.90	18.0	tr	350	0.20	1.8	-	60	250	-	2.3
Buster Bar	149	390	10	37	22	-	300	0.09	0.34	1.6	0.12	0.90	tr	-	200	0.16	0.7	-	60	150	-	1.2
DQ Chocolate Dipped Cone, sm	78	150	3	20	7	-	100	0.03	0.17	tr	0.04	0.36	tr	tr	100	0.04	tr	-	16	80	-	0.3
DQ Chocolate Dipped Cone, med	156	300	7	40	13	-	330	0.09	0.34	tr	0.08	0.60	tr	tr	200	0.08	0.4	-	24	150	-	0.6
DQ Chocolate Dipped Cone, lg	234	450	10	58	20	-	400	0.12	0.51	tr	0.12	0.90	tr	8	300	0.12	0.4	-	40	200	-	0.9
DQ Chocolate Malt, sm	241	340	10	51	11	-	430	0.06	0.34	0.4	0.16	1.20	2.4	60	300	0.08	1.8	-	40	200	-	1.5
DQ Chocolate Malt, med	418	600	15	89	20	-	750	0.12	0.60	0.8	0.20	1.80	3.6	100	500	0.12	3.6	-	60	400	-	3.0
DQ Chocolate Malt, lg	588	840	22	125	28	-	750	0.15	0.85	1.2	0.30	2.40	6.0	140	600	0.20	5.4	-	80	600	-	3.8
DQ Chocolate Sundae, sm	106	170	4	30	4	-	130	0.03	0.17	tr	0.04	0.48	tr	tr	100	0.08	0.7	-	24	100	-	0.6
DQ Chocolate Sundae, med	184	300	6	53	7	-	300	0.06	0.26	tr	0.08	6.00	tr	tr	200	0.12	1.1	-	32	150	-	0.9
DQ Chocolate Sundae, lg	248	400	9	71	9	-	430	0.09	0.43	0.4	0.12	1.20	tr	8	300	0.16	1.8	-	40	250	-	1.2
DQ Cone, sm	71	110	3	18	3	-	130	0.03	0.14	tr	0.04	0.36	tr	tr	100	tr	tr	-	8	60	-	0.3
DQ Cone, med	142	230	6	35	7	-	300	0.09	0.26	tr	0.08	0.60	tr	tr	200	0.04	tr	-	24	150	-	0.6
DQ Cone, lg	213	340	10	52	10	-	430	0.15	0.43	tr	0.12	1.20	tr	8	300	0.08	tr	-	32	200	-	0.9
Dairy Queen Parfait	284	460	10	81	11	-	430	0.12	0.43	0.4	0.16	1.20	tr	8	300	0.16	1.8	-	40	250	-	1.2
Dilly Bar	85	240	4	22	15	-	130	0.06	0.17	tr	0.04	0.48	tr	-	100	0.08	0.4	-	16	100	-	0.3
DQ Float	397	330	6	59	8	-	130	0.12	0.17	tr	-	0.60	tr	-	200	-	tr	-	-	200	-	-
DQ Freeze	397	520	11	89	13	-	200	0.15	0.34	tr	-	1.20	tr	-	300	-	tr	-	8	250	-	-
DQ Sandwich	60	140	3	24	4	-	130	0.03	0.14	0.4	tr	0.24	tr	-	60	0.04	0.4	-	8	60	-	0.3
Fiesta Sundae	269	570	9	84	22	-	200	0.23	0.26	tr	-	0.90	tr	-	200	-	tr	-	-	200	-	-
Hot Fudge Brownie Delight	266	570	11	83	22	-	500	0.45	0.43	0.8	0.16	0.90	tr	tr	300	0.20	1.1	-	40	250	-	1.5
Mr. Misty Float	404	440	6	85	8	-	120	0.12	0.17	tr	-	0.60	tr	-	200	-	tr	-	-	200	-	-
Mr. Misty Freeze	411	500	10	87	12	-	220	0.15	0.34	tr	-	1.20	tr	-	300	-	tr	-	-	200	-	-

Source: International Dairy Queen. Inc. Minneapolis, Minn. 1978. Dairy Queen stores in the State of Texas do not conform to Dairy Queen-approved products. Any nutritional information shown does not necessarily pertain to their products.

KENTUCKY FRIED CHICKEN

	Wt (g)	kcal	PRO (g)	CHO (g)	FAT (g)	Chol (mg)	Vit A (IU)	Vit B₁ (mg)	Vit B₂ (mg)	Nia (mg)	Vit B₆ (mg)	Vit B₁₂ (μg)	Vit C (mg)	Vit D (IU)	Ca (mg)	Cu (mg)	Fe (mg)	K (mg)	Mg (mg)	P (mg)	Na (mg)	Zn (mg)	Mois-ture (mg)	Crude Fiber (mg)
Original Recipe Dinner*	425	830	52	56	46	285	750‡	0.38‡	0.56‡	15.0‡	-	-	27.0‡	-	150‡	-	4.5‡	-	-	-	2285	-	-	-
Extra Crispy Dinner*	437	950	52	63	54	265	750‡	0.38‡	0.56‡	14.0‡	-	-	27.0‡	-	150‡	-	3.6‡	-	-	-	1915	-	-	-
Individual Pieces† (Original Recipe)																								
Drumstick	54	136	14	2	8	73	30	0.04	0.12	2.7	-	-	0.6	-	20	-	0.9	-	-	-	-	-	28.6	-
Keel	96	283	25	6	13	90	50	0.07	0.13	-	-	-	1.2	-	-	-	0.9	-	-	-	-	-	50.3	-
Rib	82	241	19	8	15	97	58	0.06	0.14	5.8	-	-	<1.0	-	55	-	1.0	-	-	-	-	-	37.7	-
Thigh	97	276	20	12	19	147	74	0.08	0.24	4.9	-	-	<1.0	-	39	-	1.4	-	-	-	-	-	48.3	-
Wing	45	151	11	4	10	70	-	0.03	0.07	-	-	-	<1.0	-	-	-	0.6	-	-	-	-	-	19.1	-
9 Pieces	652	1892	152	59	116	864	-	0.49	1.27	-	-	-	-	-	-	-	8.8	-	-	-	-	-	317.4	-

Source: Nutritional Content of Average Serving, Heublein Food Service and Franchising Group, June 1976.
* Dinner comprises mashed potatoes and gravy, cole slaw, roll, and three pieces of chicken, either 1) wing, rib, and thigh; 2) wing, drumstick, and thigh; or 3) wing, drumstick, and keel.
† Edible portion of chicken.
‡ Calculated from percentage of US RDA.

LONG JOHN SILVER'S

	Wt (g)	kcal	PRO (g)	CHO (g)	FAT (g)
Breaded Oysters, 6 pc	-	460	14	58	19
Breaded Clams, 5 oz	-	465	13	46	25
Chicken Planks, 4 pc	-	458	27	35	23
Cole Slaw, 4 oz	-	138	1	16	8
Corn on Cob, 1 pc	-	174	5	29	4
Fish W/Batter, 2 pc	-	318	19	19	19
Fish W/Batter, 3 pc	-	477	28	28	28
Fryes, 3 oz	-	275	4	32	15
Hush Puppies, 3 pc	-	153	1	20	7
Ocean Scallops, 6 pc	-	257	10	27	12
Peg Leg W/Batter, 5 pc	-	514	25	30	33
Shrimp W/Batter, 6 pc	-	269	9	31	13
Treasure Chest 2 pc fish, 2 Peg Legs	-	467	25	27	29

Source: Long John Silver's Seafood Shoppes, Jan 8, 1978 (nutritional analysis information furnished in study conducted by the Department of Nutrition and Food Science, University of Kentucky).

McDONALD'S

Item																							
Egg McMuffin	132	352	18	26	20	192	361	0.36	0.60	4.3	0.14	0.71	1.6	40	187	0.11	3.2	222	265	914	1.7	65.3	0.4
English Muffin, Buttered	62	186	6	28	6	12	106	0.22	0.14	6.4	0.03	0.02	<0.7	12	87	0.06	1.6	264	94	466	0.3	20.8	0.1
Hot Cakes, W/Butter & Syrup	206	472	8	89	9	36	255	0.31	0.43	4.0	0.06	0.14	<2.1	12	54	0.11	2.4	264	404	1071	0.6	95.9	0.2
Sausage (Pork)	48	184	9	tr	17	43	36	0.22	0.13	5.9	0.11	0.36	<0.5	35	13	0.04	0.9	125	55	464	1.1	21.2	0.1
Scrambled Eggs	77	162	12	2	12	301	514	0.07	0.60	0.4	0.16	0.76	<0.8	60	49	0.06	2.2	144	167	207	1.4	50.6	0.2
Big Mac	187	541	26	39	31	75	327	0.35	0.37	8.2	0.22	1.89	2.4	37	175	0.15	4.3	386	215	962	3.9	86.4	0.7
Cheeseburger	114	306	16	31	13	41	372	0.24	0.30	5.5	0.10	0.97	1.6	14	158	0.03	2.9	244	134	725	2.0	51.4	0.3
Filet O Fish	131	402	15	34	23	43	152	0.28	0.28	3.9	0.08	0.78	4.2	37	105	0.07	1.8	293	158	709	0.7	55.9	0.7
French Fries	69	211	3	26	11	10	< 52	0.15	0.03	2.9	<0.01	0.01	11.0	<3	10	0.02	0.5	570	49	113	0.1	27.8	0.6
Hamburger	99	257	13	30	9	26	231	0.23	0.23	5.1	0.11	1.03	1.8	11	63	0.08	3.0	234	88	526	1.8	44.6	0.2
Quarter Pounder	164	418	26	33	21	69	164	0.31	0.41	9.8	0.25	2.29	2.3	23	79	0.13	5.1	442	179	711	4.4	81.2	0.8
Quarter Pounder W/Cheese	193	518	31	34	29	96	683	0.35	0.59	15.1	0.25	2.42	2.9	36	251	0.15	4.6	472	257	1209	4.8	94.2	0.8
Apple Pie	91	300	2	31	19	14	< 69	0.02	0.03	1.3	0.08	0.01	2.7	5	12	0.03	0.6	39	23	414	0.1	38.3	0.2
Cherry Pie	92	298	2	33	18	14	213	0.02	0.03	0.4	0.02	0.01	1.3	<5	12	0.04	0.4	57	23	456	0.1	38.6	0.1
McDonaldland Cookies	63	294	4	45	11	9	< 48	0.28	0.23	0.8	0.02	tr	1.4	10	10	0.03	1.4	58	51	330	0.2	1.9	0.2
Chocolate Shake	289	364	11	60	9	29	318	0.12	0.89	0.8	0.12	0.85	<2.9	354	338	0.17	1.0	656	292	329	1.3	207.0	<0.3
Strawberry Shake	293	345	10	57	9	30	322	0.12	0.66	0.5	0.11	0.85	<2.9	313	339	0.09	0.2	544	298	256	1.1	214.0	<0.3
Vanilla Shake	289	323	10	52	8	29	346	0.12	0.66	0.6	0.12	0.94	<2.9	354	346	0.06	0.2	499	266	250	1.0	216.0	<0.3

Source: "Nutritional analysis of food served at McDonald's restaurants." WARF Institute, Inc. Madison, Wisc. June 1977.

PIZZA HUT*

Item																							
Thin'N Crispy																							
Beef†	-	490	29	51	19	-	750	0.30	0.60	7.0	-	-	<1.2	-	350	-	6.3	-	-	-	-	-	-
Pork†	-	520	27	51	23	-	1000	0.38	0.68	7.0	-	-	<1.2	-	350	-	6.3	-	-	-	-	-	-
Cheese	-	450	25	54	15	-	750	0.30	0.51	5.0	-	-	<1.2	-	450	-	4.5	-	-	-	-	-	-
Pepperoni	-	430	23	45	17	-	1000	0.30	0.51	6.0	-	-	<1.2	-	300	-	4.5	-	-	-	-	-	-
Supreme	-	510	27	51	21	-	1250	0.38	0.68	7.0	-	-	2.4	-	350	-	7.2	-	-	-	-	-	-
Thick'N Chewy																							
Beef†	-	620	38	73	20	-	750	0.68	0.60	8.0	-	-	<1.2	-	400	-	7.2	-	-	-	-	-	-
Pork†	-	640	36	71	23	-	750	0.90	0.77	9.0	-	-	1.2	-	400	-	7.2	-	-	-	-	-	-
Cheese	-	560	34	71	14	-	1000	0.68	0.68	7.0	-	-	<1.2	-	500	-	5.4	-	-	-	-	-	-
Pepperoni	-	560	31	68	18	-	1250	0.68	0.68	8.0	-	-	3.6	-	400	-	5.4	-	-	-	-	-	-
Supreme	-	640	36	74	22	-	1000	0.75	0.85	9.0	-	-	9.0	-	400	-	7.2	-	-	-	-	-	-

Source: Research 900 and Pizza Hut, Inc. Wichita, Kan.
* Based on a serving size of one half of a 10-inch pizza (3 slices).
† Topping mixture of ingredients.

TACO BELL

	Wt (g)	kcal	PRO (g)	CHO (g)	FAT (g)	Chol (mg)	Vit A (IU)	Vit B₁ (mg)	Vit B₂ (mg)	Nia (mg)	Vit B₆ (mg)	Vit B₁₂ (µg)	Vit C (mg)	Vit D (IU)	Ca (mg)	Cu (mg)	Fe (mg)	K (mg)	Mg (mg)	P (mg)	Na (mg)	Zn (mg)	Moisture (mg)	Crude Fiber (mg)
Bean Burrito	166	343	11	48	12	-	1657	0.37	0.22	2.2	-	-	15.2	-	98	-	2.8	235	-	173	272	-	-	-
Beef Burrito	184	466	30	37	21	-	1675	0.30	0.39	7.0	-	-	15.2	-	83	-	4.6	320	-	288	327	-	-	-
Beefy Tostada	184	291	19	21	15	-	3450	0.16	0.27	3.3	-	-	12.7	-	208	-	3.4	277	-	265	138	-	-	-
Bellbeefer	123	221	15	23	7	-	2961	0.15	0.20	3.7	-	-	10.0	-	40	-	2.6	183	-	140	231	-	-	-
Bellbeefer W/Cheese	137	278	19	23	12	-	3146	0.16	0.27	3.7	-	-	10.0	-	147	-	2.7	195	-	208	330	-	-	-
Burrito Supreme	225	457	21	43	22	-	3462	0.33	0.35	4.7	-	-	16.0	-	121	-	3.8	350	-	245	367	-	-	-
Combination Burrito	175	404	21	43	16	-	1666	0.34	0.31	4.6	-	-	15.2	-	91	-	3.7	278	-	230	300	-	-	-
Enchirito	207	454	25	42	21	-	1178	0.31	0.37	4.7	-	-	9.5	-	259	-	3.8	491	-	338	1175	-	-	-
Pintos 'N Cheese	158	168	11	21	5	-	3123	0.26	0.16	0.9	-	-	9.3	-	150	-	2.3	307	-	210	102	-	-	-
Taco	83	186	15	14	8	-	120	0.09	0.16	2.9	-	-	0.2	-	120	-	2.5	143	-	175	79	-	-	-
Tostada	138	179	9	25	6	-	3152	0.18	0.15	0.8	-	-	9.7	-	191	-	2.3	172	-	186	101	-	-	-

Sources: Menu Item Portions, July 1976. Taco Bell Co, San Antonio, Tex.
Adams CF: *Nutritive Value of American Foods in Common Units.* USDA Agricultural Research Service. Agricultural Handbook No. 456. November 1975.
Church CF, Church HN: *Food Values of Portions Commonly Used*, ed 12. Philadelphia, JB Lippincott Co, 1975.
Valley Baptist Medical Center, Food Service Department: Descriptions of Mexican-American Foods, NASCO, Fort Atkinson, Wisc.

	Wt (g)	kcal	PRO (g)	CHO (g)	FAT (g)	Chol (mg)	Vit A (IU)	Vit B₁ (mg)	Vit B₂ (mg)	Nia (mg)	Vit B₆ (mg)	Vit B₁₂ (µg)	Vit C (mg)	Vit D (IU)	Ca (mg)	Cu (mg)	Fe (mg)	K (mg)	Mg (mg)	P (mg)	Na (mg)	Zn (mg)	Caffeine (mg)	Saccharin (mg)
BEVERAGES																								
Coffee, 6 oz	180	2	tr	tr	tr	-	-	0	tr	0.5	-	-	0	-	4	-	0.2	65	-	7	2	-	100–150†	0
Tea, 6 oz	180	2	tr	-	tr	-	-	0	0.04	0.1	-	-	1	-	5	-	0.2	-	-	4	-	-	40–100†	0
Orange Juice, 6 oz	183	82	1	20	tr	-	366	0.17	0.02	0.6	-	-	82.4	-	17	-	0.2	340	18	29	2	-	0	0
Chocolate Milk, 8 oz	250	213	9	28	9	-	330	0.08	0.40	0.3	-	-	3.0	-	278	-	0.5	365	-	235	118	-	-	0
Skim Milk, 8 oz	245	88	9	13	tr	-	10	0.09	0.44	0.2	-	-	2.0	-	296	-	0.1	355	-	233	127	-	-	0
Whole Milk, 8 oz	244	159	9	12	9	27	342	0.07	0.41	0.2	-	-	2.4	100	188	-	tr	351	32	227	122	-	-	0
Coca-Cola, 8 oz	246	96	0	24	0	-	-	-	-	-	-	-	-	-	-	-	-	-	-	40	20*	-	30	0
Fanta Ginger Ale, 8 oz	244	84	0	21	0	-	-	-	-	-	-	-	-	-	-	-	-	-	-	0	30*	-	0	0
Fanta Grape, 8 oz	247	114	0	29	0	-	-	-	-	-	-	-	-	-	-	-	-	-	-	0	21*	-	0	0
Fanta Orange, 8 oz	248	117	0	30	0	-	-	-	-	-	-	-	-	-	-	-	-	-	-	0	21*	-	0	0
Fanta Root Beer, 8 oz	246	103	0	27	0	-	-	-	-	-	-	-	-	-	-	-	-	-	-	0	23*	-	0	0
Mr. Pibb, 8 oz	245	93	0	25	0	-	-	-	-	-	-	-	-	-	-	-	-	-	-	28	23*	-	38	0
Mr. Pibb Without Sugar, 8 oz	237	1	0	tr	0	-	-	-	-	-	-	-	-	-	-	-	-	-	-	28	37*	-	38	76
Sprite, 8 oz	245	95	0	24	0	-	-	-	-	-	-	-	-	-	-	-	-	-	-	0	42*	-	0	0
Sprite Without Sugar, 8 oz	237	3	0	0	0	-	-	-	-	-	-	-	-	-	-	-	-	-	-	0	42*	-	0	57
Tab, 8 oz	237	tr	0	tr	0	-	-	-	-	-	-	-	-	-	-	-	-	-	-	30	30*	-	30	74
Fresca, 8 oz	237	2	0	0	0	-	-	-	-	-	-	-	-	-	-	-	-	-	-	0	51*	-	0	80

Sources: Adams CF: *Nutritive Value of American Foods in Common Units.* USDA Agricultural Research Service. Agricultural Handbook No. 456, November 1975.

Coca-Cola Company, Atlanta, Ga. January 1977.

American Hospital Formulary Service. Washington, American Society of Hospital Pharmacists, Section 28:20, March 1978.

* The values for sodium reflect value when bottling water with average sodium content is used, 12 mg/8 oz.

† Caffeine content depends on strength.

Diabetic Exchange Lists for Meal Planning

One of the most important aspects of diabetes management is dietary care. The Food Exchanges are lists of foods grouped by similar values of carbohydrates, proteins, and fats so that they can be substituted in your daily meal plans. Foods have been divided into six categories: milks, vegetables, fruits, breads, meats, and fats. Foods in any one group can be substituted or exchanged with other foods within the same group.

BREAD EXCHANGES: One Exchange of Bread contains 15 gm of carbohydrate, 2 gm of protein, and 70 calories.

Bread		*Cereal*	
White (including French and Italian)	1 slice	Bran Flakes	½ cup
		Other ready-to-eat unsweetened cereal	¾ cup
Whole Wheat	1 slice	Puffed Cereal (unfrosted)	1 cup
Rye or Pumpernickel	1 slice	Cereal (cooked)	½ cup
Raisin	1 slice	Grits (cooked)	½ cup
Bagel, small	½	Rice or Barley (cooked)	½ cup
English Muffin, small	½	Pasta (cooked), Noodles, Spaghetti, Macaroni	½ cup
Plain Roll, bread	1		
Frankfurter Roll	½	Popcorn (popped, no fat added	3 cups
Hamburger Bun	½		
Dried Bread Crumbs	3 Tbs	Cornmeal (dry)	2 Tbs
Tortilla, 6″	1	Flour	2½ Tbs
		Wheat Germ	¼ cup

Crackers		Prepared Foods	
Arrowroot	3	Biscuit, 2" dia.	1
Graham, 2½" sq.	2	(omit 1 Fat Exchange)	
Matzoh, 4" × 6"	½ cup	Corn Bread, 2" × 2" × 1"	1
Oyster	20	(omit 1 Fat Exchange)	
Pretzels, 3-1/8" long	25	Corn Muffin, 2" dia.	1
× 1/8" dia.		(omit 1 Fat Exchange)	
Rye Wafers, 2" × 3½"	3	Crackers, round butter type	5
Saltines	6	(omit 1 Fat Exchange)	
Soda, 2½" sq.	4	Muffin, plain small	1
		(omit 1 Fat Exchange)	
Dried Beans, Peas, and		Potatoes, French Fried,	8
Lentils		length 2" to 3½"	
Beans, Peas, Lentils	½ cup	(omit 1 Fat Exchange)	
(dried and cooked)		Potato or Corn Chips	15
Baked Beans, no pork	¼ cup	(omit 2 Fat Exchanges)	
(canned)		Pancake, 5" × ½"	1
		(omit 1 Fat Exchange)	
Starchy Vegetables		Waffle, 5" × ½"	1
Corn	⅓ cup	(omit 1 Fat Exchange)	

VEGETABLE EXCHANGES: One Exchange of Vegetables contains about 5 gm of carbohydrate, 2 gm of protein, and 25 calories. One Exchange is ½ cup.

Asparagus	Greens:	Rhubarb
Bean Sprouts	Beet	Rutabaga
Beets	Chards	Sauerkraut
Broccoli	Collards	String Beans
Brussels Sprouts	Dandelion	(green or yellow)
Cabbage	Kale	Summer Squash
Carrots	Mustard	Tomatoes
Cauliflower	Spinach	Tomato Juice
Celery	Turnip	Turnips
Cucumbers	Mushrooms	Vegetable Juice Cocktail
Eggplant	Okra	Zucchini
Green Pepper	Onions	

The following raw vegetables may be used as desired:

Chicory	Lettuce
Chinese Cabbage	Parsley
Endive	Radishes
Escarole	Watercress

Starchy Vegetables are found in the Bread Exchange List

FRUIT EXCHANGES: One Exchange of Fruit contains 10 gm of carbohydrate and 40 calories.

Apple	1 small	Mango	½ small
Apple Juice	⅓ cup	Melon	
Applesauce (unsweetened)	½ cup	Cantaloupe	¼ small
Apricots, fresh	2 med.	Honeydew	⅛ med.
Apricots, dried	4 halves	Watermelon	1 cup
Banana	½ small	Nectarine	1 small
Berries		Orange	1 small
Blackberries	½ cup	Orange Juice	½ cup
Blueberries	½ cup	Papaya	¾ cup
Raspberries	½ cup	Peach	1 med.
Strawberries	¾ cup	Pear	1 small
Cherries	10 large	Persimmon, native	1 med.
Cider	⅓ cup	Pineapple	½ cup
Dates	2	Pineapple Juice	⅓ cup
Figs, fresh	1	Plums	2 med.
Figs, dried	1	Prunes	2 med.
Grapefruit	½	Prune Juice	¼ cup
Grapefruit Juice	½ cup	Raisins	2 Tbs
Grapes	12	Tangerine	1 med.
Grape Juice	¼ cup		

Cranberries may be used as desired if no sugar is added.

MEAT EXCHANGES:

LEAN MEAT: One Exchange of Lean Meat (1 oz) contains 7 gm of protein, 3 gm of fat, and 55 calories.

Beef:	Baby Beef (very lean), Chipped Beef, Chuck, Flank Steak, Tenderloin, Plate Ribs, Plate Skirt Steak, Round (bottom top), All cuts Rump, Spare Ribs, Tripe	1 oz
Lamb:	Leg, Rib, Sirloin, Loin (roast and chops), Shank, Shoulder	1 oz
Pork:	Leg (Whole Rump, Center Shank), Ham Smoked (center slices)	1 oz
Veal:	Leg, Loin, Rib, Shank, Shoulder, Cutlets	1 oz
Poultry:	Meat without skin of Chicken, Turkey, Cornish Hen, Guinea Hen, Pheasant	1 oz
Fish:	Any fresh or frozen	1 oz
	Canned Salmon, Tuna, Mackerel, Crab, and Lobster	¼ cup
	Clams, Oysters, Scallops, Shrimp	5, or 1 oz
	Sardines, drained	3

Cheeses containing less than 5 percent butterfat		1 oz
Cottage cheese, dry and 2 percent butterfat		¼ cup
Dried Beans and Peas (omit 1 Bread Exchange)		½ cup

MEDIUM-FAT MEAT: For each Exchange of Medium-Fat Meat omit ½ Fat Exchange.

Beef:	Ground (15 percent fat), Corned Beef (canned), Rib Eye, Round (ground commercial)	1 oz
Pork:	Loin (all cuts Tenderloin), Shoulder Arm (picnic) Shoulder Blade, Boston Butt, Canadian Bacon, Boiled Ham	1 oz
Liver, Heart, Kidney and Sweetbreads (these are high in cholesterol)		1 oz
Cottage cheese, creamed		¼ cup
Cheese: Mozzarella, Ricotta, Farmer's Cheese, Neufchatel, Parmesan		3 Tbs
Egg (high in cholesterol)		1
Peanut Butter (omit 2 additional Fat Exchanges)		2 Tbs

HIGH-FAT MEAT: For each Exchange of High-Fat Meat omit 1 Fat Exchange.

Beef:	Brisket, Corned Beef (Brisket), Ground Beef (more than 20 percent fat), Hamburger (commercial), Chuck (ground commercial), Roasts (Rib), Steaks (Club and Rib)	1 oz
Lamb:	Breast	1 oz
Pork:	Spare Ribs, Loin (Back Ribs), Pork (ground), Country-style Ham, Deviled Ham	1 oz
Veal:	Breast	1 oz
Poultry:	Capon, Duck (domestic), Goose	1 oz
Cheese:	Cheddar Types	1 oz
Cold Cuts		4½" × ⅛" slice
Frankfurter		1 small

MILK EXCHANGES: One Exchange of Milk contains 12 gm of carbohydrate, 8 gm of protein, a trace of fat, and 80 calories.

NON-FAT FORTIFIED MILK

Skim or nonfat milk	1 cup
Powdered (nonfat dry, before adding liquid)	⅓ cup
Canned, evaporated skim milk	½ cup
Buttermilk made from skim milk	1 cup
Yogurt made from skim milk (plain, unflavored)	1 cup

LOW-FAT FORTIFIED MILK

1 percent fat fortified milk (omit ½ Fat Exchange)	1 cup
2 percent fat fortified milk (omit 1 Fat Exchange)	1 cup
Yogurt made from 2 percent fortified milk (plain, unflavored) (omit 1 Fat Exchange)	1 cup

WHOLE MILK (omit 2 Fat Exchanges)

Whole milk	1 cup
Canned, evaporated whole milk	½ cup
Buttermilk made from whole milk	1 cup
Yogurt made from whole milk (plain, unflavored)	1 cup

FAT EXCHANGES: One Exchange of Fat contains 5 gm of fat and 45 calories.

POLYUNSATURATED		SATURATED	
Margarine, soft, tub or stick*	1 Tsp	Margarine, regular stick	1 Tsp
Avocado (4″ dia.)**	1/8	Butter	1 Tsp
Oil, Corn, Cottonseed, Safflower, Soy, Sunflower	1 Tsp	Bacon fat	1 Tsp
		Bacon crisp	1 strip
Oil, Olive**	1 Tsp	Cream, light	2 Tbs
Oil, Peanut**	1 Tsp	Cream, sour	2 Tbs
Olives**	5 small	Cream, heavy	1 Tbs
Almonds**	10 whole	Cream cheese	1 Tbs
Pecans**	2 large whole	French dressing***	1 Tbs
Peanuts, Spanish**	20 whole	Italian dressing***	1 Tbs
Peanuts, Virginia**	10 whole	Lard	1 Tsp
Walnuts	6 small	Mayonnaise***	1 Tsp
Nuts, other**	6 small	Salad dressing, Mayonnaise-type***	2 Tsp
		Salt Pork	¾″ cube

*Made with corn, cottonseed, safflower, soy or sunflower oil only.

**Fat content is primarily monounsaturated.

***If made with corn, cottonseed, safflower, soy or sunflower oil can be used on fat-modified diet.

GENERAL RULES

FREE FOODS

Seasonings: Cinnamon, celery salt, garlic, garlic salt, lemon, mustard, ming, nutmeg, parsley, pepper, sugarless sweeteners, spices, vanilla, and vinegar.

Other foods: Coffee or tea (without sugar or cream), fat-free broth, bouillon, unflavored gelatin, sour or dill pickles, cranberries (without sugar).

FOODS TO AVOID

Sugar, candy, honey, jam, jelly, marmalade, syrups, pie, cake, cookies, pastries, condensed milk, soft drinks, candy-coated gum; fried, scalloped or creamed foods; beer, wine, or other alcoholic beverages.

Source: The Exchange Lists are based on material in the *Exchange Lists for Planning,* prepared by the Committees of the American Diabetes Association, Inc., and the American Dietetic Association in cooperation with the National Institute of Arthritis, Metabolism, and Digestive Diseases and the National Heart and Lung Institute, National Institutes of Health, Public Health Service, U.S. Department of Health, Education and Welfare.

Index